DATE			

New Drugs

DRUGS AND THE PHARMACEUTICAL SCIENCES

A Series of Textbooks and Monographs

Editor

James Swarbrick

Department of Pharmacy
University of Sydney
Sydney, N.S.W., Australia

Volume 1. PHARMACOKINETICS, *Milo Gibaldi and Donald Perrier*

Volume 2. GOOD MANUFACTURING PRACTICES
FOR PHARMACEUTICALS: A PLAN FOR TOTAL
QUALITY CONTROL, *Sidney H. Willig, Murray M.
Tuckerman, and William S. Hitchings IV*

Volume 3. MICROENCAPSULATION, *edited by J. R. Nixon*

Volume 4. DRUG METABOLISM: CHEMICAL AND
BIOCHEMICAL ASPECTS, *Bernard Testa
and Peter Jenner*

Volume 5. NEW DRUGS: DISCOVERY AND DEVELOPMENT,
edited by Alan A. Rubin

Other Volumes in Preparation

New Drugs

Discovery and Development

edited by

ALAN A. RUBIN

Vice President-Research
Endo Laboratories, Inc.
Garden City, New York

MARCEL DEKKER, INC.   New York • Basel

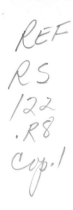

Library of Congress Cataloging in Publication Data

Rubin, Alan A
  New drugs.

  (Drugs and the pharmaceutical sciences ; v. 5)
  Includes indexes.
  1. Pharmaceutical research. 2. Drugs. I. Title.
RS122.R8   615'.1'072   77-16084
ISBN 0-8247-6634-2

MARCEL DEKKER, INC.
270 Madison Avenue, New York, New York 10016

Current printing (last digit):
10 9 8 7 6 5 4 3 2 1

PRINTED IN THE UNITED STATES OF AMERICA

PREFACE

The 1972 publication Search for New Drugs (Volume 6, Medicinal Research Series) was authored predominantly by university researchers. Its compilation represented an attempt to communicate to investigators in the field of drug research some of the more promising academic approaches to new drug discovery and evaluation.

The present volume is also concerned with the search for new drugs, but from the vantage point of the industrial researcher. All of the contributors to this volume conduct their research in pharmaceutical company settings. Their requirements for the screening and evaluation of potential drug candidates are basically similar to those of the academician insofar as predictive validity and reliability of test methods are concerned. But the industrial researcher is also accountable for high screening capacity, cost effectiveness and judicious manpower allocation. The appropriate combination of these scientific and economic components forms the basis of successful industrial research.

The nine subjects covered in this volume were selected for their broad appeal and include four on the central nervous system (major and minor tranquilizers, antidepressants, and analgesics), three on the cardiovascular system (antianginals, antiarrhytmics, and antihypertensives) and one each on allergy and arthritis. The authors have presented their personal views of (1) the advantages and shortcomings of current drug evaluation methodology, (2) the profile of an ideal drug, and (3) possible future developments in their respective areas of expertise.

Alan A. Rubin

CONTRIBUTORS

NEETI R. BOHIDAR, Department of Biometrics Research, Merck Sharp and Dohme Research Laboratories, West Point, Pennsylvania

JOHN R. CUMMINGS, Department of Pharmacology, Ayerst Research Laboratories, Montreal, Quebec, Canada

BERNARD DUBNICK,* Department of Pharmacology, Warner-Lambert/ Parke-Davis Pharmaceutical Research Division, Ann Arbor, Michigan

STEWART J. EHRREICH,† Department of Pharmacology, Schering Corporation, Bloomfield, New Jersey

WILLIAM H. FUNDERBURK, Department of Pharmacology, A. H. Robins Company, Richmond, Virginia

RALPH E. GILES,‡ Department of Pharmacology, Warner-Lambert/Parke-Davis Pharmaceutical Research Division, Ann Arbor, Michigan

FRANCIS R. GRANAT, Department of Biochemistry, Pharmaceuticals Division, CIBA-GEIGY Corporation, Summit, New Jersey

DAVID J. HERZIG, Department of Pharmacology, Warner-Lambert/Parke-Davis Pharmaceutical Research Division, Ann Arbor, Michigan

*Present affiliation: Cardiovascular and Central Nervous System Research Section, Lederle Laboratories, Pearl River, New York
†Present affiliation: Division of Cardio-Renal Drug Products, Food and Drug Administration, Rockville, Maryland
‡Present affiliation: Biomedical Research Department, ICI Americas, Inc., Wilmington, Delaware

DAVID N. JOHNSON, Department of Pharmacology, A. H. Robins Company, Richmond, Virginia

ALLAN D. RUDZIK, CNS Research, The Upjohn Company, Kalamazoo, Michigan

JEFFREY K. SAELENS, Research Department, Pharmaceuticals Division, CIBA-GEIGY Corporation, Summit, New Jersey

DEWEY H. SMITH, JR., Pharmaceuticals Division, E. I. du Pont de Nemours & Company, Inc., Stine Laboratory, Newark, Delaware

JOHN M. STUMP, Pharmaceuticals Division, E. I. du Pont de Nemours & Company, Inc., Stine Laboratory, Newark, Delaware

C. GORDON VAN ARMAN,* Department of Pharmacology, Merck Institute for Therapeutic Research, Merck Sharp and Dohme Research Laboratories, West Point, Pennsylvania

VERNON G. VERNIER, Pharmaceuticals Division, E. I. du Pont de Nemours & Company, Inc., Stine Laboratory, Newark, Delaware

---

*Present affiliation: Department of Biological Research, Wyeth Laboratories, Radnor, Pennsylvania

CONTENTS

CONTENTS

New Drugs

Chapter 1

ANTIARTHRITICS

C. Gordon Van Arman and Neeti R. Bohidar

Merck Institute for Therapeutic Research and Biometrics
Merck Sharp and Dohme Research Laboratories
West Point, Pennsylvania

1

I. INTRODUCTION

The main reason many pharmaceutical companies have had frustrating experiences in the clinical trials of their new drugs is insufficient and inadequate laboratory research.

In this chapter there is a particular philosophy of how to go about choosing a better antiarthritic drug from the abundance of compounds available for testing. Some of the assays described will become outdated within a few years because of the rapid succession of new findings about the arthritic diseases, but the basic principles of how to set up an assay can hardly change. It is not the purpose of this chapter to compare in detail the many new drug candidates that are either now in clinical trial or proposed for it by pharmaceutical companies, because most of these drugs will prove to be of temporary interest only. Nor is it appropriate here to enter into a discussion of the most fundamental aspects of arthritis, with comparisons of various theories. Some of the theories now rampant are not worth the trouble to consider; some, on the other hand, are at least partly correct, but whether or not they are makes little or no practical difference at this time. The gap between our present concepts of arthritis and the ultimate reality is surely so vast that the current theories do not help the research worker whose job is merely to find a better drug than we currently have.

In the laboratory phase of the search for any kind of drug, the first requirements for an assay are validity and reliability, in that order.

A. Validity

Validity for a human disease requires that drugs proved effective clinically should be effective in the laboratory model, that drugs effective in the model should be effective clinically, that drugs not effective clinically should not be effective in the model, and that drugs inactive in the laboratory should not be active in the clinic.[1] These requirements may seem clear and simple, but for inflammatory diseases they cannot be met at present. The model need not ostensibly resemble the clinical disease; generally, models have some points of similarity with a clinical disease, but many dissimilarities. There is no single test in vivo or in vitro that correlates well with clinical experience in the arthritic diseases over a number of different chemical structures.

With regard to chemical structure of drugs, we are forced to rely on assays that have apparent validity for some kinds of structure but not for others, even with respect to a single disease entity. The various arthritic diseases are different from one another not only in their clinical

---

[1]The term accuracy as customarily used for chemical assays means the same as validity here.

manifestations but also in their responses to drugs. It is important, therefore, to consider carefully the details of a particular disease, for example
rheumatoid arthritis, or another, such as ankylosing spondylitis, when one
is attempting either to set up a laboratory model or to choose one from the
literature.

Validity depends also on which species, sometimes even which strain
within a species, of animal is tested, and on the details of the particular
test being used with that strain. We conclude that one cannot entirely trust
any single laboratory assay alone, nor even several, to forecast quantitative
results in the arthritis clinic. The assays described herein have nevertheless shown good correlation thus far with clinical results in general, for
several of the most common arthritic diseases.

B. Reliability

Reliability is much easier to measure. Here we mean merely how reproducible a given assay method or treatment is in the laboratory.[2] If an assay
has high variability, it also has low reliability. Once the appropriate data
are in hand, sophisticated means of measuring reliability can be used with
the calculators now available, and are rapid and simple. For any new
drug, an investigator no longer has much excuse for failing to show the
dose-response line, the slope of the dose-response line, the confidence
limits at certain doses, the potency with respect to a standard, and the confidence limits of this relative potency. Certain essential terms are defined
in the section on statistical concepts. When a routine assay, especially a
new one, is running continuously, it is advisable, or even essential, to
submit one or two standard drugs at irregular intervals, in such a way that
the identity of the drug is not known to any person in direct contact with the
assay. With suitable explanations given well beforehand, there will be no
reason for the laboratory workers to feel that they are being examined; it
is the method itself on trial, and good laboratory workers welcome such
trials as proof not only of the reliability of the method but also of their skill.

C. Sensitivity

Sensitivity is a concept that is different from both validity and reliability.
The degree of response to the total amount of standard drug defines the
sensitivity. For example, the dog's knee-joint assay described herein is
quite sensitive on the basis of milligrams per kilogram of body weight,
but because a dog weighs about 10 kg, and several dogs are needed to establish an ED50, the total amount of indomethacin required is several dozen

---

[2]The term precision as customarily used for chemical assays means
the same as reliability here.

milligrams, or a few grams of aspirin. By our present definition based on
total amount, this assay must therefore be considered not sensitive. If we
use indomethacin as a standard for the five other assays described herein,
the antipyretic assay (yeast fever) is the most sensitive, because less compound is required (about 2 mg) for 50% inhibition in a group of rats. There
are many other assays sometimes called antiinflammatory that are much
more sensitive: as an example, the inhibition of prostaglandin synthetase
in vitro, for which indomethacin has a half-inhibitory concentration of 0.09
$\mu g/ml$, enough to perform the assay [1]. In screening methods, it is eco-
nomical to have good sensitivity, but in fact it is usually not necessary.
The main criterion should be validity, which at present one cannot guarantee
in any assay. The one characteristic an assay must have is a known reliability.

D. Correlations among Assays

Every biological assay method responds better to certain drugs than to
others. Assay methods may be identical or different in respect to the rank
order that they assign within a common list of several standard drugs. For
example, carrageenan-induced foot edema in the rat gives a rank order for
five drugs identical with that found by urate-induced knee-joint inflammation
in the dog [2]. In contrast, meclofenamic acid is more active than indomethacin against ultraviolet-induced skin erythema and yeast fever but less
active against cotton pellet granuloma [3]. In the mouse ear assay, certain
compounds such as ethacrynic acid are more active than indomethacin, but
are practically devoid of any effects against carrageenan foot edema in the
rat. Any assay in vivo depends on a delicate and complicated network of
cellular, humoral, neural, biochemical, and other phenomena. It is pru-
dent, therefore, to withhold conclusions about whether any assay depends
on exactly the same phenomena as some other. Among the six assays
described in this chapter, there have occurred some astonishing examples
of drugs active in one but not in another.

E. Tests In Vitro
    Compared with Tests In Vivo

Many and various are the tests in vitro used as clues to drugs for the arthritic diseases. There are methods using complement fixation, red-cell
stabilization, platelet aggregation, the Boyden chamber for cellular migration, uncoupling of oxidative phosphorylation, the Mizushima method for
protein denaturation, von Kaulla's fibrinolysis, acceleration of sulfhydryl
exchange, displacement of protein-bound uric acid, and many others. In
general, tests in vitro may be done more quickly, cheaply, and easily than
those in vivo. Swingle [4] gives references for these and other in vitro

methods, and correctly remarks that if one is going to collect irrelevant data, he may just as well do it rapidly. Tests in vitro are more likely to be valid in a series of compounds within which a prototype has been unequivocally demonstrated by other means. Furthermore, actions found in vitro may shed light upon the fundamental mechanisms relevant in vivo. Great skepticism must be used, however, and should be relented only when proof has been developed in vivo.

The foregoing comments have merely exemplified certain considerations that one should have clearly in mind before choosing which assays to use in the development of a drug. There are many other factors in the choice, and these will vary from one laboratory to another. The assays to be described here are shown merely as examples, and have been selected because they have wide applicability, and use normal laboratory species and relatively simple equipment. There are many variations of these assays presented in the literature, and there are many other methods greatly different, with particular, good reasons for their use. At present it is still necessary to have a number of assays for the selection of a drug candidate, and some of those presented here would appear essential. However, no laboratory can hope to compete in today's market without the ability to handle the statistical matters discussed in the following section.

II. STATISTICAL CONCEPTS

If the reader is not acquainted with the concepts used here, he can find better expositions in the first five chapters of the book by Finney [5]. A full understanding of the details would best be achieved by consulting a trained statistician. Here we shall merely outline the simpler tools of the pharmacologist's trade used in assay work.

The validity of laboratory assays for predicting clinical results could perhaps be quantitatively determined, but in actual practice hardly ever will be, because of the risk and cost of clinical trials. Instead, under the best conditions, the pharmacologist will carefully and laboriously select only a very few compounds by using at least five or six assay methods. These compounds will be the best he can find among perhaps thousands. After toxicology studies, still fewer of these compounds will survive to enter clinical trials. Under such conditions, certain laboratories have had a very high degree of clinical success. There have been too few published failures to allow evaluation of the comparative validity of the methods used to select these failures. At present there seems no way, therefore, in which one could measure statistically the clinical validity of any given antiinflammatory laboratory assay.

Instead, we shall describe the reliability and related measurements for six laboratory assays:

1. carrageenan foot edema of the rat

2. granuloma caused by cotton pellet

3. adjuvant-induced arthritis

4. yeast fever

5. dog's knee-joint inflammation

6. topical inflammation on the mouse's ear

A. Units of Measurement

Obviously, there are differences in the species used, in the routes of drug dosage, in the length of drug treatment, and in the affected organs and cells. The measurements for these assays are, respectively,

1. volume of rat's paw

2. weight of cotton pellet

3. volume of rat's paw

4. body temperature of rat

5. behavior of the dog

6. weight of a sample of mouse's skin

With these measurements, using suitable control values, we calculate drug effects in each assay method in the way described in the following sections. The units of the measurements are different among the several assays, except for items 1 and 3.

B. Relationship of Dose to Effect

In all these assays, as in most of those using either whole animals or isolated tissues, the relationship of the dose x to the effect y is

$$y = m \log x + b$$

This equation describes a straight line on semilogarithmic graph paper. At the extreme ends, there is always a departure of observed data from the straight-line relationship, usually below about 15% of the maximum response and above 85% of it. The slope of the line is m, which measures the rate of change in response for a unit change in the logarithm of the dose. The value of y at x = 1 is b. Since the logarithm of 1 is 0, when 1 is substituted for x in the equation, we get y = b, which is known as the intercept of the line.

C. Definition of ED50

The median effective dose is usually abbreviated as either MED or ED50. Either of these denotes the median dose required to have a certain effect which may be any value but must be clearly defined and must not be altered during computations for any set of data. We note that ED50 in textbook definitions [6] refers to a dose, i.e., to some point on the x axis, and not to any certain effect, or point on the y axis. The number 50 means that half, or 50%, of the animals at this dose will have an effect as great as (or greater than) some certain defined effect. However, there are complications. In many assays the result is best expressed as a percentage of the control value. Such expression causes no difficulty provided one can use the 50% level of inhibition, as in many antiinflammatory assays. In the granuloma assay described herein, however, the maximum achievable inhibition is only 35 or 40% of the weight gain by the control pellets. It is therefore sensible to choose 25% inhibition as the definition of the dependent variable, and to find the required ED50 for any drug to achieve this amount of inhibition. It may be confusing that the ED50 of indomethacin, for example, for 25% inhibition is 0.35 mg/kg.

In practical work we are seldom interested in any dose other than the median dose. In this chapter, therefore, we shall use the abbreviation ED to mean the dose required for an effect shown by the number following it; that is, in the granuloma assay, ED25 will denote the average dose required for a 25% decrease in the expected weight gain of the pellet. Likewise, in the yeast-fever assay, the ED1 will mean the dose required for a decrease of 1°C in fever.

D. Confidence Limits

The 95% confidence limits provide assurance that the true median will lie between these limits 19 times out of 20 repetitions of the experiment, on the average, over many, many repetitions. Nevertheless, when experiments are repeated with perhaps six or eight animals in a group, it seems amazing, and dismaying to the inexperienced, to see how often the mean for a second experiment lies beyond the estimates of the limits of the first. In such cases, one should consult a statistician to see how the data may be combined. With hundreds of animals, however, the limits tend to converge so that there comes a time when there is no practical value in any sharper definition of the median. We may be interested in either the median dose or the median effect. As an example, in the following section we find, for the dose of indomethacin needed for 50% inhibition in the carrageenan assay, limits of 2.54 and 2.92 mg/kg. Such values and the median dose itself, and the median effect, are sensitive to any changes in assay procedure. It is usually a waste of time to attempt an overfine pinpoint definition in such cases.

More useful are comparisons among different drugs in the same assay: the
rank orders of effective doses are more reproducible within and across different laboratories than are individual effective doses (for a certain effect)
or median effects (at certain doses).

E. Coefficient of Variation, λ, and R^2

The coefficient of variation expresses the variability of the assay as a percentage of the mean (100 $s/\bar{x}$). Because this number has no dimensions,
one may compare the values from one assay method to another, even though
the responses may have been measured in different units, as, for example,
degrees of fever and milliliters volume of a foot.

The lambda value (λ) is the standard deviation of the slope divided by
slope, s/b, and the smaller it is, the better. Guidelines for its interpretation are similar to those for the g value: 0.05 is excellent, 0.1 to 0.2 is
acceptable, and 0.5 or more should not be used.

R^2 is the proportion of the total variation in the response due to the
"trend" of response with log dose. It ranges from 0 to 100%, and the higher,
the better.

F. The g Value

One of the most useful concepts is the g value, a quantity that measures the
precision of an assay. The lower the g, the better. A desirable value would
be 0.05 or less. It is defined as

$$g = \frac{t^2 s^2}{b^2 [(\log x)^2]}$$

in which t is the usual familiar statistic found in t tables. The smaller the
tabular t which one must exceed, the better; tabular t decreases as the number of animals increases. s is the pooled standard deviation; it measures
variability among the individual animals in a test. If a procedure is in-
herently variable, it will have a large s. Complicated procedures have
greater s values than simple ones. b is the change in response per unit
increase in logarithm of the dose. It is also known as the slope of a dose-
response line. It is part of the measure of the sensitivity of the assay to
changes in dose. A good assay has a greater b than a poor one, i.e., a
steeper dose-response line. The quantity $(\log x)^2$ represents the spread
among the logarithmic doses used in the assay. The larger this spread in
the linear region, the better. This value is the corrected sum of squares
for the log doses, and is calculated as $\Sigma(\log x)^2 - (\Sigma \log x)^2/n$, in which n is
the number of observations.

Changes in any of these four values will change the value of g. A biological assay is considered to be of high precision if its g value is as small as 0.05, but still useful if g is 0.10 to 0.15. Values near 0.7 or higher should not be used. Note that tabular t and s should be as small as possible, whereas b and (log x)^2 should be as large as possible. The g value determines the width of the confidence limits of an ED50, and is therefore very important. The smaller the g value, the narrower will be the confidence limits.

G. Errors of Types I and II

In screening operations, there exist two dangers. The first one, known as type I error, occurs when one accepts as active a compound that in fact is not active. Such an error is not at all unusual, and can readily be tolerated, because in subsequent trials of this compound it will become clear that it is inactive. The other error, known as type II, is more serious, occurring when one fails to detect activity that is really present. The reason it is serious is that the compound will usually not be tested again, and will thus be lost. Errors of type II must therefore be minimized. The expression "power of a test" means how unlikely a certain test is to have type II errors. The power of a test is the probability of detecting an active compound. That is, an assay system may detect 99 out of 100 compounds of a certain degree of activity, and is then said to have a "power" of 0.99.

H. The Concept of Relative Potency

The primary purpose of a biological assay is to determine equally effective doses of the standard and test drugs. The ratio between these two doses estimates the potency of the test drug relative to the standard. This potency is the amount of standard drug equivalent in effect to one unit of the test drug. For the purpose of potency estimation, it is important that the standard and test drugs be analyzed by the same biological assay method.

Consider the situation in which it requires 9 mg/kg of drug A and 3 mg/kg of drug B to produce a 50% inhibition in the rat using the carrageenan-induced foot edema assay. Using the given definition, it is then inferred that drug B is three times as potent as drug A. In practice, however, it would be almost impossible to poinpoint precisely such a relationship between a given dose and its response. Therefore, one considers at least three doses of the standard drug and three doses of the test drug in the linear range (as far as possible) of their respective dose-response relationships, assigns several animals (8-12 animals) to each of the six groups (minimum number of groups) considered, and completes the experiment by measuring the response of each individual animal treated with either of the two drugs considered. The data generated by the study are subjected to the

statistical analysis outlined in detail by Finney [5, Chapter 4]. The analysis
provides a unique estimate of the relative potency and its 95% confidence
limits (or any other specified level) under the following assumptions:

1. The value of the slopes of the two drugs is the same, within the
   range of experimental variation (i.e., the two lines are parallel).

2. The lines are sufficiently steep to be of some practical value.

3. The doses fall in the linear range of the two dose-response curves,
   within the range of experimental variation.

The graph given in Figure 1 refers to an experiment (only a portion of
the data used for Tables 1 and 7) in which three doses (1, 3, and 9 mg/kg)
of a standard drug (here indomethacin) and three doses (3.3, 10, and 30
mg/kg) of diflunisal are considered. The purpose here is to estimate the
potency of diflunisal relative to indomethacin and the 95% confidence limits
of the true potency value. The following results are obtained by the application of the statistical procedure referred to earlier:

1. There was no statistically significant difference between the aver-
   ages over all three doses of the two preparations (P = 0.05), indicating that the doses of the two drugs chosen are within the comparable dose regimen (in other words, the doses were not misguessed).

2. The combined slope of the lines is highly significant (P ≪ 0.001),
   meaning that we have a useful degree of steepness in the slope.

3. The values of the two slopes are not statistically significantly different, P = 0.05 (meaning that the lines are parallel), indicating
   that a unique estimate of the potency is possible.

4. The "curvature" is not significant (P = 0.05), indicating that the
   chosen doses were, in fact, in the linear range of the dose-response
   relationships.

Now that we have met the requirements of the four tests of validity just
described, we proceed to estimate the relative potency value and the 95%
confidence limits of the true potency value. In this case the relative potency
value is 0.25 and the lower and the upper 95% confidence limits are 0.17
and 0.36, respectively. These numerical values may be interpreted as
follows: 4 mg diflunisal is equivalent to 1 mg of indomethacin, or, in other
words, diflunisal is one-fourth as potent as indomethacin. Now if we repeat
this experiment many times, then, within the chance variation, we should
find that 1 mg of diflunisal is not less potent than 0.17 mg of indomethacin
and not more potent than 0.36 mg of indomethacin. The g value provides a
measure of the overall precision of an assay. In this case, the g value is
0.04, indicating high precision.

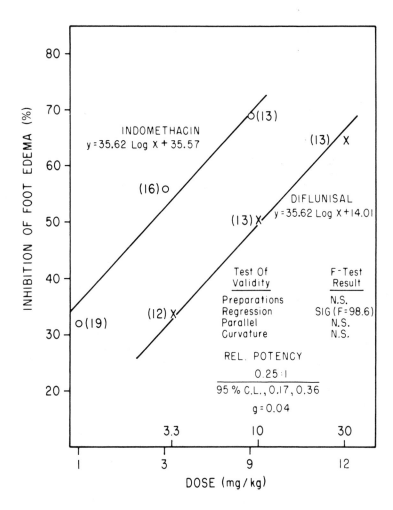

FIGURE 1. Relative potency of diflunisal compared with indomethacin, in carrageenan-induced foot edema. Numbers of six-rat groups appear beside the mean values shown.

We have not carried out the relative potency computations for most of the drugs mentioned in Table 7. This is because our primary interest here is to show the different results one obtains by using different assay methods. However, relative potency values are applicable only to compounds analyzed by the same assay method.

These simple definitions clarify the statistics used in the following sections.

III. THE LABORATORY ASSAYS

A. Carrageenan-Induced Foot Edema

The method described is that of Winter et al. [7] and Van Arman et al. [8]. Male rats of the Sprague-Dawley strain (other strains may also be used), 150 to 170 g body weight, are used in groups of at least six each. Compounds to be tested are given by stomach tube in a water solution of 0.5% Methocel[3] employed as a suspending agent; 3 ml is administered to each rat. After 1 hr, 0.1 ml of 1% carrageenan suspension[4] in saline solution, 0.85%, is injected subcutaneously under the plantar surface of the right hindfoot. The volume of the foot is then determined by immersion of the foot into a pool of mercury, up to a previously marked ink spot over the lateral malleolus; the volume of mercury displaced is determined by a pressure gauge connected to an electronic amplifier and pen-writer. For rats of the size and strain specified here, foot volumes average about 0.8 ml before swelling. After 3 hr, the volume is remeasured; the difference between the two volumes is the swelling. Drug effects are calculated as a percentage inhibition of the swelling, taking the swelling of the control group as 100%. The ED50 is defined as the dose that reduces the swelling by 50%.

The manner of preparing the drug solution or suspension is very important; if an insoluble drug is not divided finely and reproducibly enough, results may vary by factors of several-fold. One should use a VirTis "23" homogenizer[5] or equivalent for 5 min at moderate speed on drug suspensions.

Figure 2 shows foot swelling as a function of the milligram dose of carrageenan suspended in 0.1 ml of saline solution. The largest convenient

---

[3]Methocel is methylcellulose (100 cP), U.S.P.; Fisher Scientific Company, Fair Lawn, New Jersey.

[4]Carrageenan is supplied by Marine Colloids, Inc., Rockland, Maine, under the trade name Viscarin. Marine Colloids attempts to supply experimenters from a single batch of the material that the company set aside for this purpose several years ago. Batch number RE 6573 was used for several years at Merck.

[5]VirTis Company, Inc., Yonkers, New York.

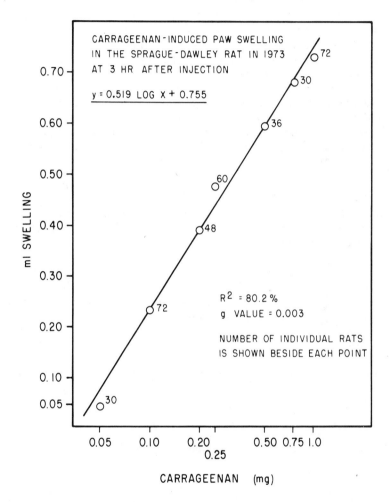

FIGURE 2. Milliliters swelling of the rat's foot as a function of amount of carrageenan injected, milligrams in 0.1 ml of saline solution.

swelling is the 0.76 ml caused by the 1-mg dose; this dose is used for routine assays.

Table 1 shows the parameters observed in this laboratory for indomethacin.

One should realize that the variability found with a certain assay method and a certain compound will probably change when a different compound is assayed by the same method; one can expect, however, that within a given series of compounds of a certain well-defined structure, the variabilities will prove to be quite similar. This fact should warn us, therefore, when screening several different families of chemical structure, not to assume without proof that the power of a test is always the same. It is not: it depends partly on the nature of the particular drug being assayed. In general, there is no way to predict how variability will be affected. Within a group of 15 acidic antiinflammatory drugs, Lombardino and Otterness [9] found that the carrageenan assay correlated fairly well with the recommended clinical dose.

TABLE 1   Carrageenan-Induced Foot Edema; Effect of Indomethacin

---

Dose-response line for indomethacin:

$$y = 38.04 \log x + 33.43,$$

in which y is percent inhibition of foot swelling, and x is mg/kg dose. Equation is based on 130 groups of six rats each.

Median effective dose for 50% inhibition (ED50):   2.73 mg/kg

95% confidence limits of ED50:   2.54, 2.92 mg/kg

$\lambda = 0.0384$

$g = 0.0058$

Coefficient of variation (st. dev./mean) = 17.9%

$R^2 = 73.2\%$

Dose-response line for carrageenan, without drugs:

$$y = 0.519 \log x + 0.755,$$

in which y is response in ml swelling, and x is mg carrageenan, in the range 0-2 mg given in 0.1 ml volume.

The upper limit of the straight-line logarithmic relationship of dose and effect is in the region of 70 to 80% inhibition for most known nonsteroid drugs tested thus far; doses greater than required for this value do not result in any further inhibition. Some few curves have had flattening in the region of only 50%. The mechanism involved in the remaining inflammation up to 100% is obviously different, and therefore needs investigation. It is interesting that the upper limit of effectiveness of steroids is approximately the same as for nonsteroids, 70 to 80%, but that the mechanisms are different, because one can achieve 100% inhibition by using, for example, indomethacin and dexamethasone together. Herein lies another clue that deserves research.

B. Granuloma Caused by Cotton Pellet

This method, derived from an earlier one by R. K. Meyer, was published by Winter and Porter in 1957 [10]. On Day 0, male rats of the Sprague-Dawley strain, 150 ± 15 g, in groups of six each are given orally the compound to be tested. Then, under hexobarbital anesthesia, two sterilized cotton pellets, from 32 to 50 mg each (same weight pellets are used in all rats in the experiment), are implanted beneath the abdominal skin, one on each side of the midline, through a single incision down the linea alba. Compounds being tested are given orally once daily through Day 6, suspended or dissolved in 0.5% methylcellulose. On Day 7, the rats are sacrificed and the pellets are dried overnight in an oven at 70°C. The mean dry weights of the two granulomas added together are approximately 124 mg if no drug is given. The mean difference in the granuloma weight between pellets from control rats and those from treated rats, when divided by the control granuloma weight, multiplied by 100, gives the percent inhibition of granuloma formation. Note, in Table 2, that the median dose is defined as the oral dose in milligrams per kilogram of body weight required to decrease the untreated granuloma weight by 25%. This decrease of 25% is approximately the most that can be achieved usefully by nonsteroid drugs; decreases beyond 30 or 35% do not lie on the linear portion of the curve of log dose versus response. Steroids, however, have yielded inhibitions as high as 63%, with inevitable effects on thymus and adrenals.

The slope of the equation for indomethacin shown in Table 2 is low relative to the slopes in other assays. This fact is reflected in the λ value of 0.12, compared with examples of 0.04 for carrageenan and 0.05 for yeast fever. On the other hand, it is better than 0.15 for adjuvant arthritis and 0.19 for the dog's knee joint.

This method discriminates well among steroids, and is extremely sensitive to some of them; hydrocortisone has an ED25 of 2.5 mg/kg, and dexamethasone 0.001 mg/kg.

TABLE 2   Cotton Pellet Granuloma; Effect of Indomethacin

Dose-response line for indomethacin:

$$y = 15.25 \log x + 32.00,$$

in which y is percent inhibition of weight gain of pellet, and x is mg/kg dose. Equation is based on 101 groups of six rats each

Median effective dose of indomethacin for 25% inhibition (ED25):

0.35 mg/kg

95% confidence limits of ED25: 0.23, 0.46 mg/kg

$\lambda = 0.12$

$g = 0.05$

Coefficient of variation (st. dev./mean) = 21.2%

$R^2 = 42.2\%$

Dose-response line for pellets without drugs:

$$y = 159.4 \log x - 188.9,$$

in which y is mg gain in weight of pellet, and x is mg weight of the pellets at implantation, in the range 30-50 mg

---

What aspects of inflammation does the granuloma assay measure? It reflects the migration of histiocytes in tissues and white cells from blood in response to the foreign material, and the consequent formation of fibrin strands in and around the cotton pellet. Macrophages, both those from the circulating blood and those from the local tissue itself, play the major role.

C. Adjuvant-Induced Arthritis

The method is essentially that of Winter and Nuss [11], differing only in slight details. Male rats of the Sprague-Dawley strain, 170 to 190 g body weight, in groups of six, are injected in the distal third of the tail with a well-ground suspension of 0.5 mg of Mycobacterium butyricum in 0.1 ml of light mineral oil. Measurements of foot volume are made on Days 0 and 14; rats are weighed and dosed daily, orally, on Days 1 through 13. A rat given no drug will have a foot swelling of about 0.75 ml, so that the measured volume will be approximately 0.8 ml normal volume + 0.75 ml swelling = 1.55 ml, or usually 1.3 to 1.9 ml. The compounds to be tested are suspended or dissolved in 0.5% methylcellulose. Rats used as adjuvant-treated controls must receive the methylcellulose solution, so that the influence, although slight, of handling the rat (adrenal stimulation through stress) is excluded. Table 3 shows the effect of indomethacin.

All drugs known to be active in rheumatoid arthritis that have been tested by this procedure have been found active; in other words, no false negatives have yet been discovered. In statistical terminology, these would be predictive errors of the second kind (β). Predictive errors of the first kind (α), i.e., wrongly finding a compound active in this test that is not active clinically against some major rheumatic disease, probably will be found eventually. Up to now, however, no certain example of this has come to light.

TABLE 3   Adjuvant Arthritis; Effect of Indomethacin
_____

Dose-response line for indomethacin:

$$y = 57.17 \log x + 84.84,$$

in which y is percent inhibition of paw swelling, and x is dose in mg/kg. Equation is based on 34 groups of six rats each.

Median effective dose of indomethacin for 50% inhibition (ED50):

0.25 mg/kg

95% confidence limits of ED50:   0.18, 0.31 mg/kg

$\lambda = 0.15$

$g = 0.10$

Coefficient of variation (st. dev./mean) = 27.23%

$R^2 = 57.6\%$

Dose-response line of adjuvant, without drugs:

$$y = 0.4 \log x + 0.75,$$

in which y is ml foot swelling and x is mg of M. butyricum in 0.1 ml mineral oil (range of x, 0-1 mg).
_____

One should note carefully that the cellular mechanisms causing adjuvant arthritis, a relatively long-term disease, are clearly distinct from those in acute assays that apparently involve only the polymorphonuclear leukocyte. There are mechanisms other than cellular ones that operate in adjuvant disease. At least some parts of the many mechanisms, both cellular and extracellular, are of an immune nature, but it is not clear what those parts may be. The obfuscating term "immunological" is too freely used by many writers. Immune mechanisms, however, are merely part of the entire complicated picture. The so-called immune suppressants, such as cyclophosphamide and 6-mercaptopurine, have no greater effectiveness than other classes, such as the usual nonsteroid antiinflammatory drugs, the glucocorticoids, and gold salts, and even agents such as thorium dioxide, sodium alginate, and polyinosinic-polycytidylic acid.

D. Yeast Fever

The method of Winter [12] is used, with a simpler calculation of results, as follows: Sprague-Dawley male rats, 170 to 190 g, in groups of six each, are injected subcutaneously with 2 ml of a 7.5% suspension of brewer's yeast in 0.5% methylcellulose solution. A rise in rectal temperature of about 2°C or more occurs and persists for more than 24 hr. It is measured by a rectal sensing probe having a rapid digital display. At 18 hr after injection, the temperature is recorded. Test compounds are then given orally, suspended or dissolved in 0.5% methylcellulose. Temperature is recorded every 30 min through 2 hr. The mean of the four readings after drug administration is calculated in degrees centigrade lowering of the fever. The ED1 is that dose causing a 1°C lowering. Note that this is also the dose causing roughtly 50% alleviation of the fever, since the usual fever is 2°C or somewhat more.

Table 4 shows that this assay is capable of excellent reliability when compared with some other assays. The difficulty is in understanding the relationship of this assay to clinical inflammatory disease. All recognized antipyretic drugs tested thus far have proved effective in this test, and the ratios of potency are in the same order found in clinical practice. All antipyretics, however, do not have a proportionate antiinflammatory potency in the other usual assays, such as carrageenan edema. Aminopyrine is an example of a good antipyretic with little antiinflammatory potency.

The mechanism of fever is complicated. The present state of research may be learned from references 13 and 14, which summarize findings and theories of the most recent few years. This assay may be useful for gaining insight into the mechanisms of fever production. For example, reduction of the circulating white blood cell count in rats down to almost zero did not seriously decrease the fever caused by yeast (Van Arman et al., unpublished observations, 1972).

TABLE 4   Yeast Fever: Effect of Indomethacin
_____

Dose-response line for indomethacin:

$$y = 1.63 \log x + 0.81,$$

in which y is degrees centigrade lowering of fever, and x is dose in
mg/kg. Equation is based on 48 groups of six rats each.

Median effective dose of indomethacin for 1°C decrease (ED1):

1.31 mg/kg

95% confidence limits of ED1:   1.23, 1.39 mg/kg

$\lambda = 0.05$

$g = 0.01$

Coefficient of variation (st.dev./mean) $= 11.9\%$

$R^2 = 83.6\%$

Dose-response line for yeast in this assay has not been established.
_____

It may be asked why this assay should be performed upon antiinflammatory candidates that will not be used primarily as antipyretics. The
answer is that it helps to classify compounds, and in some ways may lead
to understanding the mechanism. Immune suppressants such as cyclophosphamide are not antipyretic, nor are glucocorticoids.

E.   Inflammation in the Dog's Knee Joint

This technique, first used by Faires and McCarty [15] and by Rosenthale
et al. [16], was developed into a quantitative procedure by Van Arman et al.
[2]. A sterile suspension of 4 mg of sodium urate in the form of needles,
10 to 15 μ, in 0.75 ml of physiological saline solution, is injected into one
hind knee joint of a dog, never previously given any urate injections. The
dog stands quietly for 2.5-min periods on a platform which has a pivoted
board connected with an integrator; the paw of the injected leg rests on the
board. Two control readings, sometimes three, are taken in arbitrary
units on the integrator scale. These control readings usually agree within
a few percent; readings after treatment are expressed as a percentage of
the control readings. Drugs are given orally in gelatin capsules at zero

time, the time of urate injection. Readings are taken 2 hr after dosing, at which time dogs not given any antiinflammatory drug have foot pressures of zero or nearly so. Readings may be taken at other intervals also, without any disturbing effect upon the 2-hr reading usually adopted as standard for most drugs. Table 5 shows the results obtained with indomethacin.

This assay method is more variable than the others using the rat or mouse; nevertheless, there are cogent reasons for using the dog. In some pharmacologic respects the dog resembles man more closely than the rat does, especially in cardiovascular and respiratory phenomena. Certain toxic side effects, such as ulcer formation, may be more readily observed in the dog. Especially noteworthy is the fact that most antiinflammatory assay methods employ rodents, usually the rat, sometimes the mouse, less frequently the rabbit (as for the Shwartzman or Arthus phenomenon), and rarely the guinea pig (as for anaphylaxis or topical effects). The insights that one may achieve into biochemical and pharmacologic processes by using a nonrodent species may be quite valuable. The Food and Drug

TABLE 5   Dog's Knee Joint; Effect of Indomethacin

Dose-response line for indomethacin:

$$y = 54.4 \log x + 39.37,$$

in which y is percent restoration of the normal foot pressure, and x is dose in mg/kg. Equation is based on 104 dogs.

Median effective dose of indomethacin for 50% restoration (ED50):

1.57% mg/kg

95% confidence limits of ED50:   1.07, 2.08 mg/kg

$\lambda = 0.19$

$g = 0.15$

Coefficient of variation (st. dev. /mean) $= 61\%$

Dose-response line of sodium urate, without drugs:

$$y = 95.5 - 159.6 \log x,$$

in which y is percent of normal foot pressure, and x is mg urate crystals injected, in the range 1-4 mg, for a particular preparation. The potency of one crystal preparation will vary from that of another.

Administration requires data in a nonrodent species so far as toxicity is concerned, before a usual New Drug Application can be approved; why not then use the dog, and also have some antiinflammatory data in that nonrodent species? "Man's best friend" deserves that title especially in the laboratory because a careful and experienced observer can correctly infer certain information from the dog's behavior, if between the readings the dog is allowed to move freely about. A rat is not so communicative.

Much can be learned by sampling the synovial fluid. The changes in volume can be measured [17]; cellular infiltration can be quantitated by counting cell concentrations and multiplying by the volume at that time; changes in the cell population can be followed by serial sampling. The advantage of studying synovial fluid from an inflamed joint is that here one has the acute inflammatory process simplified, unencumbered by erythrocytes and metabolic effects of the various organs. The direct participation of drugs in the process can be observed by their injection into the joint. For example, local anesthetics such as xylocaine can be assayed nicely. Indomethacin (as well as other nonsteroids) has a local antiinflammatory effect in this model, so that one may infer an effect upon the function of the polymorphonuclear leukocytes, which constitute almost all of the infiltrating cells within the first few hours. There are very few publications of studies conducted for longer time periods, but see Carlson et al. [18]. The dog's knee joint obviously offers promise for fundamental research.

F. Topical Inflammation

The test animal is the female CF_1 mouse 18 to 20 g, in groups of six [19]. One-tenth milliliter of a vehicle containing 2% croton oil (N.F. VII), 20% pyridine, 73% diethyl ether, and 5% distilled water is applied in 0.05-ml aliquots, one each to the anterior and posterior surfaces of the left ear. The dose of croton oil is therefore 2 mg. The right ear is not treated. Drugs to be tested are dissolved or suspended in a vehicle containing 75% diethyl ether, 20% pyridine, and 5% water, so that each drug dose is contained in 0.1 ml of the vehicle. The drug is applied to the left ear 1 hr after application of vehicle containing the croton oil. Both applications are performed under ether anesthesia.

Three hours after drug application the mice are sacrificed with pentobarbital and both ears are removed. Circular sections are taken using a No. 4 cork borer, rinsed in ether, dried, and weighed. The increase in weight caused by the irritant is found by subtracting the weight of the untreated right ear section (usually about 10 mg) from that of the treated left ear section. Sections treated with the croton oil solution, but no drug, will have an increase of approximately 14 mg; those treated with a drug will have a lesser increase. The dose causing half inhibition of the expected increase is the ED50. Table 6 shows the results obtained with indomethacin.

TABLE 6   Topical Mouse Ear Skin; Effect of Indomethacin

Dose-response line for indomethacin:

$y = 48.22 \log x + 39.53,$

in which y is percent reduction of swelling from that measured in control mice, and x is dose in mg. Equation is based on 54 mice total.

Median effective dose of indomethacin for 50% inhibition (ED50):

1.65 mg

95% confidence limits of ED50:   1.23, 2.12 mg

$\lambda = 0.21$

$g = 0.18$

Coefficient of variation (st. dev. /mean) $= 36\%$

Dose-response line of croton oil in vehicle described, without drugs:

$y = 5.34 \log x + 12.5,$

in which y is mg weight gain of the ear, and x is mg of croton oil.

    This assay is included in this chapter because with certain compounds it yields results not parallel to those obtained with other assays. Most of the usual antiinflammatory drugs have a rank order here like that found, for example, in carrageenan edema. On the other hand, 3-chloro-4-cyclo-hexylphenylacetic acid, although 13 times as potent as indomethacin in the carrageenan assay (ED50 of 0.2 compared with 2.7 mg/kg), is almost inactive in this test; contrariwise, a compound of low activity in prevention of carrageenan edema, ethacrynic acid, has a good ED50 of 1.25 mg in the mouse's ear test, compared with 1.65 for indomethacin. Such differences probably have something to do with the transport mechanism through skin. The penetration of the skin can be affected by changes in properties resulting from apparently very slight changes in structure. For example, triamcinolone-16,17-acetonide has better topical efficacy than triamcinolone. For the steroids, the major toxic effects are common to all of them, and when given systemically these toxic effects go hand in hand with the potency. When given topically, however, a marked improvement in the ratio of therapeutic to toxic effects can often be achieved. It is likely that the same improvement may be found with suitable nonsteroid antiinflammatory drugs.

IV. COMPARISONS ACROSS ASSAY METHODS

Table 7 presents seven drugs chosen to illustrate the profiles of activity across the several assays just described. The thiadiazole is not in clinical use, nor is it considered a candidate for it, but is included here as an example to show how one might insert a compound into a table of standard drugs in order to achieve a perspective. The ED50 values are not all determined with equal reliability. Within each assay method, however, the rank order of these examples is satisfactorily fixed. Table 8 shows these rank orders within each assay. By merely adding these numbers for each drug, one can have an overall figure which can be compared with those of other drugs. The bottom line shows the rank order of potency in clinical use, assigned on the basis of general information across a number of inflammatory states such as gout, osteoarthritis, ankylosing spondylitis, and rheumatoid arthritis. In the present state of the art of medicine, opinions vary about efficacy, and there can hardly be a rigorous proof of such clinical rank orders.

In any event, potency, which means effect per unit weight of drug, is not of overwhelming consequence. What matters most is the maximum therapeutic effect that can be achieved, no matter what the required dose (up to some practical limit), without undesirable side effects. Chronic toxicity tests are therefore required. The maximum dose that can be given chronically without causing any toxicity should be determined. Also, that dose should be ascertained that will elicit the maximum possible antiinflammatory effect of that drug. If that maximum is not great enough, the drug is unlikely to be useful. Many laboratories have seen compounds otherwise desirable that have a ceiling effect considerably below those of standard drugs. Generally, then, a new candidate drug should have a ceiling effect as good as those produced by drugs already in use; the new drug should also have as great a ratio as possible between the minimum toxic dose and that required for a ceiling therapeutic effect. In five of the six assays described here, one does not measure therapeutic effects but only preventive effects, against some artificially induced disease, usually of relatively brief duration. How fortunate it is that with all these obvious dissimilarities to clinical disease, such simple laboratory models can select drugs that prove useful! They also point toward some underlying etiology. In time, basic research will reveal the etiology; but meanwhile, we should be proud of the fact that we can find excellent drugs without knowing in great detail just why they have their effects.

V. SUMMARY

Finding a better antiinflammatory drug requires first of all some acquaintance with the clinical disease selected as the target. Because laboratory experiments must be done in animals, some methods must be used that have

TABLE 7 Comparison of Seven Drugs Tested in Each of Six Different Assays

Assay	Indomethacin	Sulindac	Diflunisal	Phenylbutazone	2,5-Bis(ethylamino)-1,3,4-thiadiazole	Aspirin	Thiabendazole
Carrageenan foot edema	2.7[a]	5.5	9.8	27.7	22.4	89.2	200
Granuloma, cotton pellet	0.35	5.4	74	40	30	115	Inact.
Adjuvant arthritis	0.25	0.55	9.8	14	~50	67	217
Yeast fever	1.31	2.9	24	24	5.7	45	83
Dog's knee joint	1.57	45	24	12	8.4	72	>150
Topical, mouse's ear	1.65	6.1	3	4.3	Inact.	5.5	12.4

[a]All values represent median effective doses (MED).

24

TABLE 8 Rank Order of Potency of Seven Drugs in Six Assays

Assay	Indomethacin	Sulindac	Diflunisal	Phenylbutazone	2,5-Bis(ethylamino)-1,3,4-thiadiazole	Aspirin	Thiabendazole
Carrageenan foot edema	1	2	3	5	4	6	7
Granuloma, cotton pellet	1	2	5	4	3	6	7
Adjuvant arthritis	1	2	3	4	5	6	7
Yeast fever	1	2	4 1/2	4 1/2	3	6	7
Dog's knee joint	1	5	4	3	2	6	7
Topical, mouse's ear	1	5	2	3	7	4	6
Sum of rank orders for drug in the six assays	6	18	21 1/2	23 1/2	24	34	41
Rank order of drug in the laboratory within the group of seven	1	2	3	4	5	6	7
Rank order of drug in clinical use as an antinflammatory	1	2	3	4	Not used	5	6

as many features as possible in common with the human disease. For the arthritides, there are only imperfect animal models with varying degrees of resemblance; it is therefore best to use a number of different models. Fortunately, several assay systems have proved to be sufficiently correlated with clinical results so that they have furnished several of the drug candidates introduced into human trials in the last few years. Certain of these models have been described here in sufficient detail so that one could begin using them.

REFERENCES

1. E. A. Ham, V. J. Cirillo, M. Zanette, T. Y. Shen, and F. A. Kuehl, Jr., in Prostaglandins in Cellular Biology (P. W. Ramwell and B. B. Pharriss, eds.), Plenum Press, New York, 1972, pp. 345-352.

2. C. G. Van Arman, R. P. Carlson, E. A. Risley, R. H. Thomas, and G. W. Nuss, J. Pharmacol. Exp. Ther. 175, 459 (1970).

3. J. Wax, C. V. Winder, O. K. Tessman, and M. D. Stephens, J. Pharmacol. Exp. Ther. 192, 172 (1975).

4. K. F. Swingle, in Antiinflammatory Agents, Chemistry and Pharmacology (R. A. Scherrer and M. W. Whitehouse, eds.), Academic Press, New York, 1974, p. 84.

5. D. J. Finney, Statistical Method in Biological Assay, 2nd ed., first six chapters, Hafner, New York, 1964.

6. E. Fingl and D. M. Woodbury, in The Pharmacological Basis of Therapeutics (L. S. Goodman and A. Gilman, eds.), 5th ed., Macmillan, New York, 1975, p. 27.

7. C. A. Winter, E. A. Risley, and G. W. Nuss, Proc. Soc. Exp. Biol. 111, 544 (1962).

8. C. G. Van Arman, A. J. Begany, H. H. Pless, and L. M. Miller, J. Pharmacol. Exp. Ther. 150, 328 (1965).

9. J. G. Lombardino and I. G. Otterness, Arzneim. Forsch. 25, 1629 (1975).

10. C. A. Winter and C. C. Porter, J. Am. Pharm. Assoc. 46, 515 (1957).

11. C. A. Winter and G. W. Nuss, Arthritis Rheum. 9, 394 (1966).

12. C. A. Winter, Int. Symp. Nonsteroidal Antiinflammatory Drugs, Proc., Excerpta Medica Int. Congr. Series No. 82, Milan, 1964, pp. 198-199.

13. The Pharmacology of Thermoregulation, Proceedings of a Satellite Symposium held in conjunction with the Fifth International Congress

on Pharmacology, San Francisco, 1972 (E. Schonbaum and P. Lomax, eds.), Karger, Basel, 1973.

14. Temperature Regulation and Drug Action, Proceedings of a Symposium on Temperature Regulation and Drug Action, Paris, April 1974 (P. Lomax, ed.), Karger, Basel, 1975.

15. J. S. Faires and D. J. McCarty, Jr., Lancet 2, 682 (1962).

16. M. E. Rosenthale, J. Kassarich, and F. Schneider, Proc. Soc. Exp. Biol. Med. 122, 693 (1966).

17. C. G. Van Arman, R. P. Carlson, and P. J. Kling, Ciencia e Cultura 23, 555 (1971).

18. R. P. Carlson, G. E. Dagle, C. G. Van Arman, and P. J. Kling, Am. J. Vet. Res. 34, 515 (1973).

19. C. G. Van Arman, Clin. Pharmacol. Ther. 16, 900 (1974).

Chapter 2

ANTIALLERGICS

David J. Herzig, Ralph E. Giles* and Bernard Dubnick†

Warner Lambert/Parke-Davis
Pharmaceutical Research Division
Ann Arbor, Michigan

---

*Present affiliation: Biomedical Research Department, ICI-United States, Wilmington, Delaware.
†Present affiliation: Lederle Laboratories, Pearl River, New York.

29

I. INTRODUCTION

A. A Pharmacological View

Although discussions of allergy have usually been in the context of the field
of immunology, its manifestations (respiratory, cardiovascular, derma-
tological, gastrointestinal, etc.) are distinctly pharmacological. The diverse vasoactive autocoids which have been implicated as mediating the
adverse clinical effects are familiar to pharmacologists. These include
amines, such as histamine and serotonin, peptides such as bradykinin and
eosinophil chemotactic factor (ECF-A), and a variety of fatty acid derivatives, such as the slow reacting substance of anaphylaxis (SRS-A) and
prostaglandins.

When Dale and Laidlaw [1, 2] first studied histamine pharmacologically
they drew attention to the similarity of the immediate symptoms upon injection of the compound in animals to those symptoms resulting from injection
of a protein in previously sensitized animals. Many years later Bovet and
Staub [3, 4] reported antihistaminic activity for 2-isopropyl-5-methylphenoxy-
ethyldiethylamine in guinea pigs demonstrating protection against lethal
doses of histamine and reduced symptoms of anaphylactic shock. This observation led to the first clinically useful antihistaminic drugs, Antergan
and Neoantergan (pyrilamine maleate), and to the synthesis and testing of
many other histamine antagonists indicated for the suppression of allergic
and anaphylactic reactions.

It was expected that these compounds would control all of the important
allergic manifestations; and indeed in man, edema formation and itch were
significantly modified. But the profound fall in blood pressure and the bronchoconstriction which occur in systemic anaphylaxis as well as in bronchial
asthma (a local allergic response) were little affected, and increased gastric
secretion was not antagonized at all. The reason for some of these limitations is now known. The gastric and some of the cardiovascular responses
to histamine are of a type called H_2 which are unaffected by the classical
(H_1) antihistamines but antagonized by a new class of histamine antagonists
[5]. Other limitations of antihistamines are not clear. For example, Schild

et al. [6] showed that histamine-induced contractions of bronchiolar muscle from human asthmatic lung in vitro were about 10,000 times more sensitive to antihistamines than antigen-induced contractions. This differential sensitivity may be due to reduced access of antagonists to sites where histamine is released in intimate contact with cells, to release of other autocoids, or perhaps to a direct response of the sensitized muscle to the antigens not dependent on an autocoid. In any event, it is clear that another approach to therapy is needed, an approach which would focus on the allergic process rather than on its end result.

B. Cellular-Molecular Definitions of
    Allergy and the Choice of Laboratory Models

Often a disease is the result of a normal mechanism gone askew. A useful drug would redirect or control the deviant system without interfering with any homeostatic or protective system. Therefore, a test useful for drug development would utilize the points of uniqueness or divergence of the reactions of interest from other similar processes. In allergy, the protective mechanism in the immunological system has become deranged. Since there are components of the allergic reaction that differ significantly from those of other immunological reactions, we can construct laboratory models based on these distinguishing characteristics which do not interfere with the protective function of the immune system.

Coombs and Gell [7] have divided allergic reactions into four immunologically distinct categories (Table 1). Since Ishizaka and Ishizaka [8]

TABLE 1   Classification of Hypersensitivity Reactions[a]

Type	State of antibody	Complement requirement	Cells required	Synonyms
I	Soluble; bound to cell receptor	None	Mast cell basophil	Anaphylactic, reaginic, immediate
II	Soluble	Yes	Nonspecific	Drug sensitivity, cytotoxic, Coombs-type
III	Antigen-antibody complex	Yes	Nonspecific	Arthus, serum sickness
IV	Possibly part of lymphocyte membrane	None	T lymphocytes	Delayed, tuberculin, cell-mediated

[a]Adapted from Coombs and Gell [7].

identified IgE as a new class of immunoglobulin and, together with Johansson and coworkers [9,10], implicated IgE as the major antibody involved in type I atopic reactions (hay fever, eczema, asthma, and parasitic infections), a type I reaction is generally required for models of "allergies" [8-10]. The type I reaction has several distinguishing characteristics, such as noninvolvement of complement, requirement for the antibody to be bound to specific cells, and the noncytolytic release of defined mediators.

Uvnas and his coworkers provided a rational basis for the search for drugs which could control the release of mediators from mast cells (and basophils) and, thereby, modify the allergic process. In a series of papers beginning in 1957 [11] they described the enzymatic nature of the in vitro release process from rat mesenteric or peritoneal mast cells. Whether induced chemically by "histamine liberators" (compound 48/80) or by antigens, the release process required energy and was subject to inhibition by metabolic inhibitors.

The work of Mota [12] in rats and Ovary and Bier [13] in guinea pigs provided the basis for the use of IgE-dependent passive cutaneous anaphylaxis (PCA) in small animals as a model of human reaginic hypersensitivity. The PCA technique is precisely analogous to the clinical Prausnitz-Kustner (PK) hypersensitivity test.

This chapter is not intended to be a comprehensive review of the literature or a compilation of methods. It is, rather, a more personal approach, outlining the procedures used in our laboratory for finding and developing drugs in the treatment of allergies.

II. NONHUMAN PRIMATES

There is a twofold appeal to the use of the higher monkeys as models of human allergy. One, of course, is the phylogenetic proximity between man and monkey. The second, as a consequence of the first, is that human reaginic serum will sensitize monkey tissue and anti-human IgE will react with monkey IgE. As in man, immediate hypersensitivity reactions in monkeys can involve histamine, SRS-A, and prostaglandins. Therefore, the monkey model may not only resemble the human physiologically but can also accommodate serum factors from atopic humans. Additionally, the use of human serum in monkeys may eliminate potential problems arising from differential characteristics of primate and nonprimate IgE [14].

A. Passive Sensitization Using
Human Atopic Serum

Monkeys can be sensitized systemically or locally and then a PCA, PK, or pulmonary reaction induced with antigen. It takes 10 times as much human antibody to elicit a PCA or PK reaction in the monkey as in the human [15].

Although this may be an appropriate system for studying various compounds intended for human use, it is wasteful of human serum. Moreover, monkeys can only be used for short periods since they rapidly produce antibodies to human blood proteins and react to human serum. Finally, the cost of obtaining and maintaining monkeys is high and thereby mitigates against use of this model for extensive drug development.

B. Reversed Passive Sensitization
    Using Anti-Human IgE

A second method of inducing an immediate hypersensitivity reaction in monkeys is the reversed reaction using anti-human IgE. This involves cell-bound monkey IgE which cross-reacts with anti-human IgE [16]. It is a noncytolytic, mediator-releasing response [17]. However, the test animal becomes sensitized rapidly to the anti-human IgE since it comes from a heterologous species. Thus, one is usually limited to a short period of experimentation extending for not more than a few weeks per monkey.

C. Natural Sensitivity

A third method of inducing immediate hypersensitivity is based on a native sensitivity to environmental immunogens. Monkeys show an immediate hypersensitivity reaction to Ascaris suum, probably as the result of a previous infection by the parasite. The sensitive animal has a local cutaneous reaction as well as a pulmonary response to the antigen due to circulating anti-Ascaris IgE antibody [18,19]. Sensitized monkeys can be selected from the general population by intradermal testing; those that show cutaneous sensitivity are then tested for pulmonary sensitivity.

    Among rhesus monkeys, pulmonary Ascaris sensitivity is uncommon enough so that a large number of animals must be tested to find suitable subjects. Although skin testing has been useful to identify sensitive animals, there are few data on the response of such skin tests to drugs, especially some of the newer antiallergy compounds. Because of the wide variability found in pulmonary responses in these animals, it has been difficult to demonstrate unequivocal efficacy of these new agents. Recently Patterson and his coworkers have shown that by dissolving the Ascaris antigen in D_2O for aerosolization it is possible to induce two consecutive equivalent asthma reactions within an hour [20]. This technique appears to be extremely promising for drug testing by using each animal as his own control.

D. In Vitro Monkey and Human Lung

Patterson has removed isolated mast cells by brush biopsy of monkey lungs. The degranulation of these by anti-human IgE, compound 48/80, or Ascaris

antigen can be followed under the microscope [21]. Whether it is possible
to show drug effects on this system is not known. Thus, in the monkey we
have the potential to study drugs in several in vivo and in vitro models.
However, this has not yet been extensively investigated pharmacologically.

Schild et al. [6] first showed that isolated human lung in vitro would
release histamine anaphylactically. The use of this to study the activities
of antiasthma drugs has been most extensively developed in Austen's laboratory (see reference 22 for review). However, this test can be severely
limited by the availability of usable tissue.

III. DOGS

Dogs commonly suffer from allergic disease due to environmental aller-
gens. They are allergic to ragweed, house dust, grass, foods, and fleas.
Unlike man, the dog has a relatively high incidence of seasonal atopic der-
matitis and a low incidence of asthma and rhinitis. Nevertheless, the mere
presence of spontaneous allergic disease has spawned attempts to use this
species for the detection of potential antiallergy compounds. This approach
has been less than successful [16,23].

A. Types of Antibody

Most of the physical, chemical, and biological studies on dog reaginic antibody have been carried out with the spontaneous antiragweed antibody or that
produced by infection with roundworms, Toxacara canis [24]. The antibody
is heat labile, long-term skin fixing, and mercaptoethanol sensitive. It has
a sedimentation coefficient of 8 to 9S and chromatographs ahead of IgG on
Sephadex G-200. By chromatography on DEAE-cellulose and by immuno-
electrophoresis it appears to be different from IgG, IgM, IgD, and IgA.
Halliwell et al. [24] have been able to neutralize dog reagin with anti-human
IgE. Thus, it appears that the major reagin in dogs is of the IgE class.
However, until specific anti-dog immunoglobulins (especially to myeloma
proteins) are available, it is not possible to rule out entirely the existence
of other classes of reagins.

B. Cells and Mediators

The mast cell appears to be the cell predominantly involved in dog anaphylaxis [25]. The skin mast cell [26] and the free mast cell from the lumen of
the bronchi bind reagin and release histamine upon challenge [27].

Although histamine appears to be the major mediator released by anaphylaxis in the dog, there is evidence that bradykinin may play a role in
bronchial constriction following aerosol antigen challenge [28]. The

cholinergic system is also involved in dog bronchoconstriction, but there has not been a systematic investigation of the role of the other mediators, such as SRS-A and ECF-A, in the dog and their relative pharmacological importance is not clear at this time. Blood basophils have also not yet been evaluated in anaphylaxis or in binding dog IgE.

C. Skin Tests

Both active and passive cutaneous testing have been conducted in dogs. Generally, the light-colored skin on the abdomen is used and Evans blue is given intravenously to improve visualization of the reaction. By careful handling and preparation, it is possible to do such testing without anesthesia.

1. Roundworm infection

Dogs that have been infected with roundworms (Toxacara canis) are readily available and an active cutaneous anaphylactic reaction can be induced with a purified extract of Ascaris suum [23,29]. However, since the infection is so common, it is difficult to find negative recipients for the passive transfer of serum from these dogs. A small number of carefully bred and raised beagles from White Eagle Farm (Doylestown, Pennsylvania) are now available and these animals have been found to be negative to cutaneous testing with 0.1 ml of a 10 mg/ml solution of Ascaris extract (D. J. Herzig, unpublished results).

2. Pollen sensitivity

The major difficulty with using pollen-sensitive dogs is the limited availability of donors. A suitable supply of serum from a few such animals should provide enough material for PCA testing, especially since negative recipients are readily available. Dog cutaneous anaphylaxis is still in the early stages of development as a test system and its value in drug evaluation is not yet clear.

D. Bronchopulmonary Tests

Several parameters may be used to measure the severity of the bronchial response. These include increase in pulmonary resistance, decrease in dynamic compliance, increase in frequency of respiration, decrease in tidal volume, increase in expiratory/inspiratory ratio, decrease in peak expiratory flow rate, and increase in pCO_2. We have utilized measurements of pulmonary resistance and dynamic compliance as well as tidal volume and respiratory rate to follow changes in pulmonary mechanisms in

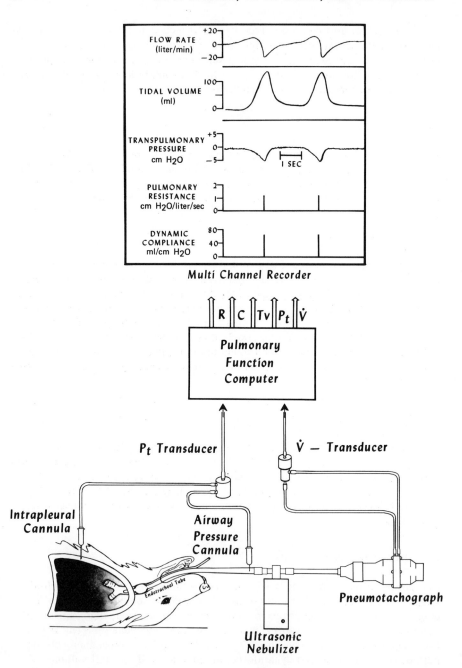

FIGURE 1.   Schematic representation of pulmonary function tests in anesthetized animals.

antigen-challenged dogs. The experimental system is schematically represented in Figure 1.

For our experiments, mongrel dogs of either sex (9-13 kg) were given morphine sulfate, 2 mg/kg, s.c., and were anesthetized 30 min later with sodium pentobarbital 30 mg/kg, i.v. Transpulmonary pressure was determined by monitoring the difference between pressure at the external end of the tracheal cannula and pressure within the pleural cavity by means of a Statham differential transducer (PM5TC 0.3 - 350). Intrapleural pressure measurements were performed with a small spearlike cannula (containing two large holes) introduced through the seventh intercostal space into the pleural cavity and held by a tight suture. A Fleisch pneumotachograph (Model 7319 No. 1) was used to monitor respiratory flow rate. Tidal volumes were obtained by electrical integration of the flow signal. Flow pressure and volume signals were fed into an on-line analog computer which performed the necessary calculations after each breath [30]. The computer output of resistance and compliance values (as well as flow, volume, and pressure) was recorded on a Beckman Dynograph.

An aqueous extract of Ascaris suum containing 1 mg protein/ml was administered via a Monaghan Ultrasonic Nebulizer into the tracheal cannula. Antigen aerosol was given for 2 breaths at zero time, for 4 breaths at 5 min, for 8 breaths at 10 min, and in certain experiments, for 16 breaths at 15 min. Animals were initially tested once every 7 days but since some dogs lost sensitivity to Ascaris during this test period, the interval was lengthened to 10 to 14 days.

Qualitatively consistent pulmonary responses to antigenic challenge included increased pulmonary resistance and decreased dynamic compliance. Changes in respiratory rate and tidal volume were less predictable. The effects of salbutamol, cyproheptadine, and cromolyn sodium in this system are summarized in Table 2 and Figure 2. Salbutamol significantly reduced the antigen-induced changes in compliance, resistance, and tidal volumes. Cyproheptadine reduced the severity of the resistance response (Table 2), suggesting the involvement of histamine or serotonin in the bronchoconstriction. Cromolyn sodium did not significantly reduce antigen-induced changes in any of the measured parameters. In a separate series of experiments even higher doses of cromolyn sodium (20 mg/ml by inhalation 5 min before challenge plus 50 mg/kg, i.v., 1 min before Ascaris challenge) afforded no protective activity. Krell et al. [31] reported that cromolyn sodium, at concentrations as high as 1×10^{-3} M, did not inhibit Ascaris-antigen-induced mediator release from canine lung fragments, whereas this same concentration of cromolyn sodium inhibited immunologically induced mediator release from both passively sensitized fragmented rat and rhesus monkey lung. The reasons for the species difference are not known. Since cromolyn sodium may be considered a standard "antiallergy" drug this raises some question as to the validity of the dog model.

TABLE 2 Percent Change of the <u>Ascaris</u>-Induced Pulmonary Response in Nine Anesthetized Dogs

Drug	Dose	Resistance (cm H_2O/liter/S)	Compliance (ml/cm H_2O)	Tidal volume (ml)	Respiratory rate (breaths/min)
Control	—	137.1 ± 19.2	-57.5 ± 2.6	-19.8 ± 8.0	96.0 ± 31.0
Salbutamol	6.25 μg/kg, i.v.	16.7 ± 2.8^a	-23.2 ± 5.5^a	3.5 ± 7.7^a	24.0 ± 23.0
Cromolyn sodium	5.0 mg/kg, i.v.	72.0 ± 21.8	-50.6 ± 9.3	-23.1 ± 11.8	103.0 ± 75.0
Cyproheptadine	20 mg/ml, aer.	44.5 ± 13.8^a	-47.6 ± 1.4	-16.8 ± 14.4	81.5 ± 38.0

[a]Significantly different from control (P < 0.05).

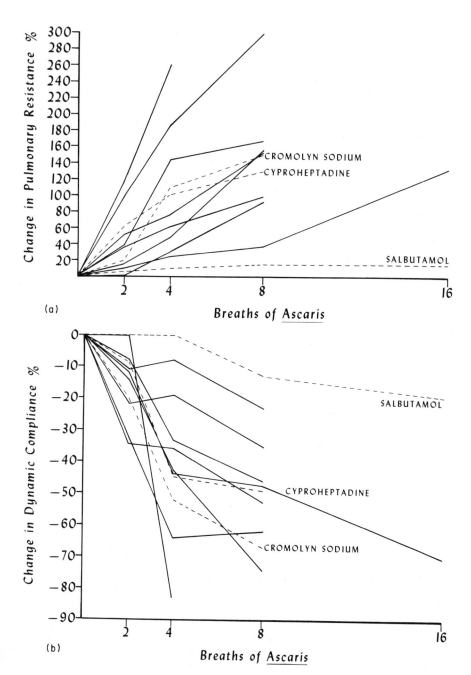

FIGURE 2. Changes in pulmonary resistance (a) and dynamic compliance (b) in a dog following cumulative doses of Ascaris antigen aerosol in the presence (----) or absence (——) of drug treatment. Each line represents the response of this animal on a particular day (test intervals, 10-14 days).

Studies on the mechanism of antigen-induced bronchospasm by Gold
and his coworkers [32-34] have implicated the cholinergic system. Increased
pulmonary resistance was abolished by vagotomy, by efferent vagal blockade
with atropine sulfate, or by afferent vagal blockade via selective cooling of
the nerves. Unilateral lung challenge with antigen resulted in bilateral
bronchoconstriction which was inhibited by cooling the vagus nerve inner-
vating the challenged lung. Gold suggested that although antigen-antibody
interaction may cause mediator release with direct local contraction of air-
way smooth muscle, a vagally mediated reflex bronchoconstriction is important in the acute phase. This reflex could be initiated by the antigen-
antibody interaction or by stimulation of irritant receptors by the released
mediators. In man, SCH 1000 (isopropyl atropine) has been reported to
have beneficial effects in acute tests in asthmatics and bronchitics [35,36],
providing some support for Gold's observations and their relevance to man.

IV. RATS

A. Types of Antibody and
    Methods of Production

The rat is the "classical" animal for laboratory study of immediate hypersensitivity. The induction of an antibody with reaginic characteristics was
described by Mota [12] almost concurrently with Ishizaka's description of
human IgE [37]. Until recently, the identification of IgE-like reagin in rat
serum was based on the following operational definitions:

1. ability to sensitize rat mast cells passively

2. ability to induce a PCA after latency of 48 hr

3. sensitivity to heating at 56°C

4. the mepyramine sensitivity of reaginic PCA

5. the lack of a requirement for complement to be effective

Isolation of this antibody and production of an antibody to it has provided direct evidence that immunochemically it is not one of the known
classes of rat immunoglobulins. Kanyerezei et al. [38] have shown that the
rat reaginic antibody has immunological determinants in common with human
IgE by absorption with anti-human ε chain. How much of the protein sequence
the IgE proteins from these two species have in common has not yet been
resolved. The recent identification of a rat IgE myeloma protein [39] may
resolve this issue by comparison with human IgE myelomas via physical and
chemical methods.

For most studies, the five criteria just cited are sufficient to assume the identity of IgE. Often, however, any single criterion is not sufficient. For instance, the sensitivity to heating appears to be a complex function of antibody concentration, its purity, and perhaps even the existence of other factors in the serum. In addition, mepyramine usually does not completely block rat PCA. This is understandable since mediators other than histamine are released. Third, the criteria as to latency are not clear-cut. Under certain conditions, especially when the titer is quite high, IgE sera will result in a short latency PCA. There is also evidence that IgGa can produce a PCA after a 24 to 48-hr latency. We have observed an antibody (IgG?) that may interfere with the 48-hr latency PCA. Similar effects have been seen in rabbits [40]. The fourth criterion can be questioned since the discovery of the alternate or nonclassical complement scheme. Generally, we have come to accept the first three criteria as evidence that what we are using for a 48-hr PCA is IgE reagin. A sixth criterion we insist on is that serial dilutions of the antibody result in a linear change in the PCA response. This is necessary because of the way we quantitate the PCA reaction (see below). Usually we have found that antisera that meet the first three criteria also meet the sixth.

Following the procedure of Mota [12], we induce reaginic antibody in rats using 1 mg of ovalbumin in saline given intramuscularly and 3×10^{10} B. pertussis organisms intraperitoneally. The resultant IgE antibody begins to appear on day 10 with peak titers of 1:40 to 1:80 occurring between days 12 and 16. We have found that by day 20 or 21 the IgE has disappeared whereas the IgG antibodies are increasing. Another approach in rats involves use of a dinitrophenylated extract of Ascaris suum (DNP-Ascaris) in saline as the immunogen and B. pertussis as the adjuvant. A peak (1:40) IgE response appears on Day 8 and by Day 12 IgE levels fall to undetectable levels. We have found that the source and age of the B. pertussis used can greatly affect the IgE response in either of these procedures. Triogen (Parke-Davis, Detroit, Michigan), a mixture of diphtheria and tetanus toxoids with pertussis, has been satisfactory. Progress has been reported on the isolation and purification of the adjuvant factor from pertussis [41], characteristics which ultimately should permit maintenance of a stable supply of the factor for routine production of antiserum.

A third method of production of IgE uses alumina gel as an adsorbent for the immunogen and no other adjuvant. In the technique of Petillo and Smith [42], three doses of alum and ovalbumin are given on alternate days. The antibody titer reaches a maximum on Day 8 and then falls precipitously. This response can be potentiated by a subsequent worm infection with Nippostrongylus brasiliensis. The antiovalbumin IgE antibody appears before the anti-worm IgE. Another variation on this theme was developed by Bloch et al. [43] in which microgram quantities of ovalbumin on alum were given on Day 0 followed by infection with Nippostrongylus on Day 14. On Day 28 a very high titer antiovalbumin IgE was obtained. In our hands,

application of this last technique has provided a serum with a 48-hr PCA
titer of greater than 1:360 and stability during storage at -80°C.

Certain strains of mice will produce IgE over several months and
respond anamnestically to subsequent challenges of antigen when microgram
quantities of immunogen on alum are given [44]. However, until recently
this was not possible in rats. It now appears that some strains of rats
respond similarly [45].

B. Cells and Mediators

In the rat, the mast cell is probably the primary receptor cell for IgE.
Most tissues have high concentrations of mast cells, especially the skin and
connective tissue [46]. Although basophils in the rat are few in number,
approximately one-fifth that found in man [47], basophilic leukemia cells
have been shown to bind rat IgE [48]. The rat mast cell sensitized with IgE
has been shown to release histamine, serotonin, SRS-A [49], and ECF-A
[50]. Histamine and serotonin, in a molar ratio of 1:20, are complexed to
heparin within the cell, forming an insoluble granule [51]. Like histamine
and serotonin, ECF-A apparently exists preformed in the mast cell [50] and
is released from the cells by IgE-mediated reaginic anaphylaxis. Although
the presence of ECF-A explains the appearance of eosinophils at the site of
a PCA reaction, its role in the pathology of the reaction is not clear.

SRS-A probably does not exist preformed in the cell [49]. Extraction
of unstimulated mast cells does not yield any measurable SRS-A. It is
possible that the SRS-A either exists as a promediator requiring enzymatic
activation or is synthesized de novo upon stimulation. The release of
SRS-A requires anaphylaxis with IgE-sensitized mast cells or IgGa antibody
and polymorphonuclear leukocytes, platelets, and complement. Since di-
ethylcarbamazine, a specific inhibitor of SRS-A, does not seem to have any
effect on rat PCA it is likely that SRS-A has little or no involvement in the
pathology of the reaction.

There exist several lines of evidence indicating that the cutaneous tissue mast cell and the peritoneal mast cell may not be identical. For one,
rat peritoneal mast cells, sensitized with rat IgE antiovalbumin and challenged with ovalbumin, will release between 20 and 30% of their total histamine [52]. Rarely can they be induced to release more than 40%. In contrast, the cutaneous tissue mast cell releases all of its histamine during
PCA. Selye et al. [53] first showed that it was possible to prepare spreads
of periosteal membranes of rat calvaria to show the mast cells (Fig. 3),
and we have adapted this technique to study tissue mast cells after passive
cutaneous anaphylaxis in the rat.

Reaginic rat antiovalbumin was injected under the skin on the top of
the head. Forty-eight hours later the rats were challenged by injecting 1
mg of ovalbumin intravenously in 1 ml of 0.25% Evans blue in saline. After
30 min the animals were decapitated, the dorsal skin on the head carefully

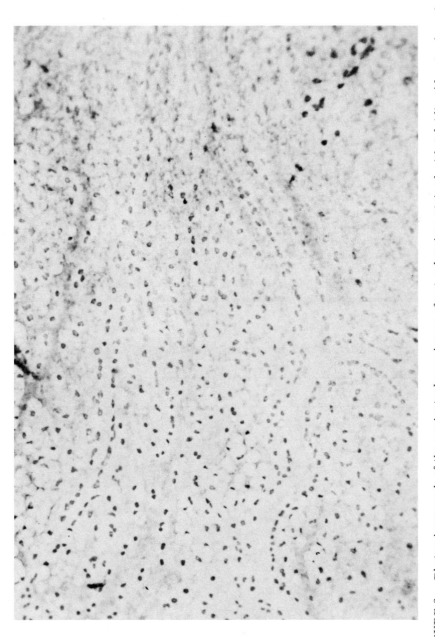

FIGURE 3. Photomicrograph of the periosteal membrane of rat calvarium stained with toluidine blue to show the densely granulated mast cells [53].

removed, and the cranium freed. After treatment for 1 hr in 95% ethanol the skulls were kept in absolute methanol overnight. The mast cells were stained in 0.18% solution of neutral red in ethanol for 30 min. After removal from the stain the skulls were washed with a stream of water, a pinhole put at the bregma for use as a landmark, and the dorsal periosteal membrane peeled off. These were then spread on a slide, dried, and mounted.

Photographs were taken of two areas of each tissue and the mast cells were counted. The results are reported as the average number of cells in these two areas per square millimeter of tissue. In those animals passively sensitized and challenged, the whole area of the top of the skull was heavily infiltrated with Evans blue, especially caudal to the coronal suture. This is indicative of the anaphylactic reaction. Table 3 illustrates that the anaphylaxis resulted in complete degranulation of the mast cells.

Another difference between the rat cutaneous tissue mast cell and the peritoneal mast cell is in the sensitivity to β-adrenergic agonists. When rat PCA was induced with rat IgE antiovalbumin and challenged after a 48-hr latency, subcutaneous doses of isoproterenol of less than 1 μg/kg effectively inhibited the reaction [54,55] (Fig. 4). This inhibition was blocked by the β-adrenergic blockers, propranolol and bunolol, and then reestablished by higher doses of isoproterenol. Histological examination of the PCA site indicated that isoproterenol prevented the degranulation of the mast cell.

TABLE 3   Mast Cell Density in the Rat Calvarium before and after Passive Cutaneous Anaphylaxis

Treatment	Animal	Mast cells/mm^2	Average
No challenge	1	291	
	2	362	346
	3	386	
Challenge	1	0	
	2	0	0
	3	0	
Isoproterenol[a] + challenge	1	336	
	2	332	360
	3	411	

[a]10 μg/kg, s.c., 5 min before challenge.

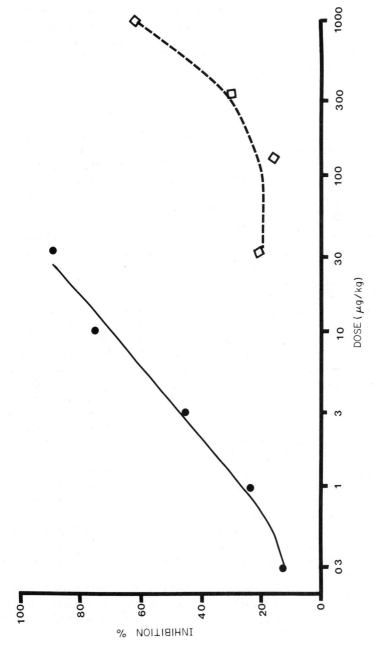

FIGURE 4. Inhibition of rat PCA by isoproterenol (——) and inhibition of isoproterenol inhibition by prior treatment with the β-adrenergic receptor antagonist bunolol (- - - -).

When peritoneal mast cells were sensitized and challenged in vitro [56], isoproterenol at levels up to 10^{-3} M did not prevent histamine release. These results confirm those reported by Johnson and Moran [57] and demonstrate that the peritoneal but not the cutaneous mast cell is insensitive to isoproterenol. Similar differences were found between pulmonary and cutaneous mast cells in the monkey [58].

C. Passive Cutaneous Anaphylaxis

IgE-mediated passive cutaneous anaphylaxis (PCA) in the rat is probably the most efficient method of screening large numbers of specific antiallergy agents. The skin of the rat is not as thin as that of the guinea pig or mouse and, consequently, it is easier to make rapid and precise intradermal injections of antiserum. Second, rats respond well to ether anesthesia with a relatively large safety margin between deep anesthesia and death. Thus, when injecting a large number of animals, the amount of time in the ether jar is not a critical factor. Third, the tail vein of the rat is not difficult to inject and five rats can be challenged with antigen and Evans blue within 2 min.

The actual procedure involves preparation of antiserum with a reaginic PCA titer of 1:40 to 1:80 by immunizing rats with 1 mg of ovalbumin, intramuscularly, and 2 ml of B. pertussis vaccine (Triogen, Parke-Davis) intraperitoneally. Fourteen days later the animals are bled, and serum, prepared in the usual way, is stored at -20°C. For PCA, dilutions of antiserum are chosen such that the diameters will fall between 7 and 19 mm. Within this range the mean orthogonal diameter is a linear function of the antiserum concentration. If antiserum concentration A with a PCA diameter of 12.6 mm is one-half the concentration B with a PCA diameter of 16.8, then any drug which reduces the PCA diameter from 16.8 mm to 12.6 mm will have inhibited the reaction by 50%. Rats are anesthetized with ether and then sensitized by intradermal injections on the back with 0.1 ml of suitable dilutions of antiserum. Each dilution is injected at similar sites on all animals. Forty-eight hours later, the test compounds are administered and under light ether anesthesia, 1 ml of physiological saline containing 1 mg of ovalbumin and 2.5 mg of Evans blue is injected into the tail vein. After 30 min, the animals are sacrificed in ether, the dorsal skin reflected, and the mean orthogonal diameter recorded. The blue spot appears rapidly, within several minutes, and does not change significantly over 40 min. Moreover, the doses of antigen between 0.5 and 20 mg result in little variation in the reaction.

The statistical significance of treatment effects on PCA is determined by Student's t-test. Since the standard error of the mean diameters in the control reactions is about 5 to 6%, drug inhibition greater than 15 to 20% is usually significant.

D. Active Cutaneous Anaphylaxis

There are advantages and disadvantages in using rat active cutaneous ana-phylaxis (ACA) to detect antiallergic compounds. Immunization in the rat induces antibodies other than IgE, some of which may be analogous to the non-IgE anaphylactic antibodies found in humans [59]. ACA may more closely mimic dermal allergies in atopic individuals and accordingly repre-sents a test model of high physiological validity. Limitations of ACA include wide variations in the level of sensitivity from rat to rat, the need for prior immunization of 8 to 14 days before the test day, and the relatively large amounts of adjuvant (e.g., B. pertussis) and immunogen needed. In con-trast, a small number of animals donating sera for PCA provide enough antibody to sensitize several hundred recipients, and serum pooling sub-stantially reduces variability.

Another limitation of ACA is the basic insensitivity of the response to changes in the amount of challenging antigen. For a change of 3 mm in diameter, for example (a change often seen by one twofold antiserum dilu-tion in PCA), one would have to dilute the antigen tenfold. In drug terms, this would require an inhibition of the ACA reaction by more than 90% [60].

We have eliminated some animal to animal variability in ACA by using each animal as his own control. Actively sensitized rats receive intrader-mal injections of logarithmic doses of antigen in 0.1 ml along one side of the dorsal midline and 1 ml of 0.25% Evans blue intravenously. Thirty minutes later they are treated with test compound and receive identical injections of antigen along the other side of the dorsal midline. After an additional 30 min, the rats are sacrificed in ether and the reaction measured as for PCA. We have been able to show inhibition of this reaction by drugs found effective in PCA [60].

E. Bronchopulmonary Tests

The rat has long been considered a poor choice for the study of pulmonary responses. However, recent studies have demonstrated a significant decrease in tracheal airflow and an increase in inflation pressure after intravenous injection of antigen following appropriate immunization [61-63]. Since antibodies responsible for this sytemic anaphylaxis in rats are rea-ginic and of the IgE type, it is conceivable that this anaphylactic broncho-constriction is immunologically similar to extrinsic human asthma. Phar-macologic tests in this model indicated that intravenous cromolyn sodium antagonized the bronchoconstriction, inducing a bell-shaped dose-response curve with peak activity at 1 mg/kg [63,64]. Meclofenamate, mepyramine, atropine, propranolol, or adrenalectomy did not significantly modify the response. Methysergide was an effective inhibitor, suggesting that serotonin is one of the major mediators of the bronchospasm.

Dexamethasone also blocked bronchospasm in the rat in a dose-related manner. In human asthma, the rationale for the therapeutic use of steroids has been based on their antiinflammatory efficacy. However, the effect of dexamethasone in the rat studies cannot be rationalized easily with its anti-inflammatory activity and may reflect some other action of the drug. Tozzi et al. have also used this system to test antiallergy compounds, specifically SCH 15,280 [64].

F. In Vitro Tests

1. Isolated peritoneal mast cells

The ready availability of free-floating mast cells in the rat peritoneal cavity has facilitated the use of an excellent in vitro system for detecting antial-lergic activity. Mast cells are obtained by lavage of the rat peritoneum, sensitized in vitro, and challenged with antigen after washing the cells. Thus, drug effects are observed under well-controlled conditions.

In all procedures of peritoneal lavage, Hank's Balanced Salt Solution is used without phenol red (Gibco, Grand Island, New York). Its buffering capacity is increased by the addition of 5% (v/v) 0.1 M phosphate buffer, pH 6.9. For the initial stages of cell preparation, the buffer contains 0.1% human serum albumin and 0.005% heparin. The cells from each animal are kept separate until they are centrifuged and washed once; then they are combined.

To isolate pure mast cells, we have found the procedure of Lagunoff [65] using 35% albumin (Pathocyte IV, Pentex Labs, Kankakee, Illinois) to be the easiest and most reliable. The purified cells are passively sensi-tized by incubating them in rat reaginic serum for 2 hr at 37°C followed by dilution with buffer and washing. The cells are suspended in buffer and ovalbumin is added to a concentration of 20 μg/ml. The variation in release as a function of antigenic concentration is minimal over the range 5 to 80 μg/ml [56]. After incubation at 37°C for 5 min, the cells are chilled and centrifuged and the supernatant assayed for histamine. Because of the vari-ation in the number of cells and the histamine content from day to day we routinely measure the total histamine in an aliquot of the cell suspension by boiling it for 5 min and centrifuging. The histamine release is then ex-pressed as the percentage of total available histamine. Aliquots of the cell suspension are carried through all procedures except that buffer is added instead of antigen. These samples are used to measure the antigen-inde-pendent or "spontaneous" histamine release. The latter, never more than 5% of the total, is subtracted from the amount of histamine released by antigen to obtain the net release due to anaphylaxis.

In most studies (run in duplicate) the net anaphylactic histamine release is between 20 and 30%, occasionally reaching 45%. We consider experiments unacceptable if the net histamine release is less than 20%. Acceptable release levels can usually be achieved by using fresh serum as already described for PCA. We have found that the activity of the serum declines in about 1 week, even when stored at -80°C, to the point where one cannot release sufficient (20%) histamine. Although its in vitro activity disappears, the PCA activity of the serum is not affected. We do not know if this reflects a change in the ability of the antibody to bind to the cell or a change in the interaction between antigen and antibody. Dilution of the antiserum with fresh normal rat serum does not restore the in vitro activity.

If the loss of in vitro sensitizing ability is due either to a change in the structure of the antibody or to some competitive substance, it is obviously reversible since the 48-hr latency PCA in vivo is not changed. As previously mentioned, peritoneal mast cells and tissue mast cells do not respond in the same way to certain pharmacological agents, such as isoproterenol. However, cromolyn sodium is active in vitro in blocking anaphylactic histamine release [56], an effect similar to that observed in rat PCA. Since it is possible to use up to 0.13% (v/v) acetone in the buffer without affecting histamine release, many insoluble compounds may be studied by first dissolving them in acetone.

Histamine may be reacted directly with o-phthaldialdehyde in base without extraction for fluorimetric assay since no interfering substances are released. An automated assay based on this procedure has been developed for the Technicon AutoAnalyzer [66].

V. MICE

A homolog of human IgE reagin has been described in the mouse [67–70] which will fix to both mouse and rat skin [70, 71]. Interestingly, cromolyn sodium, which is effective in man (and in the rat sensitized with homologous rat or heterologous mouse antiserum), was ineffective in the mouse [72].

VI. GUINEA PIGS

A. Skin Tests

An IgE-like antibody to ovalbumin has been described in the guinea pig [73] affording the possibility to carry out PCA in this species. However, we have found that this system does not lend itself readily to large-scale testing of compounds. There is the difficulty in anesthetizing guinea pigs rapidly as is necessary for rapid PCA injections and also the problem of obtaining reproducible PCA reactions.

B. Bronchopulmonary Tests

Guinea pigs have been classical test animals for the evaluation of pulmonary insults from both immunologic and pharmacologic sources. Characteristically, animals are actively sensitized and then challenged with the appropriate antigen at a later period. Response to antigenic treatment includes dyspnea, cough, and collapse.

Active anaphylactic bronchoconstriction in the guinea pig, as it was classically used in pharmacological laboratories (e.g., Herxheimer "microshock"), is probably mediated by IgG precipitating antibodies, not by reaginic antibodies [74]. However, the time period between sensitization and subsequent challenge with an antigen aerosol as well as the adjuvant used are important determinants of the type of antibody formed and present. Mota and Perini [75] reported that guinea pigs produced a "reaginic antibody" 10 to 17 days after immunization with ovalbumin and B. pertussis which disappeared by day 30. Its short existence probably contributed to the fact that it was not recognized in past experiments. We were able to adapt this procedure to induce a reaginic antibody in guinea pigs, to produce a reaginic anaphylaxis at the proper time, and to demonstrate a prophylactic effect of cromolyn sodium.

For these experiments, 200 to 250 g Hartley inbred guinea pigs (Springville Farms, Staten Island, New York) were sensitized as already described for rat IgE. The presence of reaginic antiovalbumin antibody was confirmed using the criteria of skin fixation for 48 hr and heat lability. On the 13th or 14th day after sensitization, the guinea pigs were exposed to an aerosol of ovalbumin (5% v/v in water) in a closed chamber. Guinea pigs were observed for dyspnea, cough (severe labored breathing with forceful expulsion of air), and collapse. Drugs were evaluated for their protection against each of the responses by means of a three-point scoring system. A score of 1 indicated dyspnea only; 2, dyspnea and cough; and 3, dyspnea, cough, and collapse. Total scores for a group were averaged to obtain a mean score. Cromolyn sodium was administered by two routes simultaneously, intraperitoneally (75 mg/kg) 3 min before challenge and by aerosol (20 mg/ml) for 2 min (using the Monaghan Ultrasonic Nebulizer) immediately before challenge with albumin.

The results shown in Table 4 indicate that 80% of the guinea pigs treated with a gum tragacanth vehicle responded to aerosolized ovalbumin with dyspnea and cough and 40% collapsed. Cromolyn sodium protected against dyspnea and cough. It did not protect against antigen-induced collapse in the Herxheimer microshock model at doses of 80 or 250 mg/kg, i.p., but did potentiate the protective effect of mepyramine at 40 and 160 mg/kg [76]. Thus, microshock is probably not a purely reaginic form of anaphylaxis.

We believe that a reaginic antibody is involved in the test for bronchospasm based on the work of Mota and Perini [75] although such an assumption is still speculative and proof requires appropriate immunochemical definition of the antibody. Furthermore, the protective activity of cromolyn sodium cannot, of itself, be taken as proof of a reaginic mechanism since (a) Morse et al. [77] found that cromolyn sodium also suppressed

TABLE 4   Effect of Cromolyn Sodium on the Response of
Sensitized Guinea Pigs to Aerosolized Ovalbumin

Treatment	Dose	Dyspnea	Cough	Collapse	Score
Vehicle	—	$80/80^a$	65/80	30/80	2.19
Cromolyn sodium	75 mg/kg, i.p. + 20 mg/ml, aer.	$14/80^b$	$10/18^b$	3/18	1.50

a Number responding/number in sample.
b Significantly different from vehicle (P < 0.05, 2 × 2x^2 test).

histamine release from mast cells sensitized with a heat-stable (nonrea-
ginic) IgGa antibody and (b) Orr et al. [78] have reported inhibition by cromolyn sodium of 4-hr PCA and associated histamine release in the rat,
mediated by a heat-stable anti-DNP IgG_2 antibody fraction. It is apparent
that the action of cromolyn sodium is not as specific for reagins as was at
first supposed.

Sensitive, sophisticated systems yielding reproducible data are now
available for the measurement of pulmonary mechanics in smaller animals
such as guinea pigs. Techniques to measure resistance and compliance
utilizing flow rate and pleural pressure in spontaneously breathing subjects
were first described by von Neegard and Wirz [79]. The principles of their
method were utilized by Amdur and Mead [80] to measure resistance and
compliance in spontaneously breathing, unanesthetized guinea pigs. Unfortunately, time-consuming manual calculations from three different tracings
(i.e., flow, tidal volume, and transpulmonary pressure) required the selection of only certain breaths for analysis and did not permit continuous monitoring. To overcome this difficulty both Dennis et al. [81] and Giles et al.
[30] developed on-line analog computer systems which provided resistance
and compliance values on a permanent record immediately after each breath.
Both of the computer systems can be used for guinea pigs as well as for
larger animals. A sample trace for this computer system applied to the
guinea pig is shown in Figure 5.

Responses to drugs in anaphylactic bronchoconstriction in guinea pigs
are not identical to those observed in human asthma. Although the bronchospasm in guinea pigs is attenuated by β-adrenergic agonists and potentiated
by β-adrenergic antagonists (similar to man), antihistamines are more
effective in blocking anaphylactic bronchospasm in the guinea pig than in
relieving human asthma. Also, steroids do not seem to markedly alleviate
anaphylactic bronchospasm in the guinea pig.

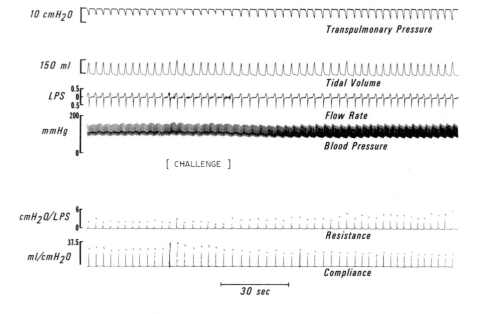

FIGURE 5. Representative tracing from the on-line computer showing the pulmonary and cardiovascular characteristics of a sensitized guinea pig before and after aerosolized antigen challenge.

VII. SCHEME FOR ANTIALLERGIC DRUG EVALUATION

Quantitative PCA in rats has served as a useful primary screen in our laboratory for many years and has enabled us to find compounds suitable for development as clinical candidates. Figure 6 outlines our route for the development of antiallergic candidates but which also identifies antimediator and bronchodilator drugs.

VIII. CONCLUSIONS

Although we would like to have more complete information about human disease before setting up counterpart laboratory models, this is often not possible. As a result, we frequently learn as much about the disease from testing new drugs in man as about the drug itself.

    The approach we have outlined here to search for new antiallergic agents is necessarily based on a simplistic view of allergy. There is

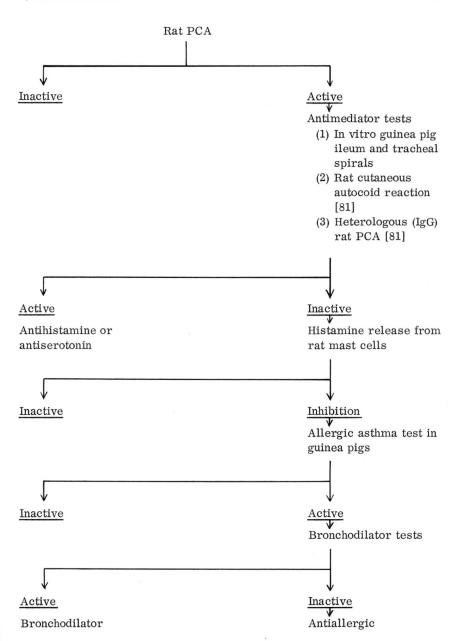

FIGURE 6.   Scheme for antiallergic drug evaluation.

evidence that in man (and rat) IgE is not the only reaginic antibody and that the basophils and mast cells are not the only allergized cells. Moreover, although the immediate response is important, there may be a later or secondary response that is also important. However, as pharmacologists searching for new therapies, we require a laboratory model that (a) is related to certain specific aspects of the disease, (b) is well controlled and reproducible, (c) lends itself to the testing of large numbers of compounds with some selectivity in the response, and (d) shows some predictability for clinical efficacy.

The scheme we have outlined fits all of these criteria except that no compound first discovered in rat PCA has been successfully developed for clinical use. Only a few compounds have even started to travel this road and the signposts are still blurred. We look forward to successful drug development in the antiallergy field in the years ahead and to validation of the techniques described in this chapter.

REFERENCES

1. H. H. Dale and P. P. Laidlaw, J. Physiol. (London) 41, 318 (1910).

2. H. H. Dale and P. P. Laidlaw, J. Physiol. (London) 43, 182 (1911).

3. D. Bovet and A. Staub, C. R. Seance Biol. 124, 547 (1937).

4. A. Staub and D. Bovet, C. R. Seance Biol. 125, 818 (1937).

5. J. W. Black, W. A. W. Duncan, C. J. Durant, C. R. Ganellin, and E. M. Parsons, Nature (New Biol.) 236, 385 (1972).

6. H. O. Schild, D. F. Hawkins, J. L. Mongar, and H. Herxheimer, Lancet 2, 376 (1951).

7. R. R. A. Coombs and P. G. H. Gell, in Clinical Aspects of Allergy (P. G. H. Gell, R. R. A. Coombs, and P. J. Lachmann, eds.), 3rd ed., Blackwell, Oxford, 1975, p. 761.

8. K. Ishizaka and T. Ishizaka, Ann. Allergy 28, 189 (1970).

9. S. G. O. Johansson, Lancet 2, 951 (1967).

10. S. G. O. Johansson, T. Mellbin, and B. Vohlquist, Lancet 2, 1118 (1968).

11. B. Uvnas and I. L. Thon, Exp. Cell Res. 23, 45 (1961).

12. I. Mota, Life Sci. 2, 917 (1963).

13. Z. Ovary and O. G. Bier, Proc. Soc. Exp. Biol. Med. 81, 584 (1952).

14. R. Patterson, in Progress in Allergy (P. Kallos and B. Waksman, eds.), Vol. 13, Karger, Basel, 1969, pp. 332-408.

15. R. Patterson, J. N. Fink, E. T. Nishimura, and J. J. Pruzansky, Clin. Invest. 44, 140 (1965).

16. R. Patterson and J. F. Kelly, Annu. Rev. Med. 25, 53 (1974).

17. K. Ishizaka and T. Ishizaka, J. Immunol. 103, 588 (1969).

18. R. Patterson, C. H. Talbot, and M. Roberts, J. Clin. Exp. Med. 10, 267 (1972).

19. R. Patterson and C. H. Talbot, J. Lab. Clin. Med. 73, 924 (1969).

20. R. Patterson, J. Irons, and K. Harris, Int. Arch. Allergy 48, 412 (1975).

21. R. Patterson, I. M. Suszko, and C. R. Zeiss, Jr., J. Allergy Clin. Immunol. 50, 7 (1972).

22. K. F. Austen, Fed. Proc. 33, 2256 (1974).

23. B. H. Booth, R. Patterson, and C. H. Talbot, J. Lab. Clin. Med. 76, 181 (1970).

24. R. E. W. Halliwell, R. M. Schwartzman, and J. H. Rockey, Clin. Exp. Immunol. 10, 399 (1972).

25. J. R. Battisto, D. Budman, and R. Freedman, J. Exp. Med. 134, 381 (1971).

26. R. E. W. Halliwell, J. Immunol. 110, 422 (1973).

27. R. Patterson, Y. Tomita, S. Oh, I. M. Suszko, and J. J. Pruzansky, Clin. Exp. Immunol. 16, 223 (1974).

28. H. Wilkins and N. Back, Arch. Int. Pharmacodyn. Ther. 190, 14 (1971).

29. D. J. Herzig, Immunol. Methods 5, 219 (1974).

30. R. E. Giles, M. Finkel, and J. Mazurowski, Arch. Int. Pharmacodyn. Ther. 194, 213 (1971).

31. R. D. Krell, L. W. Chakrin, J. Mengel, D. Young, C. Zaher, and J. R. Wardell, Pharmacologist 16, 570 (1974).

32. W. M. Gold, G. F. Kessler, and Y. C. Yu, J. Appl. Physiol. 33, 719 (1972).

33. A. B. DuBois, A. W. Brody, D. H. Lewis, and B. F. Burgess, J. Appl. Physiol. 8, 587 (1956).

34. A. B. Fisher, A. B. DuBois, and R. W. Hyde, Clin. Invest. 47, 2045 (1968).

35. H. Poppius and Y. Salorinne, Br. Med. J. 4, 134 (1973).

36. A. Lakdensus, A. A. Vilsanen, and A. Muittari, Scand. J. Clin. Lab. Invest. 31 (Suppl. 13), 16 (1971).

37. K. Ishizaka and T. Ishizaka, J. Allergy 42, 330 (1968).

38. B. Kanyerezei, J. C. Katon, and K. J. Bloch, J. Immunol. 106, 1411 (1971).

39. H. Bazin, A. Becker, and P. Querinjean, Eur. J. Immunol. 4, 44 (1974).

40. R. Revoltella and Z. Ovary, J. Immunol. 111, 698 (1973).

41. S. B. Lehrer, J. H. Vaughan, and E. M. Tau, J. Immunol. 114, 34 (1975).

42. J. P. Petillo and S. R. Smith, Int. Arch. Allergy 44, 309 (1973).

43. K. J. Bloch, J. L. Ohrman, Jr., J. Waltin, and R. W. Cygan, J. Immunol. 115, 197 (1973).

44. E. M. Vaz, N. M. Vaz, and B. B. Levine, Immunology 21, 11 (1971).

45. S. M. Murphy, S. Brown, N. Miklos, and P. Fireman, Immunology 27, 245 (1974).

46. P. Constantinides, Science 117, 505 (1953).

47. Blood and Other Body Fluids (D. S. Ditman, ed.), Fed. Am. Soc. Exp. Biol., Washington, D.C., 1961, pp. 125-127.

48. A. Kulczycki, C. Isersky, and H. Metzger, J. Exp. Med. 139, 600 (1974).

49. R. P. Orange, D. J. Stechschulte, and K. F. Austen, J. Immunol. 105, 1087 (1970).

50. S. I. Wasserman, E. J. Goetzl, and K. F. Austen, J. Immunol. 112, 351 (1974).

51. R. Keller, in Tissue Mast Cells in Immune Reactions, American Elsevier, New York, 1966, p. 25.

52. D. J. Herzig and E. J. Kusner, J. Pharmacol. Exp. Ther. 194, 457 (1975).

53. H. Selye, G. Gabbiana, and K. Hielsen, Proc. Soc. Exp. Biol. 112, 460 (1963).

54. B. Dubnick, L. J. Robichaud, and D. J. Herzig, Pharmacologist 13, 236 (1971).

55. E. S. K. Assem and H. O. Schild, Br. J. Pharmacol. 42, 620 (1971).

56. E. J. Kusner, B. Dubnick, and D. J. Herzig, J. Pharmacol. Exp. Ther. 184, 41 (1973).

57. A. R. Johnson and N. C. Moran, J. Pharmacol. Exp. Ther. 175, 632 (1970).

58. R. Patterson, C. H. Talbot, and M. Brandfonbrener, Int. Arch. Allergy 41, 592 (1971).

59. W. E. Parish, in Progress in Immunology II (L. Brest and J. Holborow, eds.), Vol. 4, American Elsevier, New York, 1974, p. 1.

60. D. J. Herzig, in Immunopharmacology (M. E. Rosenthal and H. C. Mansmann, eds.), Spectrum Press, New York, 1976, p. 108.

61. M. K. Church, H. O. J. Collier, and G. W. L. James, Br. J. Pharmacol. 46, 56 (1972).

62. L. M. Stotland and N. M. Share, Can. J. Physiol. Pharmacol. 52, 1114 (1974).

63. L. M. Stotland and N. M. Share, Can. J. Physiol. Pharmacol. 52, 1119 (1974).

64. S. Tozzi, F. E. Roth, and I. I. A. Tabachnik, Agents and Actions 4, 264 (1974).

65. D. Lagunoff, Biochem. Pharmacol. 21, 1889 (1972).

66. E. J. Kusner and D. J. Herzig, in Advances in Automated Analysis, Vol. 2, Thurman Associates, Miami, 1971, p. 429.

67. I. Mota and J. M. Peixoto, Life Sci. 5, 1723 (1966).

68. P. Provoust-Davon, J. M. Peixoto, and M. Queiroz-Javierre, Immunology 15, 217 (1968).

69. R. Revoltella and Z. Ovary, Immunology 17, 45 (1969).

70. Z. Ovary, S. Caiazza, and S. Kojima, Int. Arch. Allergy 48, 16 (1975).

71. M. K. Bach and J. R. Brashler, Immunol. Commun. 2, 85 (1973).

72. R. J. Perper, A. L. Oronsky, and V. Blancuzzi, J. Pharmacol. Exp. Ther. 193, 594 (1975).

73. A. Perini and I. Mota, Immunology 22, 915 (1972).

74. H. Herxheimer, J. Physiol. (London) 117, 251 (1952).

75. I. Mota and A. Perini, Life Sci. 9, 923 (1970).

76. J. S. G. Cox, in Advances in Drug Research (C. N. Harper and A. B. Simmonds, eds.), Vol. 5, Academic Press, New York, 1970, p. 115.

77. H. C. Morse, K. F. Austen, and K. J. Bloch, J. Immunol. 102, 327 (1969).

58   D. J. HERZIG, R. E. GILES, AND B. DUBNICK

78. T. S. C. Orr, J. G. William, and J. S. G. Cox, Immunology 19, 469 (1970).

79. K. von Neegard and K. Z. Wirz, Klin. Med. 105, 51 (1927).

80. M. O. Amdur and J. Mead, Am. J. Physiol. 192, 364 (1958).

81. M. W. Dennis, J. S. Douglas, J. W. Casby, J. A. J. Stolwyk, and A. Bouhuys, J. Appl. Physiol. 26, 248 (1969).

Chapter 3

ANTIHYPERTENSIVES

Stewart J. Ehrreich*

Schering Corporation
Bloomfield, New Jersey

*Present affiliation: Division of Cardio-Renal Drug Products, Food
and Drug Administration, Rockville, Maryland.

I. INTRODUCTION

Cardiovascular disease is at present the leading cause of death in the United States. An important component of this disease complex which impacts on other cardiovascular areas is essential hypertension. It has been determined, for example, that elevated arterial blood pressure is a causal or contributing factor in stroke, myocardial infarction, cerebral vascular, and peripheral vascular disease.

The underlying interrelationships associated with the onset and maintenance of hypertension were described by Page in 1949 [1]. Not only is there a mosaic of factors which contribute to elevated arterial pressure but pressure per se seems to play a self-sustaining role ultimately leading to reversible and irreversible pathologic changes.

Current medical practice advocates treatment of hypertension. However, method of treatment, time of initiation, and duration of treatment remain subjective. Antihypertensive drugs are usually effective, and only in limited cases, such as renal and adrenal hypertension or vascular lesions, is surgery indicated. Low sodium diets have been successful only when rigorously maintained.

When the pathological consequences of elevated blood pressure became apparent, various pressure-reducing procedures were attempted. Initially, reduction of patient anxiety was emphasized, imputing an emotional base to hypertension. Sedatives were commonly used but found to be only partially successful in lowering blood pressure. To be sure, there are some individuals whose hypertension is a manifestation of emotional stress and others whose blood pressures rise in consequence of the measurement itself. But these phenomena are of relatively minor significance in the treatment of essential hypertension.

The sedative approach was followed by the low sodium diet which in turn was essentially replaced by its pharmacological counterpart, the diuretic. Other types of antihypertensive drugs are now available which reduce blood pressure by such diverse mechanisms as selective central nervous system activity and direct peripheral vascular dilatation.

High blood pressure is a symptomless disease for an extended period of time, and most hypertensive patients are unaware of their condition. At present, there is a strong drive to monitor blood pressure throughout the general population. Such facilities as free clinics, hospital outpatient services, nurses, and dentists, to name a few resources, are being tapped for this purpose. The pressing need is to measure blood pressure in patients who do not visit physicians regularly.

Since a substantial segment of the hypertensive population is not yet optimally treated, the development of new antihypertensive drugs has been accorded a high priority. All major pharmaceutical companies are committed to this effort. The challenge lies not in finding an active antihypertensive compound but in demonstrating its safety, efficacy, and ultimately, mode of action. Equally important is the need to compare the new agent with existing drugs in order to establish its comparative efficacy. These and other objectives are explored in the succeeding sections.

The purpose of this chapter is to describe, in general, and give some background on the various approaches used in the pharmaceutical industry for finding new antihypertensive agents.

The first consideration in a pharmaceutical drug development program is to utilize simple and direct research approaches which are closely related to the treatment of the clinical condition. Other concerns are selectivity of action, desirable mode of action, long-term safety, patentability, and the likelihood that the agent will be successful from the points of view of cost, formulation, stability, and competitiveness with existing agents. The methodology and conclusions regarding a "typical" approach to the search for antihypertensive agents naturally reflect the author's views, but discussions held with other investigators regarding models and procedures used by the pharmaceutical industry tend to support the approaches described herein.

II. EXPERIMENTAL MODELS
OF HYPERTENSION

Many animal models of hypertension are available for drug screening and evaluation. Investigators have experimentally elevated blood pressures in rats, mice, rabbits, cats, dogs, and monkeys; a thorough review of the literature may be found in the monograph by Schlittler [2]. These models mimic human hypertension and provide a tool for developing safe and efficacious antihypertensive drugs.

A. Hormonal

Hormonal models of hypertension are produced by endogenous or naturally occurring exogenous substances, and are exemplified by renal and steroidal hypertension.

1. Renal hypertension

Renal hypertension has been produced in rats using clips placed around the renal artery [3-6] in procedures modified from the initial work of Goldblatt et al. [7] in dogs. We have used the method of Page [8] which involves wrapping one dog kidney with cellophane and removing the contralateral kidney 1 week later. Both methods produce an accelerated hypertension which leads to decreased survival time and blindness.

Renal involvement in homeostasis has been demonstrated by the fact that intact tissue from normally functioning kidneys can reduce blood pressure in hypertensive rats [9]. Blood pressure lowering substances are also found in renal venous blood [10] and are suspected to be prostaglandins. Infusion of prostaglandin A into patients with essential hypertension lowered blood pressure [11].

It is not yet clear whether the renal factor involved in hypertension develops as a consequence of renin production, reduced output of prostaglandin-like substances, or both [12]. Pettinger's group found no suppression of renin output in the spontaneously hypertensive rat (SHR) at 40 weeks of age, a stage similar to the malignant phase of human essential hypertension [13]. DeJong et al. indicated that onset of hypertension in the SHR may not be renin related since renin levels in renal venous blood were normal during the development phase of hypertension (8-12 weeks of age) and only increased at about 15 to 16 weeks [14]. In contrast, Sen and coworkers demonstrated elevated plasma and kidney renin levels in SHR before and during the initial phase of hypertension and normal or below-normal levels during the established phase [15]. These investigators believe that renin may play a primary role, possibly along with other factors, in the initiation of hypertension in SHR.

The importance of the renin-angiotensin system in the development of experimental and naturally occurring hypertension cannot be overemphasized. Peart [16] reviewed the field over a decade ago and the complexities seem to have increased since that time. It is known that angiotensin I, a decapeptide precursor of the powerful vasoconstrictor angiotensin II, is derived from a plasma tetradecapeptide through the action of the enzyme renin. Angiotensin II (or simply angiotensin) is formed by removal of two amino acids from angiotensin I by converting enzyme. In addition to vasoconstriction, angiotensin stimulates aldosterone secretion, causing sodium and water retention and increased blood volume.

In renal hypertensive rats, sodium retention caused "waterlogging" of the vascular smooth muscle [17-20]. Aortae from renal hypertensive rats produced greater tension than aortae from normal rats when exposed to constrictor agents [21] and have a higher wall/lumen ratio [22,23]. However, rat femoral artery studies did not confirm these observations [24]. Renal hypertensive rats fed high salt diets reached high pressures more rapidly than those on low salt diets [25-27] but leveled off at the same pressure as rats on normal sodium diets [28].

Sodium turnover is increased in renal hypertensive rats [29]. These animals tend to increase their sodium intake as evidenced by a preference for saline over fresh water [30]. Cats made hypertensive by renal artery stenosis had lower blood pressures during sleep, suggesting a central influence [31]. Likewise, pithing or ganglionic blockade reduced blood pressure in renal rats [32]. In renal hypertensive dogs, increased cardiac output may contribute to the elevated pressure [33].

Though renal hypertension is classically thought to be due to activation of the renin-angiotensin system causing water retention [34], some workers found only modest elevation of plasma renin activity [35]. Others have implicated the kallikrein-kinin system [36].

2. DOCA hypertension

Perhaps the most popular experimental model of hypertension is that induced by desoxycorticosterone acetate (DOCA) in rats. DOCA pellets (50-
500 mg/kg) are implanted subcutaneously and rats are offered 1% saline
instead of water for at least 3 weeks [37]. Those animals which remain
hypertensive long after all traces of steroid are gone are considered "meta-
corticoid." Our experience indicates that both DOCA-influenced and meta-
corticoid rats respond similarly to antihypertensive agents. Vascular
lesions and permeability changes have been observed in these animals [38]
as well as increased vascular norepinephrine concentrations [39].

   Variations of the standard DOCA rat procedure have been attempted
with other steroids and other laboratory animals. For example, methyl-
testosterone has been used successfully in nephrectomized rats [39a,39b]
as has aldosterone [39c], but progesterone failed to elevate blood pressure
in rabbits [39d]. Dogs chronically exposed to mineralocorticoid developed
hypertension sensitive to drug intervention [39e]. Mice also were made
experimentally hypertensive but their relatively small size rendered blood
pressure measurements technically difficult [39f].

3. Angiotensin and Triiodothyronine

Intravenous injections of angiotensin administered for 1 week produced elevated pressures in rats [40,41]. Formanek [42] and Tanz [43] have used
angiotensin-induced hypertension in rats and dogs, respectively, to test
antihypertensive agents.

   Triiodothyronine in combination with dinitrophenol and sodium chloride
caused hypertension in rats [44]. Likewise, triiodothyronine and sodium
chloride treatment of rats raised blood pressure and increased catecholamine turnover, resembling DOCA hypertension [45].

B. Neurogenic

Neurogenic hypertension can be produced in animals by surgical procedures
which remove or modify neural homeostatic mechanisms. The usual approach involves removal of the carotid sinuses, one vagosympathetic trunk,
and the contralateral aortic depressor nerve. Dogs [46] are the species of
choice but rabbits [47] have also been used. A review of most of these
methods may be found in the monographs by Kezdi [48] and Boura and
Green [49].

   More recently, behavioral techniques have been used to produce neurogenic hypertension in monkeys [50-52]. The monkeys, trained to press a
key in order to diminish noxious stimuli, were also monitored continuously
for blood pressure changes. As training progressed, elevated blood pressure correlated positively with increased key-pressing frequency. At the
end of the training period, keys were removed from the apparatus and the
schedule altered so that increased blood pressure per se suppressed noxious

stimuli. Mean arterial blood pressure rose during each session. In other experiments in rats, complete removal of sound resulted in blood pressure elevations of 30 mmHg which, in turn, were responsive to antihypertensive agents [53]. Both the monkey and the rat experiments indicated that change of environmental conditions produced a stressful situation which resulted in elevated arterial blood pressure. The monkey studies further demonstrated that high blood pressure per se is "recognizable" by the animal and can be consciously controlled.

We have used neurogenic hypertensive dogs for many years in our laboratory. Their elevated arterial blood pressures are due to increased vascular resistance and increased cardiac output [54]. Sympathetic outflow is enhanced and a persistent, though labile, hypertension develops. Because pressures and heart rates are highly labile in this model, the dogs are handled by the same individuals under controlled laboratory conditions.

C. Genetic

Okamoto [55,56] has successfully bred a strain of rats with markedly elevated blood pressures. These spontaneously hypertensive rats (SHR) are now commercially available and are ideal for screening purposes because of their sensitivity to standard antihypertensive agents.

Considerable evidence is available to support the contention that the onset of hypertension in SHR and in humans is accompanied by adaptive structural changes in the vasculature. Increases in the wall/lumen ratio of SHR can account for the approximately 50% increase in blood flow resistance over that of normotensive rats at comparable degrees of smooth muscle shortening [57-59].

Immunosympathectomized SHR and normotensive rats had 40 and 25% reductions in blood pressure, respectively, indicating higher sympathetic tone in SHR [60-62]. Moreover, immunosympathectomized SHR had a more rapid vascular response to norepinephrine, supporting the higher SHR wall/lumen ratio concept [63-65]. Other studies have implicated catecholamines as possible etiologic factors in the hypertension of SHR. Norepinephrine synthesis appears to be increased in SHR [66], even though reduced catecholamine levels were found in heart and spleen [67,68]. On the other hand, Mizogami et al. found that neither sensitivity to catecholamines nor uptake mechanisms were important features of SHR hypertension [69].

A "resetting" of the baroreceptor mechanism has been proposed for SHR [70-72], but this may not be a primary factor [73,74].

The sensitivity of SHR to environmental factors such as stress [75] and high sodium diet [76,77] parallels comparable aspects of human essential hypertension. Even effects on the eye [78] and age of onset [79] seem similar. Substrains of genetic hypertensive rats have been produced which are exceptionally sensitive to salt administration [80,81] in respect to elevated

blood pressures [82], cardiovascular lesions [83,84], or both. It is clear
that sensitivity to salt ingestion is genetic in nature [85,86]. There is also
evidence that the ratio of 18-hydroxydesoxycorticosterone to corticosterone
may be controlled by one of the several genes involved in rat blood pressure regulation [87,88].

One drawback of an SHR screening program is the acknowledged difficulty in reproducing experimental data from one laboratory to another.
This may be due to genetic drift accentuated by the large number of separate
SHR breeding sites. Systolic blood pressures vary among populations as
do hemodynamic profiles and dose-response curves for standard antihypertensive drugs. Accordingly, a conservative screening approach is suggested
whereby emphasis is placed on data generated within one's own laboratory.

D. Miscellaneous

The heavy metal cadmium, implicated in the development of human hypertension, has caused hypertension in dogs when administered intraperitoneally
at 2 mg/kg in 24 injections spaced over a 9-month period [89]. In rats, too,
cadmium produced elevated arterial pressures [72,90]. In mice, hypertension was observed after feeding high fat diets [1] and in young rats after
choline-deficient diets [91].

III. DRUG EFFECTS IN
      EXPERIMENTAL MODELS

A. Spontaneously Hypertensive Rats

Table 1 illustrates the effects of various antihypertensive agents administered parenterally to spontaneously hypertensive rats (SHR). Most clinically
used agents lower blood pressure in this model. The single exception may
be β-adrenergic blockers [92-94], but one group has claimed antihypertensive
efficacy for propranolol in SHR when administered intravenously [96].

Freis et al. [97] have shown that the course of blood pressure elevation
and end-organ lesions in the SHR is significantly altered by chronic administration of antihypertensive agents during the development phase of hypertension and exacerbated by salt administration. The implications of this
finding are that early diagnosis and treatment of hypertension may provide
a favorably altered course of the disease [98], and that reduced salt intake
is recommended along with appropriate therapy.

The apparent similarity of the SHR model to (essential) hypertensive
man and its sensitivity to most clinically effective drugs recommend it
highly as an initial screening tool.

TABLE 1   Effect of Some Antihypertensive Agents in the
Spontaneously Hypertensive Rat

Drug	Dose (mg/kg, i.p.)	Systolic blood pressure (mmHg)	Peak effect (hr)	Reference
Clonidine[a]	0.01	-32	0.2	127
	0.10	-50	0.2	
Chlorisondamine	10	-50	3	92
Chlorothiazide	10	-30	2	92
	20	- 8	2	128
L-Dopa	200	-60	5	129
Guanethidine	40	-55	4	128
Hydralazine	2	-50	1	128
6-Hydroxydopamine	200	-50	24	130
Methyldopa	200	-50	5	131
		-50	4	128
Methyltyrosine ethyl ester	200	-35	4	92
Pargyline	75	-50	1	92
Phentolamine	5	-40	2	92
Pronethalol	10	+40	1.5	92
Reserpine	0.1	-45	5	128

[a]Injected intravenously into urethane anesthetized rats.

B.   DOCA Rats

In studies carried out over many years in our own laboratory [94] and that
of Pharmakon of Scranton, Pennsylvania [99], we have tested a large number of compounds in the DOCA hypertensive rat.   Tables 2 to 5 summarize
the oral effects of various antihypertensive agents in this model.   For purposes of convenience, the drugs are tabulated according to their pharmacological actions, i.e., diuretics, vasodilators, and neurogenic agents.

TABLE 2 Effect of Diuretics in the DOCA Hypertensive Rat

Drug	Dose (mg/kg, p.o.)	N	Systolic blood pressure (mmHg ± SEM)			Ref.	Ratio[a]
			0	4 hr	24 hr		
Vehicle[b]		456	188 ± 9.7	188 ± 10.3 >0.8[c]	189 ± 10.4 >0.8	99	
Acetazolamide	10	12	190 ± 2.8	182 ± 3.5 >0.05	185 ± 3.2 >0.2	99	5
	50	12	193 ± 4.8	172 ± 5.5 <0.01	178 ± 5.1 >0.05	99	
	100	12	185 ± 2.4	166 ± 4.7 <0.01	186 ± 4.3 >0.8	99	
Chlorothiazide	50	10	175 ± 6.0	159 ± 7.6 >0.05	—	94	
	250	5	149 ± 5.1	147.4 ± 6.7 >0.8	—	94	
Furosemide	25	12	193 ± 3.5	179 ± 4.9 >0.05	187 ± 4.2 >0.3	99	42
	50	12	189 ± 2.5	171 ± 2.7 <0.001	175 ± 5.7 >0.05	99	
	100	12	190 ± 3.4	170 ± 3.4 <0.01	186 ± 3.2 >0.5	99	

TABLE 2 (Cont.)

Drug	Dose (mg/kg, p.o.)	N	Systolic blood pressure (mmHg ± SEM)			Ref.	Ratio[a]
			0	4 hr	24 hr		
Hydrochlorothiazide	5	24	184 ± 1.8	170 ± 3.9 <0.01	187 ± 2.2 >0.4	99	1.3
	25	24	194 ± 2.9	174 ± 3.5 <0.001	186 ± 3.2 >0.05	99	
	100	24	192 ± 3.2	166 ± 5.8 <0.01	191 ± 4.0 >0.5	99	
Mercuhydrin[d]	20	12	196 ± 4.0	153 ± 3.0 <0.001	181 ± 4.0 <0.05	99	
Triamterene	100	12	196 ± 3.9	182 ± 5.3 >0.2	185 ± 4.2 >0.4	99	

[a] Effective rat dose/effective human dose.
[b] Methylcellulose, 0.25%.
[c] Probability, compared to pretreatment value.
[d] Injected intramuscularly.

Table ... of Systemic Vasodilator Agents in the DOCA Hypertensive Rat

Drug	Dose (mg/kg, p.o.)	N	Systolic blood pressure (mmHg ± SEM)				Ref.	Ratio[a]
			0	Day 1		Day 2, 4 hr		
				4 hr	24 hr			
Diazoxide	10	45	199 ± 3.0	180 ± 3.2 <0.001[b]			94	
	20	20	199 ± 3.4	173 ± 3.9 <0.001			94	
	40	23	191 ± 4.3	153 ± 6.2 <0.001			94	
Hydralazine	1.5	26	179 ± 2.5	159 ± 4.9 <0.005			94	
	3.0	10	199 ± 4.4	173 ± 6.1 <0.001	188 ± 48 >0.1	170 ± 5.6 <0.001	99	
	6.0	10	198 ± 3.5	146 ± 6.5 <0.001	178 ± 5.5 <0.02	138 ± 6.3 <0.001	99	
Isoxuprine	50	5	192 ± 3.1	168 ± 4.8 <0.01	184 ± 3.0 <0.1	175 ± 3.4 <0.1	99	50
Papaverine	50	5	190 ± 3.0	167 ± 2.8 <0.01	182 ± 2.6 <0.1	174 ± 3.3 <0.01	99	17
Prazosin	0.1	5	169 ± 2.6	157 ± 3.4 <0.05			94	
Nylidrin	12.5	5	190 ± 2.5	176 ± 2.8 <0.01	188 ± 2.8 >0.8	175 ± 4.7 <0.05	99	20
	25	5	186 ± 2.1	169 ± 4.7 <0.01	179 ± 5.6 >0.1	171 ± 4.8 <0.01	99	

[a] Effective rat dose/effective human dose.
[b] Probability, compared to pretreatment value.

TABLE 4 Effects of Neurogenic Agents

| Drug | Dose (mg/kg, p.o.) | N | Systolic blood pressure (mmHg ± SEM) | | | | | Ratio[a] |
			0	Day 1 4 hr	Day 1 24 hr	Day 2, 4 hr		
Bretylium	80	4	158 ± 1.5	118 ± 5.2 <0.01b	141 ± 5.0 <0.01	126 ± 4.0 <0.01	94	
Clonidine	0.100	15	205 ± 2.9	178 ± 4.9 <0.001			94	25
	0.250	12	186 ± 2.9	146 ± 5.6 <0.001	174 ± 7.5 >0.2		99	
	0.500	4	165 ± 1.7	121 ± 3.5 <0.01	136 ± 3.5 <0.01	118 ± 1.5 <0.001	94	
Guanethidine	12.5	10	194 ± 2.7	176 ± 4.9 <0.02	191|± 2.6 >0.5	178 ± 2.8 <0.01	99	12
	25	10	194 ± 2.7	171 ± 3.6 <0.001	181 ± 3.5 <0.02	164 ± 4.0 <0.001	99	
	50	12	195 ± 4.3	154 ± 4.67 <0.001			99	
Methyldopa	30	5	190 ± 4.0	169 ± 4.3 <0.01			94	
	100	5	190 ± 4.0	159 ± 11.9 <0.01			94	
	200	12	189 ± 2.5	152 ± 6.0 <0.001	170 ± 8.0 <0.05		99	

Phentolamine	20	5	188 ± 2.3	172 ± 4.3 <0.05	182 ± 1.9 >0.1	173 ± 3.1 <0.05	99
	80	5	194 ± 3.7	174 ± 4.1 <0.05	196 ± 3.4 >0.8	172 ± 4.6 <0.05	99 · 20
Propranolol	80	4	160 ± 1.6	144 ± 8.5 >0.1	156 ± 7.9 >0.1	133 ± 7.5 <0.1	94 · 80
Reserpine	12.5	5	199 ± 5.7	162 ± 6.9 <0.05	177 ± 2.9 <0.05	158 ± 5.5 <0.01	99 · 15
	25	5	195 ± 3.8	151 ± 4.6 <0.01	176 ± 5.5 >0.05	154 ± 5.7 <0.01	99
	50	5	196 ± 4.9	144 ± 8.2 <0.01	170 ± 7.4 >0.05	146 ± 9.8 <0.02	99
Sotalol	400	5	196 ± 3.6	172 ± 6.7 >0.5	187 ± 8.4 >0.4	172 ± 9.8 >0.1	99

[a] Effective rat dose/effective human dose.
[b] Probability, compared to pretreatment value.

TABLE 5 Effect of Miscellaneous Agents in the DOCA Hypertensive Rat

Drug	Dose (mg/kg, p.o.)	Systolic blood pressure (mmHg ± SEM)				Ref.	Ratio[a]
		0	Day 1 4 hr	24 hr	Day 2, 4 hr		
Mebutamate	100	186 ± 1.5	168 ± 7.0 <0.001[b]			99	
Metaraminol	5	166 ± 1.8	160 ± 13.9		141 ± 8.1 <0.02	94	
Pargyline	100	186 ± 1.5	156 ± 5.2 <0.01			99	200
p-Hydroxy-norephedrine	5	169 ± 2.6	158 ± 4.7 <0.05	159 ± 7.3 >0.1	156 ± 11.1 >0.2	94	

[a] Effective rat dose/effective human dose.
[b] Probability, compared to pretreatment value.

All diuretics which are potassium wasting, that is, produce a low urinary Na^+/K^+ ratio, are antihypertensive. These include acetazolamide, chlorothiazide, furosemide, hydrochlorothiazide, and mercuhydrin (Table 2). The ratio of effective rat dose to effective human dose gives some indication of the relative sensitivity of the animal model to man. The effective rat dose is defined as the lowest, single antihypertensive dose (mg/kg), and the effective human dose, the manufacturer's recommended average daily dose (mg/kg). The ratio is most favorable for hydrochlorothiazide and least for furosemide. Triamterene, a potassium sparing agent which is very valuable in combination with other diuretics, is ineffective alone in man and is ineffective in the DOCA rat at doses up to 300 mg/kg.

Table 3 illustrates the effects of various vasodilators, some of which are potent blood pressure lowering agents in the DOCA rat. Dose-response curves for diazoxide and hydralazine shown in Figure 1 are derived from composite data obtained in two laboratories. Nevertheless, the linear relationship of dose and response at time of peak effects suggests a desirable consistency for the DOCA rat model as a reliable test procedure. Table 3 also contains data on vasodilators (isoxuprine, papaverine, and nylidrin) primarily used to increase blood flow in obstructive vascular disease.

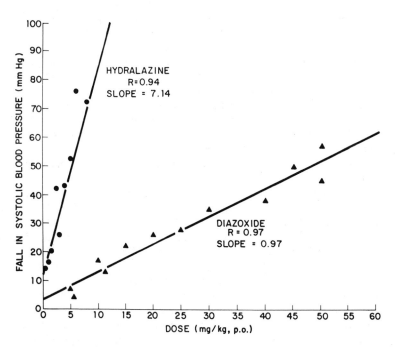

FIGURE 1.   Effect of hydralazine and diazoxide in DOCA hypertensive rats.

These drugs can usually be distinguished from antihypertensives by their
side effects (hyperemia of ears, face, and legs) and their relatively weak
blood pressure lowering effects in other models of hypertension. Prazosin,
a new antihypertensive agent, is active at very low doses in the DOCA rat.
In addition to its vasodilator activity, prazosin is known to possess adrenergic neuron and α-receptor blocking actions as well as CNS effects.

Table 4 shows the effects of agents acting primarily on the autonomic
and central nervous systems of the DOCA rat. The most potent by far is
clonidine, but other standard agents such as guanethidine, methyldopa,
phentolamine (which is not used clinically as an antihypertensive), and reserpine are all active. Propranolol may be active in this model [100] but the
dose required relative to the human dose is very high.

C. Neurogenic, Renal, and
    Normotensive Dogs

In the experiments described in this section, all neurogenic hypertensive
dogs were previously tested with placebo to eliminate labile reactors. Statistical analyses involved paired comparisons versus the animals' last six
control readings prior to drug [101].

Figure 2 illustrates, from top to bottom, the responses of two normotensive, three renal hypertensive, and three neurogenic hypertensive dogs
to oral hydrochlorothiazide. Hydrochlorothiazide was administered once a
day for 3 consecutive days at 10 or 20 mg/kg. In only one of eight dogs (a
neurogenic hypertensive dog) did hydrochlorothiazide lower blood pressure
to statistically significant levels. Figure 3 summarizes the relative effects
of oral hydralazine in normotensive, renal, and neurogenic hypertensive
dogs. At doses of 5 to 20 mg/kg hydralazine is most effective in the neurogenic hypertensive dog and slightly more effective in the normotensive than
in the renal hypertensive dog. In each experiment, tolerance occurred to
repeated administration. Reflex tachycardia is readily apparent in the intact
normotensive dog, less so in the debuffered neurogenic dog, and variable in
the renal dog.

Figure 4 illustrates the effect of oral reserpine in each of the dog
models. A single dose of 0.05 mg/kg is sufficient to lower blood pressure
and induce bradycardia for 3 to 4 days in the neurogenic dogs. Only incon-
sistent effects are observed in the normotensive and renal hypertensive dogs.
The effects of oral phenoxybenzamine, shown in Figure 5, indicate relative
efficacy in the normotensive and neurogenic hypertensive dogs at 5 to 20 mg/
kg but inconsistency in the renal hypertensive dogs.

The ganglionic blocking agent mecamylamine was tested in normotensive and neurogenic hypertensive dogs. Figure 6 illustrates the marked
oral effectiveness of this compound in neurogenic dogs only, bradycardia
closely tracking the hypotensive curve. Since neurogenic hypertension is a
high cardiac output condition [54], reduction of cardiac output alone, through

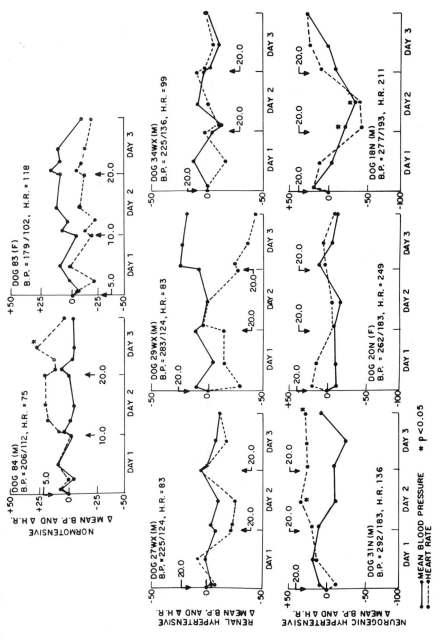

FIGURE 2. Effect of hydrochlorothiazide in normotensive and hypertensive trained dogs.

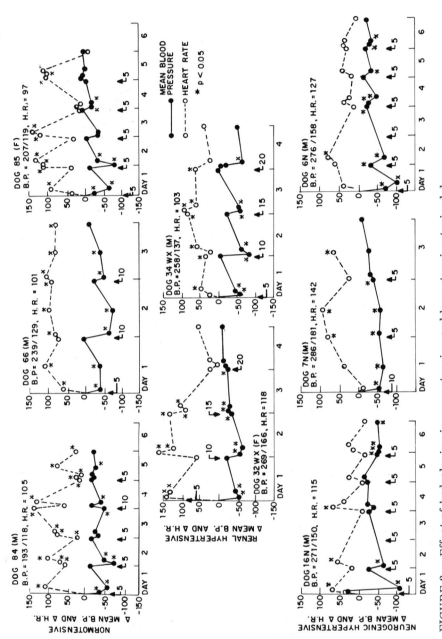

FIGURE 3.   Effect of hydralazine in normotensive and hypertensive trained dogs.

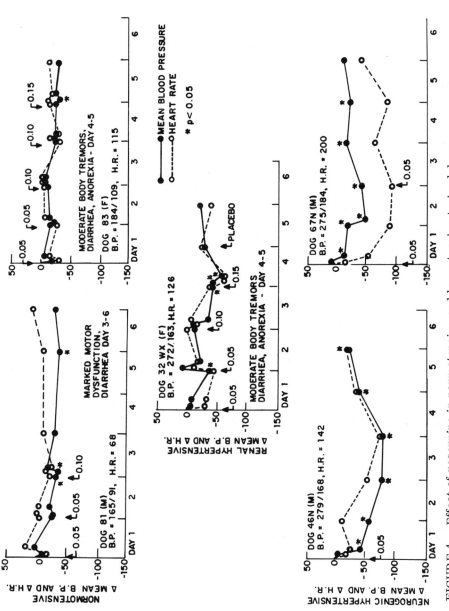

FIGURE 4. Effect of reserpine in normotensive and hypertensive trained dogs.

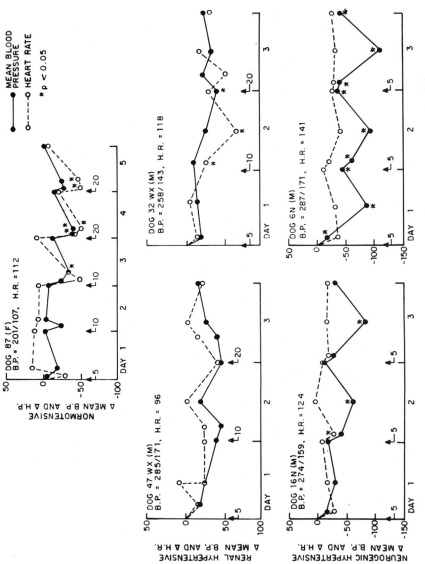

FIGURE 5.   Effect of phenoxybenzamine in normotensive and hypertensive trained dogs.

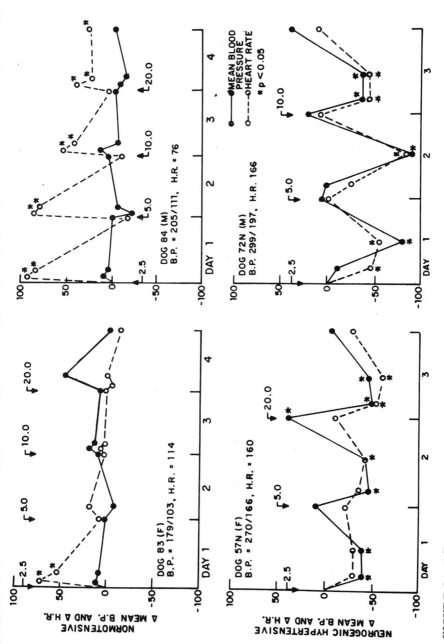

FIGURE 6.   Effect of mecamylamine in normotensive and neurogenic hypertensive trained dogs.

S. J. EHRREICH

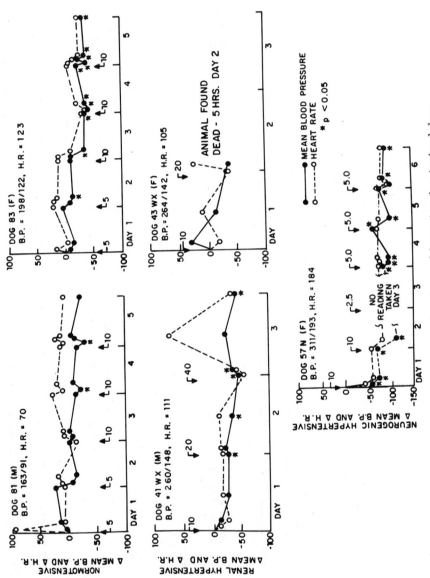

FIGURE 7.   Effect of guanethidine in normotensive and hypertensive trained dogs.

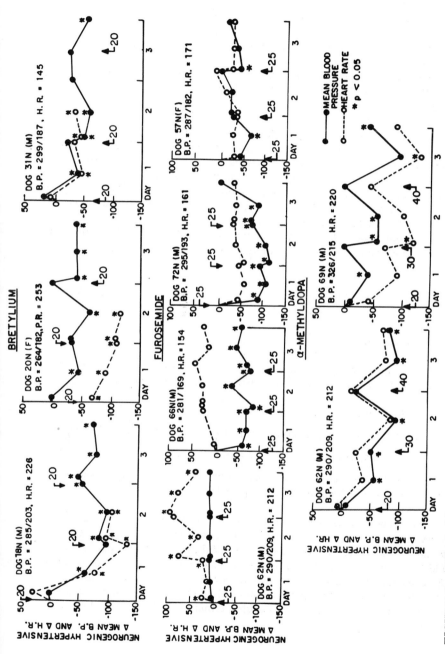

FIGURE 8.   Effect of bretylium, furosemide, and α-methyldopa in neurogenic hypertensive trained dogs.

bradycardia, may explain the entire hypotensive response. Guanethidine lowers blood pressure in all three dog models (Fig. 7), although toxicity was observed in one renal hypertensive dog at a dose of 20 mg/kg. Oral administration of this antihypertensive proved more effective in neurogenic hypertensive dogs than in normotensive or renal hypertensive animals.

Several other compounds were tested in the neurogenic dog only. These are illustrated in Figure 8. Bretylium, furosemide, and methyldopa were all active in this preparation. It should be noted that furosemide is the only diuretic agent tested which is active in the neurogenic dog; ethacrynic acid has not yet been tested. The order of sensitivity of these hypertensive preparations to standard antihypertensive drugs is as follows: neurogenic dog > normotensive dog > renal hypertensive dog [102]. The neurogenic dog in particular provides a useful nonrodent model for the evaluation of anti-hypertensive drugs, and although it cannot detect all clinically useful agents it is an extremely valuable tool for secondary or tertiary evaluations. Activity in this model provides, at the very least, an impetus to continue testing a compound which may have shown little or no activity in an anesthetized animal or in conscious normotensive or renal hypertensive models.

IV. SCREENING AND
EVALUATION PROCEDURES

A. Concepts and Criteria

One of the most important aspects of a development program is the primary screening test. This test should fulfill the following criteria:

1. Resemble the appropriate disease condition.

2. Detect currently useful therapeutic agents at reasonable dose levels.

3. Be relatively inexpensive and simple to carry out.

4. Accommodate large numbers of small animals and minimal quantities of investigational compounds.

The experimental model should not be limited in its detection characteristics to a novel mode of action or to an otherwise specific class of compounds. Wide range application is essential for screening purposes. In addition, either the screening test or a secondary procedure should have the capability of multiple dose evaluation. Much of the costly "discrepancies" noted between animal responses and clinical effects may not be due to species or model differences but to acute (animal) effects versus chronic (human) effects.

B. Indirect Blood Pressure
    Measurement

The rat is an ideal test model because of its size and ease of handling.
Moreover the rat tail allows for blood pressure measurements to be made
by indirect means utilizing a tail cuff. Bunag [103] has shown that there is
a direct correlation between the systolic blood pressure taken by indirect
means and direct aortic blood pressures. Regardless of the type of rat
model used, the animal must be restrained and placed in an environmental
temperature of at least 32°C in order to obtain a tail pulse. Several methods are available [104] but the usual approach is first to place the animals
in a warming chamber at 40 to 42°C and then at a lower temperature for the
remainder of the experiment. In most systems, the operator observes the
falling pressure in the tail cuff manometrically and the appearance of the
tail pulse oscillographically. Heart rate may be obtained with a cardio-
tachometer, but generally no hard-copy records are available for either
blood pressure or heart rate.

The author uses an automated recording device to obtain permanent
pressure and heart rate records of large numbers of animals in a relatively
short period of time [105]. In this system, rats are heated to a temperature
of 32 to 33°C or just above the critical temperature required. Animals
remain in the warming box, each in its own restrainer, for up to 5 hr after
dosing while systolic blood pressures and heart rates are taken at intervals
preset by a timer controller. In this way, heat stress is minimized and
discontinuous determinations follow the time course of drug effects. Some
measure of stress and exaggerated toxicity are present due to the warming
and restraining conditions inherent in this procedure. Therefore, it is not
possible to determine precisely the actual therapeutic ratios of experimental
compounds until their toxicity components are assessed in a normal environment.

C. Primary Screening Technique

In our primary screening procedure, compounds are administered orally
to hypertensive rats for 2 days at 100 mg/kg/day. The vehicle is 0.4%
methylcellulose. Blood pressures and heart rates are not measured during
the first 24 hr postdosing. After the second dose, rats are placed in their
restraining cages and pressure and heart rate readings are taken at 0, 1,
2, 3, and 4 hr postdosing. A compound is considered active if it reduces
systolic blood pressure by at least 20 mmHg.

The 2-day dosing schedule would miss compounds that are active on
Day 1 but inactive on Day 2. Such compounds probably induce rapid tolerance and consequently are of no interest as development candidates. However,

the compound with little or no antihypertensive activity on Day 1 but significant activity on Day 2 would be detected and further evaluated by virtue of
its cumulative action.

If an active compound is identified in the primary screen, its effect
on heart rate is then evaluated. Although this parameter is relatively variable in the rat, it is often useful in confirming weak antihypertensive activity.
Duration of antihypertensive action should exceed 3 hr. An active compound
of acceptable duration is generally retested to corroborate the initial results.

D. Secondary and Tertiary Tests

If the retest in the rat confirms activity, the next stage in evaluation is to
determine whether the compound has an undesirable mode of action. Some
of the latter may include blockade of α-adrenergic, β-adrenergic, ganglionic, and adrenergic neuron systems as well as histaminergic or cholinergic activity.

1. The anesthetized dog
    challenge test

In this procedure, compounds are administered intravenously (or intradu-
odenally) to anesthetized dogs (or cats) in order to determine effects on
blood pressure, heart rate, and the autonomic nervous system. Animals
are challenged with various autonomic procedures prior to and immediately
following administration of experimental compounds. We have found the
following series useful to characterize autonomic activity:

1. epinephrine/norepinephrine

2. isoproterenol

3. dimethylphenylpiperazinium (DMPP)

4. bilateral carotid occlusion

5. peripheral vagal stimulation

6. angiotensin

7. acetylcholine or furtrethonium

The challenge procedure requires that the anesthetized animal preparation last for approximately 3 to 5 hr. Most agents acting on autonomic
effectors will be detected by their action on one or more of the challenges.
It should be noted that many clinically useful agents do not affect blood
pressure, heart rate, or challenges in the autonomic procedure. Therefore,
the primary purpose of this test is to identify undesirable actions rather

than to determine mode of action. Even if all results in the challenge procedure are negative, it is entirely possible that a compound is not active in the anesthetized dog because of insolubility or lack of absorption. We have often solubilized compounds in polyethylene glycol-200 only to find that they precipitate when in contact with an aqueous solution (such as saline or blood). One must be careful to test with a blank, especially with those compounds made soluble at nonphysiological pH. Highly acidic or basic solutions have dramatic effects on blood pressure, heart rate, and even some challenges.

2. Preliminary toxicity test

The next step in evaluation is an overt effects/subacute toxicity procedure in conscious dogs and cats. This is easy to do and extremely important because serious side effects (e.g., vomiting, convulsions) cannot be observed in rodents or anesthetized animals. A preliminary toxicity test also serves to protect a valuable colony of hypertensive dogs (or other tertiary test model) from debilitating side effects or even death. We routinely test all compounds at this stage by administration of multiples of the "therapeutic" dose for several days orally to cats and dogs and observe these animals immediately, and at periodic intervals after dosing. This includes careful observation for signs of emesis during the night.

3. Hypertensive and normotensive dogs

At this stage of development, the experimental compound is assessed for blood pressure lowering activity in the various hypertensive and normotensive dog models described previously. A special effort is made to determine whether tolerance or side effects occur during multiple-dose experiments.

Marked tachycardia is typical of many hypotensive agents whose modes of action include peripheral vasodilatation or α-adrenergic blockade. Heart rate increases do not accompany the hypotension induced by β-adrenergic or ganglionic blocking agents. Nor does tachycardia occur following certain nervous system effects or direct cardiac depression.

4. Cardiovascular dynamics

All active compounds are routinely tested in anesthetized dogs for effects on cardiovascular dynamics. The latter include measurements of cardiac output, cardiac contractility (strain gauge arch and/or left ventricular pressure), and first derivatives necessary for assessing the contractile element velocity of shortening. Regional blood flows, pressures, and resistances are also measured and/or calculated. Also important is the analysis of coronary flow dynamics. An otherwise promising compound may be shelved if it reduces coronary flow or increases coronary vascular resistance beyond that which would be expected from changes in systemic blood pressure or heart rate. Venous pressures, especially central venous or right atrial pressures, are measured to assess pooling of blood in capacitance vessels.

V. FUTURE TRENDS

The ideal antihypertensive agent is one which would be useful in all forms of hypertension replacing most or all currently used drugs. It would possess the following clinical features:

1. orally effective at relatively low doses

2. long-lasting action of at least 8 hr per dose

3. blood pressure reduced to normal or near-normal levels

4. no undesirable side effects

5. inexpensive to the manufacturer and to the patient

The most desirable mechanism for an antihypertensive agent would be one mimicking the normal homeostatic mechanisms for maintaining blood pressure. A veratrum alkaloid-like drug which did not cause emesis would reduce blood pressure by a physiological mechanism, i.e., increased discharge of buffer nerves with compensatory vasodilatation and bradycardia. Another desirable mechanism would operate via the medullary vasomotor center to produce hypotension with minimal tachycardia.

The antihypertensive actions of reserpine, hydralazine, and methyldopa are at least partially due to a central effect [106]. L-Dopa, used to treat Parkinson's disease, also causes centrally mediated hypotension [107]. The centrally acting antihypertensive, clonidine, apparently causes no orthostatic hypotension because venoconstrictor reflexes are left intact [108]. Certain oxazolines appear to reduce blood pressure by a central mechanism [109]. Inhibition of sympathetic tone occurs with an aminoguanidine [110,111] while adrenergic blockade accounts for the hypotension induced by a series of isoquinolines [112].

Some of the newer investigational drugs are direct vasodilators. Among these are diaminopyridines [102,113], piperidines, and others [114]. Guancydine has vasodilator and other properties [115] and minoxidil may be especially effective when combined with a β-adrenergic blocker to reduce reflex tachycardia. Diazoxide has found important use in hypertensive crises [116].

But what will the future bring? What new approaches will lead us closer to the ideal agent? Some readers may feel that no new agents could surpass the large number of currently available or investigational drugs. Nevertheless, each of these agents has specific side effects and precautions which limit its usefulness.

Research emphasis on the immunological approach to hypertension may lead to new and different drugs. Rats immunized against angiotensin II are resistant to the pressor effects of this agent [1,60,117-119]; animals can also be immunized against renin [120,121]. In addition, the antibody to angiotensin is now being used as a tool to dissect the etiology of renal hypertension [122,123].

A renin inhibitor, pepstatin, is available [124] as is the angiotensin antagonist saralasin [125,126]. The latter, an octapeptide, is not orally absorbed but does lower blood pressure when administered intravenously to renal hypertensives.

Future hypertension research in industry may well be influenced by new immunologic discoveries and by improved angiotensin-renin antagonists. Meanwhile, the standard procedures outlined in this chapter are practical, productive, and applicable to the search for new antihypertensive drugs.

ACKNOWLEDGMENTS

The author gratefully acknowledges the assistance of Carol Zych in gathering the references for this chapter and of Smith Kline & French Laboratories for permission to use the data in Figures 1 to 8. The author also wishes to thank Emma Eynon for some of the data used in Tables 2 to 5.

REFERENCES

1. I. H. Page, JAMA 140, 451 (1949).

2. E. Schlittler, Antihypertensive Agents, Academic Press, New York, 1967.

3. F. H. Leenen and W. DeJong, J. Appl. Physiol. 31, 142 (1971).

4. B. Brooks and E. E. Muirhead, Appl. Physiol. 31, 307 (1971).

5. J. Burns and B. G. Robbins, J. Pharm. Pharmacol. 24, 86 (1972).

6. K. Aoki, Y. Yamori, and A. Ooshima, Jap. Circ. J. 36, 539 (1972).

7. H. Goldblatt, J. Lynch, R. Hanzol, and W. Summerville, J. Exp. Med. 59, 347 (1934).

8. I. H. Page, Science 89, 273 (1939).

9. E. E. Muirhead, G. B. Brown, G. S. Germain, and B. E. Leach, J. Lab. Clin. Med. 76, 641 (1970).

10. C. S. Sweet, P. J. Kadowitz, E. L. Forker, and M. J. Brody, Arch. Int. Pharmacodyn. Ther. 198, 229 (1972).

11. E. E. Westura, H. Kanegresser, J. D. O'Toole, and J. B. Lee, Circ. Res. 27 (Suppl. I), 131 (1970).

12. A. Nekrasova and L. Lantsber, Kardiologiya 9, 86 (1969).

13. L. B. Czyzewski and W. A. Pettinger, Am. J. Physiol. 225, 234 (1973).

14. W. DeJong, W. Lovenberg, and A. Sjoerdsma, Proc. Soc. Exp. Biol. Med. 139, 1213 (1972).

15. S. Sen, R. R. Smeby, and F. M. Bumpus, Circ. Res. 31, 876 (1972).

16. W. S. Peart, Pharmacol. Res. 17, 143 (1965).

17. L. Tobian, R. Olson, and G. Chesley, Am. J. Physiol. 216, 22 (1968).

18. R. Tarazi, J. Huano, H. Dustan, and E. Masson, Union Med. Can. 97, 1387 (1968).

19. L. Tobian, K. Coffee, and P. McCrea, Am. J. Physiol. 217, 458 (1969).

20. L. Tobian and M. Duke, Am. J. Physiol. 217, 522 (1969).

21. D. D. McGregor and F. H. Smirk, J. Am. Physiol. 219, 687 (1970).

22. F. P. Field, R. A. Janis, and D. J. Triggle, Can. J. Physiol. Pharmacol. 51, 344 (1973).

23. H. Wolinsky, Circ. Res. 30, 301 (1972).

24. N. R. Bandick and H. V. Sparks, Am. J. Physiol. 219, 340 (1970).

25. H. Ueda, J. Iwai, and H. Yasuda, Jap. Heart J. 10, 149 (1969).

26. J. Fujii, H. Kurihara, H. Yamaguchi, and M. Ikeda, J. Exp. Med. 97, 191 (1969).

27. J. Conway, Proc. Soc. Exp. Biol. Med. 132, 318 (1969).

28. A. Ebihara, B. L. Martz, and A. Grollman, Jap. Heart J. 11, 36 (1970).

29. H. Brunner, Naunyn Schmiedebergs Arch. Pharmacol. 267, 278 (1970).

30. P. Kramer and B. Ochwadt, Pfluegers Arch. Eur. J. Physiol. 332, 56 (1972).

31. M. Guazzi, O. T. Ellsworth, and E. D. Freis, Cardiovasc. Res. 5, 71 (1971).

32. L. Finch, Pharmacology 5, 245 (1971).

33. C. M. Ferrario, I. H. Page, and J. W. McCubbin, Circ. Res. 27, 799 (1970).

34. K. M. Koch, H. S. Aynedjian, and N. Bank, J. Clin. Invest. 47, 1696 (1968).

35. U. Helmchen, U. Knessler, P. Churchill, L. Peters-Haefeli, G. Schaechtelin, and G. Paters, Pfluegers Arch. Eur. J. Physiol. 332, 232 (1972).

36. S. Margolius, R. Geller, W. DeJong, J. Pisano, and A. Sjoerdsma, Circ. Res. 30, 358 (1972).

37. H. S. Ormsbee and C. F. Ryan, J. Pharm. Sci. 62, 255 (1973).

38. H. Ueda, Jap. Heart J. 8, 42 (1967).

39. H. Thoenen, Naunyn Schmiedebergs Arch. Pharmacol. 268, 125 (1971).

39a. A. Milteni, A. C. Brownie, and F. R. Skelton, Lab. Invest. 21, 129 (1969).

39b. H. D. Colby, F. R. Skelton, and A. C. Brownie, Endocrinology 86, 1093 (1970).

39c. M. J. Fregly, K. J. Kin, and C. I. Hood, Toxicol. Appl. Pharmacol. 15, 229 (1969).

39d. M. Winter, B. Velduyzen, and E. J. Dorhout Mees, Lancet 1, 1263 (1972).

39e. J. T. Higgins, Proc. Soc. Exp. Biol. Med. 134, 768 (1970).

39f. T. D. Clarke, A. D. Ashburn, and W. L. Williams, Am. J. Anat. 123, 429 (1968).

40. M. Karoabata, Jap. Circ. J. 34, 587 (1970).

41. F. Olsen, Acta Pathol. Microbiol. Scand. 78, 451 (1970).

42. K. Formanek, A. Lindner, and H. Selzer, Wien. Klin. Wochenschr. 80, 185 (1968).

43. R. D. Tanz, Proc. Soc. Exp. Biol. Med. 136, 867 (1971).

44. P. W. Willard, Proc. Soc. Exp. Biol. Med. 132, 181 (1969).

45. R. A. Mueller, P. Willard, and J. Exelrod, Pharmacology 5, 153 (1971).

46. L. Grimson, Arch. Surg. 43, 284 (1941).

47. N. Alexander and M. Decur, Am. J. Physiol. 219, 107 (1970).

48. P. Kezdi, Baroreceptors and Hypertension, Pergamon Press, Oxford, 1967.

49. A. Boura and A. Green, in Evaluation of Drug Activities (D. R. Lawrence and A. L. Bacharach, eds.), Chap. 19, Academic Press, New York, 1964.

50. H. Benson, J. A. Herd, W. H. Morse, and R. T. Kelleher, Am. J. Physiol. 217, 30 (1969).

51. H. Benson, J. A. Herd, W. H. Morse, and R. T. Kelleher, Circ. Res. 27 (Suppl. 1), 121 (1970).

52. J. A. Herd, W. H. Morse, R. T. Kelleher, and L. G. Jones, Am. J. Physiol. 217, 24 (1969).

53. J. F. Marwood and M. F. Lockett, J. Pharm. Pharmacol. 25, 42 (1973).

54. C. M. Ferrario, J. W. McCubbin, and I. H. Page, Circ. Res. 24, 911 (1969).

55. K. Okamoto, Spontaneous Hypertension, Igaku Shoin Ltd., Tokyo, 1962.

56. K. Okamoto and K. Aoki, Jap. Circ. J. 27, 282 (1963).

57. B. Folkow, M. Hallback, Y. Lundgren, and L. Weiss, Acta Physiol. Scand. 79, 373 (1970).

58. F. P. Field, R. A. Janis, and D. J. Triggle, Can. J. Physiol. Pharmacol. 50, 1072 (1972).

59. R. Swertson, Acta Physiol. Scand. Suppl. 3, 435 (1970).

60. A. R. Christlieb and R. B. Hickler, Endocrinology 91, 1064 (1972).

61. B. Folkow, M. Hallback, Y. Lundgren, and L. Weiss, Acta Physiol. Scand. 84, 512 (1972).

62. L. Finch and G. D. H. Leach, Br. J. Pharmacol. 39, 317 (1970).

63. B. Folkow, Clin. Sci. 41, 1 (1971).

64. B. Folkow, M. Gurevich, M. Hallback, Y. Lundgren, and L. Weiss, Acta Physiol. Scand. 83, 532 (1971).

65. B. Folkow, M. Hallback, Y. Lundgren, and L. Weiss, Acta Physiol. Scand. 83, 96 (1971).

66. B. Nikodijevic, T. Trajkov, E. Glavas, S. Gudeska, and D. Vetadzokoska, Naunyn Schmiedebergs Arch. Pharmacol. 268, 185 (1971).

67. T. Trajkov, E. Glavas, S. Gudeska, D. Vetadzokoska, and B. Nikodijevic, Iugosl. Physiol. Pharmacol. Acta 7, 197 (1971).

68. T. Trajkov, E. Glavas, S. Gudeska, D. Vetadzokoska, and B. Niko-
    dijevic, Acta Biol. Iugosl. Ser. C, Iugosl. Physiol. Pharmacol. Acta
    7, 197 (1971).

69. S. Mizogami, M. Suzuki, and H. Sokabe, Jap. Heart J. 13, 428 (1972).

70. S. Nosaka and L. Okamoto, Jap. Circ. J. 34, 685 (1970).

71. S. Nosaka and S. C. Wang, Am. J. Physiol. 222, 1079 (1972).

72. H. M. Perry, Jr., M. Erlanger, A. Yunice, A. Schoepfle, and
    E. Perry, Am. J. Physiol. 219, 755 (1970).

73. Y. Yamori and K. Okamoto, Jap. Circ. J. 33, 509 (1969).

74. M. Thant, Y. Yamori, and L. Okamoto, Jap. Circ. J. 33, 501 (1969).

75. Y. Yamori, M. Matsumoto, H. Yamabe, and K. Okamoto, Jap. Circ.
    J. 33 (1969).

76. J. A. Barsanti, H. R. Pillsbury, III, and E. D. Freis, Proc. Soc.
    Exp. Biol. Med. 136, 565 (1971).

77. G. T. Smith-Vaniz, A. D. Ashburn, and W. L. Williams, Yale J.
    Biol. Med. 43, 61 (1970).

78. S. Takahashi and J. Watanabe, Acta Soc. Ophthalmol. Jap. 73, 1429
    (1969).

79. A. Nagaoka, H. Kawaji, Y. Imai, and H. Fukui, Jap. J. Pharmacol.
    20, 509 (1970).

80. D. Jaffe, L. E. Sutherland, D. M. Barker, and L. K. Dahl, Arch.
    Pathol. 90, 1 (1970).

81. K. D. Knudsen, L. K. Dahl, K. Thompson, J. Iwai, H. Heine, and
    G. Leitl, J. Exp. Med. 132, 976 (1970).

82. D. M. Barker, L. E. Sutherland, D. Jaffe, and L. K. Dahl, Arch.
    Pathol. 89, 247 (1970).

83. K. Okamoto, Y. Yamori, A. Ooshima, and T. Toshinari, Jap. Circ.
    J. 36, 461 (1972).

84. A. Ooshima, Y. Yamori, and K. Okamoto, Jap. Circ. J. 36, 797
    (1972).

85. G. Shlager, J. Hered. 63, 35 (1972).

86. H. Tanase, Y. Suzuki, A. Ooshima, Y. Yamori, and K. Okamoto,
    Jap. Circ. J. 34, 1197 (1970).

87. J. P. Rapp and L. K. Dahl, Endocrinology 88, 52 (1971).

88. J. P. Rapp and L. K. Dahl, Endocrinology 90, 1435 (1972).

92 S. J. EHRREICH

89. G. S. Thind, D. N. Biery, and K. C. Bovee, J. Lab. Clin. Med. 81, 549 (1973).'

90. H. M. Perry, Jr. and M. Erlanger, Am. J. Physiol. 220, 808 (1970).

91. A. Leth, Circulation 42, 479 (1970).

92. R. Tabei, S. Spector, W. J. Louis, and A. Sjoerdsma, Clin. Pharmacol. Ther. 11, 269 (1970).

93. B. Folkow, Third International Symposium on Hypertension, Milan, Italy, 1974, in press.

94. S. J. Ehrreich, unpublished data.

95. J. Roba, G. Lambelin, and A. F. DeSchaepdryver, Arch. Int. Pharmacodyn. Ther. 200, 182 (1972).

96. B. E. Leach, F. B. Armstrong, Jr., G. S. Germain, and E. E. Miurhead, J. Pharmacol. Exp. Ther. 185, 479 (1973).

97. E. D. Freis, D. Gagen, H. R. Pillsbury, III, and M. Mathews, Circ. Res. 31, 1 (1972).

98. B. Folkow, M. Hallback, Y. Lundgren, and L. Weiss, Acta Physiol. Scand. 83, 280 (1971).

99. R. Matthews and R. Panesevich, Pharmakon Laboratories, Scranton, Pennsylvania.

100. A. Pirrelli and R. Deceasaris, Bull. Soc. Ital. Biol. Sper. 48, 229 (1972).

101. S. Free and J. Pauls, Smith, Kline & French Laboratories, Biostatistics Dept., unpublished data.

102. S. J. Ehrreich, J. E. Heringslake, F. R. Warren, J. Weinstock, and R. E. Tedeschi, Arch. Int. Pharmacodyn. Ther. 179, 284 (1969).

103. R. D. Bunag, J. Appl. Physiol. 34, 279 (1973).

104. E. D. Frohlich, M. A. Pfeffer, A. K. Weiss, and G. A. Brecher, Proc. Soc. Exp. Biol. Med. 140, 145 (1972).

105. B. Vaynovsky, Am. Lab. 5, 79 (1973).

106. T. Baum, A. T. Shropshire, and L. L. Varner, J. Pharmacol. Exp. Ther. 182, 135 (1972).

107. M. Henning and A. Rubenson, J. Pharm. Pharmacol. 22, 553 (1970).

108. D. M. P. Li and G. A. Bentley, Eur. J. Pharmacol. 12, 24 (1970).

109. R. Giudicelli and H. Schmitt, J. Pharmacol. (Paris) 1, 339 (1970).

110. T. Baum and A. T. Shropshire, Neuropharmacology 9, 503 (1970).

111. T. Baum, A. T. Shropshire, G. Rowles, R. Van Pelt, S. O. Fernandez, D. K. Eckfeld, and M. I. Gluckman, J. Pharmacol. Exp. Ther. 171, 276 (1970).

112. P. J. Privitera, T. Blickenstaff, T. E. Gaffney, and S. Mohammed, J. Pharmacol. Exp. Ther. 176, 655 (1971).

113. S. J. Ehrreich, J. E. Heringslake, R. Jablonski, J. Weinstock, and R. E. Tedeschi, Arch. Int. Pharmacodyn. Ther. 179, 303 (1969).

114. K. K. Midha, R. T. Coutts, J. W. Hubbard, and K. Prasad, Eur. J. Pharmacol. 11, 48 (1970).

115. J. R. Cummings, A. N. Welter, J. L. Grace, Jr., and W. D. Gray, J. Pharmacol. Exp. Ther. 170, 334 (1969).

116. W. G. Nayler, I. McInnes, J. B. Swann, D. Race, V. Carson, and T. E. Love, Am. Heart J. 75, 223 (1968).

117. I. Eide, Circ. Res. 30, 149 (1972).

118. G. J. MacDonald, W. J. Louis, V. Renzini, G. W. Boyd, and W. S. Peart, Circ. Res. 27, 197 (1970).

119. Y. Ohkusu, Jap. Circ. J. 35, 1175 (1971).

120. R. Hill, J. Chester, and P. Weisenbaugh, Lab. Invest. 22, 404 (1970).

121. R. A. Weiser, A. G. Johnson, and S. W. Hoobler, Lab. Invest. 20, 326 (1969).

122. H. R. Brunner, J. D. Kirshman, J. E. Sealy, and J. H. Laragh, Science 174, 1344 (1971).

123. J. Bing and K. Neilsen, Acta Pathol. Microbiol. Scand. 81, 254 (1973).

124. R. D. Miller, C. J. Poper, C. W. Wilson, and E. DeVito, Biochem. Pharmacol. 21, 2941 (1972).

125. D. T. Pals, F. D. Masucci, G. S. Denning, Jr., F. Sipoz, and D. C. Fessler, Circ. Res. 29, 673 (1971).

126. H. W. Overbeck, Am. J. Physiol. 223, 1358 (1972).

127. I. H. Page, JAMA 113, 2046 (1939).

128. A. Ebinhara and B. L. Martz, Am. J. Med. Sci. 259, 257 (1970).

129. Y. Yamori, W. DeJong, H. Yamabe, W. Lovenberg, and A. Sjoerdsma, J. Pharm. Pharmacol. 24, 690 (1972).

130. Y. Yamori, H. Yamabe, W. DeJong, W. Lovenberg, and A. Sjoerds-
      ma, Eur. J. Pharmacol. 17, 135 (1972).

131. M. D. Day, A. G. Roach, and R. L. Whiting, Eur. J. Pharmacol.
      21, 241 (1973).

Chapter 4

ANTIANGINALS

John M. Stump and Vernon G. Vernier

Pharmaceuticals Division
E. I. du Pont de Nemours & Company, Inc.
Stine Laboratory
Newark, Delaware

I. ANGINA PECTORIS

William Heberden recognized angina pectoris (from the Latin angina meaning a choking and pectoris the chest) as a clinical entity over 200 years
ago [1]. He clearly described it in a paper entitled "Some Account of a

Disorder of the Breast" published in the Medical Transactions of the Royal
College of Physicians in 1772.

Heberden and many others since have intensively studied the anginal
syndrome, and now Friedberg [2] says it is a glamor subject in every aspect
of diagnosis, treatment, and pathophysiology.

Imbalance between myocardial oxygen demand and myocardial oxygen
delivery resulting in myocardial ischemia causes angina pectoris. It is
precipitated by many situations which require increased coronary flow beyond the capability of the disease-narrowed coronary arteries.

Angina patients complain of substernal pain often described as that
which would be produced by a heavy weight being placed on the chest. They
also complain of pain radiating to the left arm and shoulder although the
right arm or both may be involved. Some are only aware of a rather vague
form of discomfort frequently attributed to indigestion [3]. Physical exer-
tion most commonly triggers an anginal attack but food, cold, emotion, and
other events may also precipitate an attack.

Although angina has long been suspected of being induced by a large
meal only recently have controlled experiments demonstrated this. Goldstein et al. [4] evaluated the circulatory response to upright bicycle exercise in a group of angina patients before and after a 1000-calorie meal.
Over 90% of these patients developed angina and ischemic electrocardiographic findings sooner than they had before eating. These investigators
found the hemodynamic response to exercise in the postprandial state resulted in a significantly higher heart rate and blood pressure. The double
product, mean blood pressure and heart rate, which has been shown to correlate reasonably well with myocardial oxygen consumption [5], was the
same at the onset of angina in the preprandial and postprandial conditions.
Thus, the increased susceptibility to anginal attacks after meals was due to
an increase in myocardial oxygen requirement brought about by a more
rapid heart rate and blood pressure response to exercise.

Epstein et al. [6] showed that cold caused higher blood pressure and
peripheral resistance in a group of angina patients at rest and during upright
exercise on a bicycle. These alterations increased myocardial oxygen demand which further increased the likelihood of an anginal attack during exercise. Ansari and Burch [7] have shown that a hot, humid environment can
also precipitate angina.

Emotional upset triggers angina. Anger and fear increase heart rate
and blood pressure at rest [8]. The resultant increase in myocardial oxygen
demand exceeds the capacity of the coronary system to deliver sufficient
oxygen, thus producing myocardial hypoxia and angina. Angina attacks may
also occur in patients during sleep. Goldstein and Epstein [9] have suggested that an increase in left ventricular volume results when the patient
assumes the supine position upon retiring. The volume increase accentuates
systolic ventricular wall stress and produces an increase in myocardial
oxygen consumption. The latter may be sufficient to precipitate angina in

individuals with very limited coronary reserve. Increased ventricular volume during sleep may also result from an increase in venous return due to absorption of intestinal fluid. Still another mechanism suggested for nocturnal angina is increased heart rate and blood pressure during rapid eye movement (REM) sleep [10].

The precipitation of angina by cigarette smoking may be prevented by abstention. Aronow et al. [11] showed that when angina patients smoke one high-nicotine-content cigarette before exercise, there is a significant reduction in the duration of exercise required to produce an anginal attack. These investigators concluded that reduction in exercise capacity was due to increased myocardial oxygen consumption which resulted from nicotine-induced catecholamine release in the adrenal medulla and other chromaffin tissue [12,13]. In subsequent studies, the same authors [14,15] found that both high- and low-nicotine-content cigarettes reduced exercise capacity and increased heart rate and blood pressure but that lettuce leaf cigarettes (containing no nicotine) did not affect these parameters.

Kannel and Feinleib [16] in the Framingham, Massachusetts study reported on the occurrence of angina pectoris in a general population sample of over 5000 persons. During 14 years of biennial cardiovascular surveillance, 492 persons had clinical evidence of coronary artery disease for the first time. The study showed that the majority of angina pectoris cases, 53% of men and 85% of women, were of the uncomplicated type, i.e., those in which angina was the initial sign of coronary artery disease and in which myocardial infarction, coronary insufficiency syndrome, or coronary death did not occur within 6 months of initial diagnosis. The higher percentage in women could be due to a greater percentage of false-positive clinical diagnoses since angiographic studies of patients with chest pain show women have a higher proportion of normal coronary arteriograms.

Angina occurred in men with myocardial infarction in 37% of the cases and in only 10% after a myocardial infarction. In contrast, angina occurred together with or subsequent to a myocardial infarction in only 15% of the women. The Framingham study also revealed that about 50% of the men over 45 years of age had a myocardial infarction within 8 years after the onset of angina, double the probability of the normal population.

It is important to note that the contention that a myocardial infraction may "cure" angina pectoris was not supported since it was found that the rate of spontaneous remission of angina was 30% whereas that after infarct was only 15%.

The annual mortality of the angina patients in the Framingham study was approximately 4% with about 60% of the patients surviving at 10 years. Approximately 45% of the deaths were so-called sudden deaths, an incidence triple that of the general population but similar to that seen in victims of myocardial infarction and in those who die of coronary heart disease without prior evidence of disease.

Reeves et al. [17] attempted to determine the fate of a large number of angina patients by combining the data from several studies. They compensated for the considerable heterogeneity in diagnostic techniques, referral protocols, and follow-up patterns by calculating a weighted average mortality. Their data show that patients with disease limited to either the circumflex or right coronary artery have an annual mortality of slightly more than 2%. When the single diseased vessed is the left anterior descending coronary artery, annual mortality may be as high as 7.4%. Patients with disease involving two and three coronary vessels had annual mortalities of 6.8 and 11.4%, respectively. Reeves et al. [17] found that the presence of cardiac enlargement or congestive heart failure, or both, markedly increased mortality.

II. PHARMACOLOGY OF ANTIANGINAL DRUGS

A. Nitroglycerin (Glyceryl Trinitrate)

$$
\begin{array}{l}
H_2C-O-NO_2 \\
\ \ \ | \\
HC-O-NO_2 \\
\ \ \ | \\
H_2C-O-NO_2
\end{array}
$$

(1)

Almost 100 years ago Murrel [18] recommended nitroglycerin (1) in the treatment of angina pectoris. Today, many clinicians feel no single drug is more effective than nitroglycerin despite exhaustive efforts to find one.

How does nitroglycerin cause its favorable effect on angina? The effect of nitroglycerin on coronary blood flow, as reported in the literature, yields an overwhelming amount of conflicting data in both man and animals. Much of the disagreement results from dissimilarities in (a) technique used for measuring myocardial blood flow: flowmeter, radioisotopes, etc.; (b) route of administration of the drug: intracoronary, sublingual, intravenous; and (c) type of experimental subjects: ischemic or nonischemic dog or man.

1. Effects on coronary circulation in dogs

Early studies performed by Essex et al. [19] showed that intravenously administered nitroglycerin produced a transient increase in coronary flow of

unanesthetized dogs. Wegria et al. [20] confirmed these results and found
that when nitroglycerin was given orally the increase in coronary flow persisted for up to 15 times longer. Others using similar measurement techniques were unable to demonstrate consistent changes in coronary blood
flow.

Melville et al. [21] found transient dose-dependent increases in coronary flow of anesthetized dogs after intravenous nitroglycerin lasting about
20 sec. This transient effect was confirmed by Vyden et al. [22]. Later
Gillis and Melville [23] found that doses of nitroglycerin of 0.22 to 1.95 mg
sublingually did not significantly alter coronary flow although significant
blood pressure reduction was produced at the 0.65- and 1.95-mg doses.
They concluded that nitroglycerin administered by different routes produced
qualitatively and quantitatively different effects (i.e., coronary flow increased after intravenous but not after sublingual administration and blood
pressure decreased to a greater extent but for a shorter duration on intravenous as compared to sublingual administration) and that the beneficial
effect of nitroglycerin in angina pectoris was unrelated to increases in
coronary flow. However, Fam and McGregor [24] showed that sublingual
nitroglycerin caused a significant increase in coronary collateral flow in
dogs with chronic myocardial ischemia but they did not observe this effect
in normal nonischemic dogs. They also showed that dipyridamole, which
is capable of increasing total coronary flow of normal dogs, did not affect
the coronary collateral flow of ischemic dogs. This is very important
since dipyridamole is reportedly ineffective in angina pectoris.

The conclusions of Gillis and Melville [23] can be criticized on the
grounds that their dog model (nonischemic myocardium) is not representative of angina pectoris in man. Also, changes in blood flow through the
circumflex coronary artery do not reflect changes in flow to ischemic areas
such as those found in the myocardium of angina patients. Bernstein et al.
[25] using a radioisotope method (^{133}Xe) found that intravenous nitroglycerin
decreased myocardial blood flow in dogs but that intracoronary administration increased it.

Other indirect methods (radioactive ^{85}Kr, nitrous oxide, and ^{84}Rb
coincidence counting) have been used to examine the effect of nitroglycerin
on coronary blood flow. Results are conflicting and not definitive primarily
because these methods fail to detect transient changes in blood flow.

Winbury et al. [26], using a polarographic method for the determination of oxygen tension, showed that nitroglycerin selectively increased the
subendocardial oxygen tension of dogs with both normal and compromised
coronary circulations. This occurred in the absence of any increase in
total coronary blood flow and was particularly marked in the dogs that had
coronary blood flow compromised by a Goldblatt clamp around the anterior
descending coronary artery. Fam and McGregor [24] found similar changes
in chronically ischemic dogs.

In contrast, Forman et al. [27] found that intravenous or intracoronary nitroglycerin caused a significant reduction of subendocardial blood flow in anesthetized dogs with partially occluded left coronary arteries. They suggested that occlusion activated the autoregulatory mechanism to dilate subendocardial vessels fully. In these circumstances, nitroglycerin reduced vascular resistance in the subepicardium more than in the subendocardium, resulting in what these authors term a "steal" of blood flow from deep to superficial myocardium. This redistribution of coronary blood flow away from the subendocardium was evidenced by a reduction of contractile force of deep layers in the ventricular wall.

Thus, the long-standing disagreement among investigators concerning the effect of nitroglycerin on coronary blood flow of dogs has not yet been resolved.

2. Effect of coronary
    circulation in man

Considerable data are available on the effect of nitroglycerin on coronary blood flow in man. They are as conflicting as those obtained in animals and are complicated by the fact that the methods used to determine myocardial blood flow in man are largely indirect. However, the studies in man are more pertinent since they can be performed on subjects with angina pectoris, a considerable advantage over those in animals.

Early studies by Gorlin et al. [28] using the nitrous oxide method for determining myocardial blood flow showed that sublingual nitroglycerin produced no significant change in either myocardial blood flow or oxygen consumption of patients with angina pectoris. Bing et al. [29], using [84]Rb, showed that sublingual nitroglycerin produced a marked increase in the coronary flow of normal subjects although it did not alter that of the angina patient. However, the flow measurements were not made until 3 min after nitroglycerin administration so early effects were not detected. When the same investigators [30] later used a technique which allowed more rapid measurement of coronary flow, sublingual nitroglycerin produced a significant increase in myocardial blood flow in both normal subjects and those with coronary artery disease 45 sec after administration. Bernstein et al. [25], using ^{133}Xe, found that nitroglycerin injected directly into the coronary artery caused an increase in myocardial blood flow in patients with and without coronary artery disease. In contrast, sublingual nitroglycerin caused a decrease in myocardial blood flow.

One explanation for the disparity in results in man is that the clearance techniques usually employed vary considerably in their ability to detect transient changes in myocardial flow. Cohn and Gorlin [31] have pointed out that myocardial blood flow is nonuniformly distributed when coronary artery disease is present and what is being measured by clearance techniques reflects primarily muscle perfused by normal coronary arteries. Obstructed coronary arteries show slow clearance rates whereas nonobstructed vessels show more rapid rates. Thus the clearance values obtained in patients with coronary artery disease predominantly reflect flow in normal vessels, and the critical obstructed vessels are poorly represented.

These studies in man have primarily yielded data concerning the effect of nitroglycerin on total myocardial blood flow and have neglected effects that nitroglycerin may have on regional blood flow. The previously discussed investigations of Fam and McGregor [24] and Winbury et al. [26] in dogs have demonstrated nitroglycerin-induced effects on regional flow.

Horwitz et al. [32] examined the effects of sublingual nitroglycerin on regional myocardial blood flow of 10 patients with coronary artery disease using ^{133}Xe clearance techniques. These investigators found that 0.4 mg of nitroglycerin sublingually significantly increased slow phase flow which they associated with an increase in collateral blood flow. They concluded that under the conditions studied nitroglycerin improved perfusion in regions of diseased myocardium of patients with coronary artery disease. Knoebel et al. [33], using the ^{84}Rb coincidence technique, found that sublingual nitroglycerin increased nutrient myocardial blood flow of patients with severe coronary artery disease during right atrial pacing. Interestingly, atrial pacing alone in these patients caused a decrease in nutrient myocardial flow. These authors point out that the directional changes in myocardial blood flow were unrelated to perfusion pressure or pressure work and that their findings in man are consistent with observations in experimental animals indicating that nitroglycerin produced a redistribution of myocardial blood flow.

In contrast, Ganz and Marcus [34] found intracoronary administered nitroglycerin ineffective in alleviating pacing-induced angina. Nitroglycerin was injected into both the left and right coronary arteries during pacing-induced angina but did not relieve the pain or reduce the intensity even though 14 of the 25 patients studied had an increase in coronary sinus blood flow. When nitroglycerin was given intravenously to six of these patients angina was relieved within 40 to 80 sec. This was preceded by a fall in arterial blood pressure and coronary sinus blood flow.

The variable results obtained with nitroglycerin can probably be ascribed to the techniques used for measuring myocardial blood flow in man. These techniques rely on indirect assessments of flow and do not measure the same parameters. Some do not detect transient changes in flow, some measure total coronary flow without distinguishing between nutritional and nonnutritional flow, and others measure regional flow. The discrepant results found with nitroglycerin in man, like those in the dogs, must be primarily ascribed to dissimilar measurement techniques. Analysis of results is further complicated by the application of various diagnostic and/or surgical procedures and the concomitant administration of a wide variety of drugs.

The increasing use of aortocoronary bypass surgery for the treatment of severe angina has afforded investigators the opportunity of examing the effect of nitroglycerin on coronary blood flow using more direct measurement techniques.

Goldstein et al. [35] studied the effect of nitroglycerin on coronary collateral function of patients with severe multivessel coronary occlusive disease undergoing saphenous vein bypass surgery. This study is significant because the effect of nitroglycerin on coronary collateral flow was determined directly by measuring retrograde flow collected from a catheter inserted into the saphenous vein graft. The coronary artery proximal to the graft was mechanically occluded to prevent antegrade flow. Experiments were conducted in which (a) aortic pressure was allowed to fall in response to nitroglycerin and (b) aortic pressure was maintained near control level. Nitroglycerin was administered into the ascending aorta as a bolus followed by an infusion.

When aortic pressure was allowed to fall in response to nitroglycerin there was no significant effect on retrograde flow; however, coronary collateral resistance showed a significant decrease. The authors point out that assessment of drug effects should be made with constant aortic pressure. In patients with aortic pressure held constant they found that nitroglycerin significantly increased retrograde flow and reduced collateral resistance. These data indicate that nitroglycerin can increase collateral flow in patients with severe occlusive coronary artery disease. They are supported by the Horwitz et al. [32] studies in man in which an indirect method was used for flow determination and by those of Fam and McGregor [24] in which an animal model of coronary artery disease was used.

Barner et al. [36] used an electromagnetic flowmeter to measure the effect of nitroglycerin on the blood flow of human coronary bypass grafts at the time of surgery. They found that intravenously administered nitroglycerin (0.4 mg) produced a significant increase in coronary flow at 15 and 30 sec but as arterial blood pressure fell the coronary flow decreased significantly below control. Sublingual administration of the same dose produced only a reduction in coronary flow and blood pressure. In a similar study Greenfield et al. [37] using a lower intravenous dose of nitroglycerin (0.15 mg) observed an increase in blood flow in only one of their five patients.

3. Mechanism of action
    in angina pectoris

It is generally accepted that angina pectoris results from an imbalance
between myocardial oxygen demand and myocardial oxygen delivery.
Thus, the anginal state could be relieved by improving coronary blood flow
and by reducing myocardial oxygen consumption, or by a combination of
these.

Though nitroglycerin has been used extensively and effectively in the
treatment of angina pectoris for over 100 years, the mechanism of this
relief is still debated. The coronary blood flow studies described herein
do not conclusively establish that nitroglycerin improves flow, although
the evidence is suggestive.

Nitroglycerin can relieve angina pectoris by reducing myocardial
oxygen consumption. This mechanism is reasonably well accepted. Nitroglycerin does this primarily by producing hemodynamic changes that decrease systolic wall stress, a major determinant of myocardial oxygen
consumption.

Mason and Braunwald [38] have shown in man that sublingual nitroglycerin produced an increase in venous distensibility which resulted in
pooling of blood in the peripheral veins. They suggested that this reduction in venous return would reduce ventricular size and intramyocardial
tension with resultant reduction in myocardial oxygen consumption. Several investigators have recently confirmed this, reporting that nitroglycerin
does indeed reduce left ventricular end–systolic and end-diastolic volume
in normal subjects and in patients with coronary artery disease [39,40].
The reduction in ventricular preload decreases systolic wall stress,
thereby helping correct the imbalance between myocardial oxygen demand
and delivery.

In addition, sublingual nitroglycerin inconsistently decreases peripheral vascular resistance by a direct action on arteriolar smooth muscle
[40]. In those individuals in whom this occurs the reduction in ventricular
afterload allows for a further reduction in heart size by lowering the resistance to systolic emptying. This additional reduction in ventricular
dimension further reduces myocardial oxygen consumption.

The hemodynamic changes that decrease myocardial oxygen consumption also lead to a reflex increase in heart rate and cardiac contractile force, both of which increase myocardial oxygen consumption.
However, the net effect is a reduction in myocardial oxygen consumption
due to a decrease in systolic wall stress.

In summary, the relief of angina pectoris by nitroglycerin appears
to be due to a combination of (a) a reduction in myocardial oxygen demand
by reduction in heart size and systolic wall tension, and (b) improvement

of coronary blood flow to ischemic areas of the myocardium. The exact importance of either one of these probably varies from patient to patient although the reduction in myocardial oxygen demand probably plays the major role in most individuals.

B. Isosorbide Dinitrate

$$
\begin{array}{l}
\text{H}_2\text{C} \\
\quad | \\
\text{HC}-\text{O}-\text{NO}_2 \\
\quad | \qquad\qquad \text{O} \\
\quad\quad \text{CH} \\
\quad | \\
\quad\text{HC} \\
\text{O} \quad | \\
\text{O}_2\text{N}-\text{O}-\text{CH} \\
\quad | \\
\quad\quad \text{CH}_2
\end{array}
$$

(2)

This organic nitrate is one of the presumed long-acting nitrates. Isosorbide dinitrate (2) and other organic nitrates have been widely used on the presumption that they provide longer duration of protection than nitroglycerin. The clinical evidence is controversial.

Russek [41] states that isosorbide dinitrate sublingually offers distinct advantages over sublingual nitroglycerin in the prophylactic therapy of angina. He supports this claim with data obtained in a double blind study in which isosorbide dinitrate 5 mg sublingually relieved angina induced by a relatively simple exercise tolerance test for up to 2 hr whereas sublingual nitroglycerin 0.4 mg was not beneficial for even 30 min after administration.

In contrast, Goldstein et al. [42] found that most of their patients receiving 5 to 10 mg of isosorbide dinitrate sublingually were not protected against exercise-induced angina 60 min after dosing. Significantly, sublingual nitroglycerin in the same individuals afforded them a prolonged protection. Goldstein et al. [42] developed an extremely well-designed protocol for this study. They used an exercise test that was particularly sensitive and reliable in identifying alterations in exercise capacity, chose drug dosages on an individual basis depending on physiologic responses in the resting state, and directly measured critical circulatory parameters allowing for a comparison of clinical performance with those hemodynamic changes most closely associated with angina pectoris. Chronic administration of isosorbide dinitrate did not alter the responsiveness to acutely administered sublingual isosorbide dinitrate, indicating that nitrate tachyphylaxis does not appear to be a significant problem when 5 to 10 mg is administered sublingually four times a day for as long as 7 months.

Klaus et al. [43] found that exercise-induced angina could only be relieved for 45 min after sublingual administration of 5 mg of isosorbide dinitrate.

In a recent study Brunner et al. [44] have shown that oral administration of one 40-mg sustained-action isosorbide dinitrate tablet relieved exercise-induced angina for at least 3 hr. In one group of patients that were exercised for up to 8 hr after receiving the drug almost 85% had prevention of angina for 6 hr and 34% for 8 hr after dosing. However, this study had neither a double blind design for control nor a crossover design for comparison with nitroglycerin.

Analysis of available data indicates that the duration of protection offered by sublingual isosorbide dinitrate is not longer than that afforded by sublingual nitroglycerin. However, special preparations of isosorbide dinitrate may give more prolonged protection than the regular sublingual form.

C. Pentaerythritol Tetranitrate

$$\text{H}_2\text{C}-\text{O}-\text{NO}_2$$
$$\text{O}_2\text{N}-\text{O}-\text{CH}_2-\overset{|}{\underset{|}{\text{C}}}-\text{CH}_2-\text{O}-\text{NO}_2$$
$$\text{H}_2\text{C}-\text{O}-\text{NO}_2$$

(3)

Pentaerythritol tetranitrate [PETN (3)] has been shown to increase the coronary arterial blood flow of dogs [45], although it is less potent than nitroglycerin. Winbury [46] using a ^{86}Rb clearance technique found that it increased the nutritional circulation of anesthetized dogs without increasing total coronary flow. Thus, an improvement in myocardial oxygenation should occur. Weiss and Winbury [47] found PETN did indeed selectively increase subendocardial pO_2, did not increase subepicardial pO_2, and produced only a transient increase in total coronary blood flow. They concluded that PETN increased subendocardial pO_2 by a redistribution of blood flow to the endocardium from the epicardium and a reduction in myocardial metabolism.

The clinical effectiveness of PETN is controversial. A few studies have reported efficacy but most of the well-designed studies have been negative. Russek [41] found that PETN 20 mg orally or sublingually did not significantly improve exercise tolerance in angina patients but 40 mg orally did and also reduced the magnitude of electrocardiographic changes produced by exercise. The beneficial effect of PETN was not manifest until 60 to 80 min after ingestion and persisted for 4 to 5 hr. In order to be orally effective PETN had to be administered on an empty stomach.

In a double blind study Dewar et al. [48] found PETN 30 or 60 mg
orally three times a day was no more effective than placebo in reducing the
frequency of anginal attacks or the number of nitroglycerin tablets consumed. Similar findings were reported by Oram and Sowton [49] with 30
mg orally three times a day. No significant improvement in exercise duration or electrocardiographic indication of ischemia was reported by Dagenais et al. [50] with either 20 or 40 mg of PETN.

Klaus et al. [43] found that 45 min after 10 mg sublingual PETN there
was a significant increase in the duration of exercise that a group of angina
patients could perform, but the duration observed 100 min after dosing was
not significantly different from placebo. Sublingual nitroglycerin increased
the duration of exercise 2 min but not 55 min after dosing. These investigators concluded that PETN had a longer duration of action than nitroglycerin,
a questionable conclusion since dose-response curves were not established
for the drugs and stress testing for each drug was not performed at comparable times after administration. Since Goldstein et al. [42] found that
when drug dosages were matched to produce similar circulatory changes
nitroglycerin provided the same duration of action as isosorbide dinitrate,
it is unlikely that PETN if evaluated in this manner would be longer lasting
than nitroglycerin.

D.   Erythrityl Tetranitrate

$$H_2C-O-NO_2$$
$$|$$
$$HC-O-NO_2$$
$$|$$
$$HC-O-NO_2$$
$$|$$
$$H_2C-O-NO_2$$

(4)

Erythrityl tetranitrate (4) is another of the organic nitrates synthetized in
the expectation of providing a more prolonged effect than nitroglycerin in
the treatment of angina pectoris. As with PETN, the clinical efficacy of
erythrityl tetranitrate is controversial. In the 1930s Evans and Hoyle [51]
found that 30 mg orally three times a day was actually worse than placebo
in a group of 20 angina patients. Cole et al. [52] reported that 15 mg sublingually four to eight times a day was of little benefit in reducing the frequency of anginal attacks. In contrast, Dagenais et al. [53] found that 10
mg significantly decreased the frequency of anginal attacks and reduced the
magnitude of the electrocardiographic changes associated with exercise-
induced myocardial ischemia.

Riseman et al. [54] in a group of 20 angina patients found that erythrityl tetranitrate 15 mg when administered sublingually was comparable in efficacy to 0.3 mg of nitroglycerin sublingually in nine patients, somewhat less effective in eight, and of no value in three. They found that the onset of effect was 6 to 10 min whereas that of nitroglycerin was 2 min. In contrast, erythrityl tetranitrate 30 mg three times a day orally was ineffective. Similarly, when an effective sublingual dose of nitroglycerin was given orally it was also ineffective. An almost tenfold increase in the sublingual dose of nitroglycerin was required to produce beneficial effects orally. The clinical evidence available at present seems to indicate that erythrityl tetranitrate in the treatment of angina is ineffective orally but effective sublingually.

E. Propranolol

$$\text{O-CH}_2\text{-}\overset{\overset{\text{OH}}{|}}{\underset{\underset{\text{H}}{|}}{\text{C}}}\text{-CH}_2\text{-N}\overset{\diagup \text{H}}{\diagdown \underset{\underset{\text{CH}_3}{|}}{\text{CH-CH}_3}}$$

(5)

The rationale for the use of propranolol (5) in angina pectoris arises from its ability to directly block the sympathetically mediated increases in heart rate and myocardial contractility that accompany exercise and precede the onset of angina. Since this heightened sympathetic activity is associated with increases in myocardial oxygen consumption, propranolol and other β-adrenergic receptor blockers exert their beneficial effects primarily by reducing this increased myocardial oxygen consumption. However, β-receptor blockade also produces hemodynamic changes that partially antagonize the beneficial alterations. It increases ventricular ejection time and ventricular volume, both of which increase myocardial oxygen consumption. However, the beneficial effects of propranolol (those which reduce myocardial oxygen consumption) predominate, yielding a net reduction in myocardial oxygen consumption.

Although the increase in ventricular volume and ejection time produced by β-receptor blockade have been reported to cause congestive heart failure in angina patients [55], it is not a major drawback [56]. The combination of β-receptor blockers with nitrates has been reported to be particularly beneficial in the treatment of angina. Battock et al. [57] found that based on subjective evaluations their patients improved significantly more when receiving a combination of propranolol and isosorbide dinitrate than they did when administered either drug alone. However, these investigators did not find a significant difference between the various drug regimens when only objective evaluation was used. This is in contrast to the data of Goldstein and Epstein [9] who found a combination of propranolol and nitroglycerin to be superior to either drug alone.

Considering the hemodynamic effects of propranolol and the nitrates it is not surprising that these drugs complement one another in the treatment of angina pectoris. As previously mentioned, β-adrenergic receptor blockade produces an increase in ventricular volume and prolongs ejection time, both of which increase myocardial oxygen consumption. These effects can be counteracted by the concomitant administration of nitrates which reduce ventricular volume and decrease ejection time. In addition, the sympathetically mediated increase in heart rate and myocardial contractility produced by the nitrate can be reduced or abolished by β-receptor blockade. Thus, the reduction in myocardial oxygen consumption produced by a combination of a β-receptor blocking agent and a nitrate should be greater than that produced by either drug alone.

In support of this concept, Goldstein and Epstein [9] found that the pressure-rate product, which with some reservations can be used as an indicator of myocardial oxygen consumption [5], was reduced in angina patients receiving propranolol primarily by a reduction in heart rate. The addition of nitroglycerin further reduced the pressure-rate product by reducing blood pressure and produced an additional increase in exercise capacity. These investigators also noted that the reflex tachycardia normally observed with nitroglycerin administration was not found in patients receiving the drug combination, presumably the result of β-receptor blockade.

Thus the combination of a β-receptor blocking agent such as propranolol and a nitrate offers distinct advantages over either drug alone in the treatment of angina pectoris.

F. Chromonar

(6)

Chromonar (6) administered to anesthetized dogs in doses of 2.5 and 5 mg/kg, i.v., produced a marked and prolonged increase in coronary blood

flow while not significantly altering blood pressure [58]. Charlier [59]
showed that chromonar 5 mg/kg, i.v., increased coronary blood flow
in the anesthetized dog fourfold, with flow remaining elevated for over
60 min. Grayson et al. [60] found that chromonar 2 mg/kg, i.v.,
increased myocardial blood flow of anesthetized dogs by 67% without
altering blood pressure or heart rate. In a group of dogs with acute
coronary artery ligation these investigators found that chromonar increased
myocardial flow only 23%. They concluded that chromonar exerts its
effect predominately on the resistance vessels in the myocardium and thus
abolishes autoregulation which can reduce irrigation in ischemic regions
of the heart.

Parratt et al. [61], using a ^{133}Xe clearance technique in anesthetized
dogs, found that chromonar increased blood flow in normal areas of myocardium but failed to increase flow after coronary artery ligation, and in
some of the dogs there was a decrease in flow. In spite of this there was
a marked increase in the pO_2 of the coronary venous blood draining from
the ischemic area combined with a reduction in oxygen extraction. These
investigators concluded that chromonar and other arteriolar dilators dis-
proportionately increase total flow but not nutritive flow in the ischemic
myocardium. Their conclusions suggest that chromonar may not be
clinically effective in the treatment of angina pectoris.

Nevertheless, several investigators have indicated that chromonar
is effective in the treatment of angina [62-64] based on subjective improvement. In a double blind test Conway et al. [65] were unable to show objective improvement in exercise tolerance of angina patients given chromonar.
Similarly, Hunscha et al. [66] found that intravenous chromonar had no
effect on electrocardiographic indications of myocardial ischemia induced
by exercise.

Recently Bing et al. [67] published a study of chromonar which included 187 patients from 12 clinical departments in North America all of
which followed the same double blind crossover test protocol. They found
that patients receiving chromonar 150 mg three times daily had fewer
anginal attacks and required fewer nitroglycerin tablets than while on
placebo. However, the results are difficult to interpret since patients
receiving 225 mg three times daily had fewer anginal attacks but required
as many nitroglycerin tablets as they did on placebo. Chromonar produced
an improvement in exercise tolerance in only 22% of the patients where
placebo produced a 7% improvement. The majority of patients (71%) had
no improvement in exercise tolerance. Although these data suggest that
chromonar can produce an improvement in the frequency of anginal attacks
and nitroglycerin requirements, the minimal effect on exercise tolerance
is not encouraging. The value of chromonar in the long-term management
of angina pectoris remains to be established.

G. Perhexiline

(7)

Perhexiline (7) is a relatively new antianginal drug that is currently undergoing widespread clinical evaluation. The pharmacology has recently been
reviewed by Hudak et al. [68]. These authors report that in animal experiments perhexiline produced vasodilatation that appears to be due to a direct
action predominately on resistance but not capacitance vessels. Perhexiline reduced the heart rate of several species and prolonged conduction
time in the dog heart. The reduction in heart rate was not the result of
β-receptor blockade, stimulation of cholinergic receptors, or direct myocardial depression. Utilizing a dog coronary flow preparation in which
regional myocardial blood flow was measured with radioactive microspheres
Klassen et al. [69] found that perhexiline produced a favorable profile of
actions including increased coronary perfusion pressure with unchanged
systemic arterial pressure, reduced myocardial oxygen consumption, and
increased lactate extraction. The endocardial/epicardial ratio increased
after perhexiline, indicating a favorable redistribution of blood flow.

Perhexiline was effective in relieving angina in a number of clinical
trials. Morledge [70] found in a double blind evaluation that perhexiline
300 mg daily produced an increase in exercise tolerance in a group of 30
angina patients. It also reduced the frequency of anginal attacks and the
number of nitroglycerin tablets consumed. Cherchi et al. [71] in a small
double blind study in anginal patients found perhexiline 200 mg daily increased the work load required to produce electrocardiographic changes
indicative of myocardial ischemia. Martins de Olivera et al. [72] found
that perhexiline administered over an 18-month period to angina patients
progressively increased the work performance of 22 of the 34 treated.

Pepine et al. [73] examined the effects of perhexiline on symptomatic
and hemodynamic responses to exercise stress in patients with coronary
artery disease and angina. Perhexiline, 200 mg/day for at least 10 days,
significantly increased exercise tolerance in over 70% of the patients. It
also reduced the frequency of anginal attacks and the number of nitroglycerin
tablets consumed. The increase in heart rate due to exercise was significantly reduced by perhexiline. Pepine et al. [73] suggest that the antianginal and hemodynamic effects of perhexiline closely resemble those observed with a combination of nitroglycerin and propranolol. Perhexiline

and nitroglycerin both reduce left ventricular filling pressure, but the reduction in cardiac output, the decrease in systemic blood pressure, the
reflex increase in heart rate, and myocardial contractility produced by
nitroglycerin are not observed with perhexiline. The increase in heart
rate and myocardial contractility produced by nitroglycerin increases myocardial oxygen consumption, thereby partially countering its beneficial
oxygen-sparing effects. The reduction of these undesirable effects of
nitroglycerin by propranolol is the primary basis for the combination of
the two drugs. However, accompanying the beneficial effects, propranolol
produces undesirable myocardial depression. Since the reduction in
exercise-induced tachycardia produced by perhexiline is not accompanied
by myocardial depression it appears to offer the advantages of both nitroglycerin and propranolol in the treatment of angina pectoris without the
disadvantages. Although these results are promising the ultimate value of
perhexiline awaits further clinical evaluation.

H, Dipyridamole

(8)

Dipyridamole (8) markedly increased coronary blood flow and coronary
sinus oxygen content of the anesthetized dog. Kadatz [74] found that an infusion of 0.3 mg/kg/min increased coronary flow by 113% whereas the same
dose of papaverine increased flow 60%. In contrast, dipyridamole was
three times less potent than papaverine in producing an increase in blood
flow in the extremities. The duration of the increased flow was twice that
of papaverine. Grabner et al. [75] found that 1 mg/kg, i.v., in anesthetized dogs significantly increased coronary blood flow and improved oxygen
extraction. Arterial blood pressure and heart rate were unchanged and
cardiac output was slightly reduced. Similar findings were reported by
Hockerts and Bögelmann [76] with 0.5 mg/kg, i.v.
     Even though total coronary flow was increased, Fam and McGregor
[24] found in anesthetized dogs that dipyridamole, unlike nitroglycerin, did
not increase collateral flow to the myocardium distal to a chronically

occluded coronary vessel. These data stimulated Fam and McGregor [77] later to examine the effect of dipyridamole and nitroglycerin on regional coronary resistance in the anesthetized dog to see if their site of action differed. Dipyridamole produced a significant reduction in total coronary resistance but did not significantly alter the resistance of large conductance vessels. In contrast, nitroglycerin reduced conductance vessel resistance and did not affect total resistance. These data suggested that the large coronary arteries are responsible for maintenance of collateral circulation and that nitroglycerin by selective dilatation of these larger arteries redistributes the blood flow to ischemic areas via the collateral vessels. In contrast, dipyridamole produced only dilatation of the small resistive coronary arteries which produced in turn a diversion of blood away from the collateral channels in what has been termed an inappropriate redistribution of blood flow. Winbury et al. [58] reported similar results and conclusions.

Supporting this conclusion of inappropriate redistribution of blood flow Weiss and Winbury [47] found in anesthetized dogs that dipyridamole produced a decrease in the subendocardial pO_2, a slight increase in subepicardial pO_2, and a prolonged significant increase in coronary flow. In contrast, nitroglycerin produced a selective increase in subendocardial pO_2, confirming that the large conductance vessels must supply this region. Since dipyridamole reduced subendocardial pO_2 it is unlikely to be clinically effective in angina pectoris if this model is predictive.

In fact, a number of clinical investigators do consider dipyridamole ineffective in the treatment of angina [78-80]. Newhouse and McGregor [81] administered 50 mg three times a day to patients for 1 year and found that in most patients dipyridamole did not improve exercise tolerance or reduce the magnitude of electrocardiographic changes associated with exercise. However, in a double blind test Igloe [82] found that with a slightly higher dose, 200 mg daily for 5 months, 81% of the patients had improved exercise tolerance, reduction in the frequency of anginal attacks, and required fewer nitroglycerin tablets. Igloe [82] concluded that dipyridamole, although not intended to abort acute anginal attacks, was an effective drug for the long-term management of patients with angina pectoris.

III. PHARMACOLOGICAL TESTING
      METHODS FOR ANTIANGINAL DRUGS

In the search for new drugs that would reduce the severity and/or the frequency of anginal attacks, cardiovascular pharmacologists have over the last 75 years developed many techniques to examine the effects of various chemicals and procedures on the coronary circulation.

Until recent years the most frequently used methods involved measurement of coronary venous outflow from the coronary sinus by different techniques. These methods were popular because they were convenient. The coronary sinus can be reached easily for flow measurement without the elaborate surgery required for some direct measures of coronary arterial flow. It was also believed by many investigators that compounds that substantially increased coronary venous outflow would be beneficial in the treatment of angina pectoris. Unfortunately, the coronary sinus outflow represents only about 60% of the total coronary venous drainage [83] and, more important, it has been shown that it can be a poor index of total coronary blood flow [84]. Thus, the evaluation of compounds for antianginal activity using only an increase in coronary sinus outflow as the sole indicator of efficacy was often misleading and did not predict clinical efficacy.

From coronary sinus flow procedures many investigators moved to techniques measuring coronary arterial blood flow. Cannulation was used frequently in past years but has been superseded by noninvasive techniques, i.e., the electromagnetic flow transducer. However, evaluation of drugs for antianginal activity using as the only criterion an increase in coronary arterial blood flow or coronary sinus blood flow has poor predictive validity for efficacy in man. Thus dipyridamole produces a sustained increase in coronary flow but may not relieve angina pectoris in man [24]. Therefore, only pharmacological testing procedures which can differentiate an effective antianginal agent from an ineffective one are discussed here. Charlier [59] in an excellent review has discussed the many methods that have been used for measurement of coronary flow and evaluation of drugs for antianginal activity.

A. Collateral Coronary
   Circulation Method

Fam and McGregor [85] recommend that in the search for an antianginal drug a retrograde flow technique be used. This technique allows the investigator to measure the volume of blood delivered to the distal end of an obstructed coronary artery through interarterial collateral channels, i.e., the retrograde flow. The peripheral coronary pressure, which is the pressure driving the collateral flow, is also measured. For this procedure dogs with experimental myocardial ischemia are used. The ischemia is produced by gradual chronic occlusion of the anterior descending and circumflex branches of the left coronary artery with ameroid constrictors [86]. Normal dogs have poor collateral circulation while the ameroid-constricted animals develop numerous collateral vessels in a 3-week period and exhibit either complete or 90% occlusion of the involved coronary arteries.

After the development of collaterals the dogs are anesthetized and a left thoracotomy performed. The pericardium is incised and sutured to the chest wall to form a cradle. The circumflex branch of the coronary is then isolated immediately distal to the ameroid constrictor, cannulated, and connected through a stopcock system to the femoral artery. This system

allows the myocardium to be perfused during periods when retrograde flow
or peripheral coronary pressure measurements are not being made. The
measurement of retrograde flow is made by collecting for 30-sec periods
the blood which exits the circumflex cannula. The latter is held at the level
of the anterior surface of the heart. After obtaining a number of successive
retrograde flow values in close agreement they are averaged and serve as
the control value. Drugs may be given intravenously or sublingually and
data on flow, pressure, etc., are usually recorded every few minutes until
the values become stable. In this preparation it is necessary to maintain
systemic arterial pressure at control level since many drugs being evaluated for antianginal activity produce systemic hypotension and retrograde
flow is linearly related to aortic pressure [87]. This is easily accomplished
by connecting a height-adjustable blood reservoir to the femoral artery for
infusion of the appropriate amount of blood.

In their retrograde flow preparation Fam and McGregor [24] found that
both nitroglycerin and dipyridamole produced a fall in systemic arterial
blood pressure. Dipyridamole produced a significant reduction in retrograde flow and peripheral coronary pressure although these parameters
were not significantly altered by nitroglycerin despite a greater fall in systemic pressure. In the animals in which systemic pressure was maintained
at control level nitroglycerin produced an approximately 50% increase in
retrograde flow whereas dipyridamole did not.

The data obtained using this technique provide an explanation of why
dipyridamole is considered to be clinically ineffective in the relief of angina
pectoris. Since coronary flow is not increased, ischemic areas within the
myocardium are not irrigated to any greater degree. Thus, the hypoxia
present is not altered and the anginal attack is not alleviated. The increase
in total coronary flow produced by dipyridamole must therefore be due to
vasodilatation of the resistance vessels of nonischemic areas.

B.   Pacing-Induced S-T
     Segment Depression

Lee and Baky [88] have devised a method for inducing S-T segment depression in unanesthetized atherosclerotic rabbits by electrical pacing. The
coronary circulation is significantly compromised by extensive atheroscloro-
sis induced by the addition of 2% cholesterol to the diet. Impairment of the
coronary circulation, as evidenced by S-T segment depression during pacing,
occurs as early as 6 weeks after beginning the high cholesterol diet. After
8 to 12 weeks Lee and Baky [88] found that 80% of their rabbits exhibited
S-T segment depression during pacing. The duration of the high cholesterol
feeding determines how these animals respond to drugs. Rabbits fed the
high cholesterol diet for 1.5 to 3 months are optimally sensitive to nitroglycerin. At autopsy these rabbits exhibit a reasonable degree of atherosclerotic involvement and are most representative of the patient with

coronary artery disease. Rabbits fed for 4.5 to 7 months, although readily
exhibiting S-T segment depression during pacing and occasionally even
during the nonpaced state, were unresponsive to nitroglycerin; those fed
for longer periods exhibited extensive atheromatous deposits in the aorta
and in some cases coronary ostium occlusion. Thus, it appears that long-
term treatment with cholesterol critically compromised the coronary circulation which Lee and Baky [88] suggest may be analogous to patients with
severe coronary artery disease and intractable angina who are unresponsive to nitroglycerin.

The pacing procedure is carried out without the need for general
anesthesia since rabbits can be put in a so-called hypnotic state while being gently restrained [89]. A heparinized saline-filled 14-gauge polyvinyl
catheter is inserted under local anesthesia 6 to 7 cm into the superior vena
cava via the anterior facial branch of the external jugular vein. A bipolar
pacing electrode which has platinum stimulating electrodes is passed
through the indwelling catheter until it is in the right atrium. If forelimb
muscle twitching or involvement of the normal movement of the diaphragm
occurs, this must be eliminated by repositioning the pacing electrode.
Stimuli are delivered at 1.5 times threshold voltage with a pacing rate of
at least 100 beats/min above the resting rate. A maximum rate of 410
beats/min is used since stimulus artifact makes electrocardiographic
evaluation impossible at higher rates. At least two successive reproducible
episodes of S-T segment depression at a given pacing rate are obtained
before administration of drugs, which can either be given intravenously
usually through the marginal ear vein or placed in the buccal cavity. With
this procedure Lee and Baky [88] found that the buccal administration of
nitroglycerin 0.6 mg significantly attenuated the S-T segment depression
induced by pacing. Intravenous administration of nitroglycerin 0.02 to
0.07 mg/kg attenuated whereas 0.1 mg/kg abolished the S-T segment depression and 0.5 mg/kg actually potentiated the depression.

Winbury et al. [90] produced S-T segment depression via an anoxic
episode produced by allowing the rabbits to breathe only 10% oxygen. Although the incidence of S-T segment depression was high the animals were
unresponsive to nitroglycerin. Thus, pacing-induced S-T depression in
the atherosclerotic rabbit appears to be a good procedure for the evaluation
of drugs for antianginal activity. It offers the same advantage as the previously described coronary collateral flow procedure, namely, that coronary vasodilators that are not effective clinically are also ineffective in this
model.

C. Measurement of Intramyocardial
Oxygen Tension

Winbury et al. [26] have successfully used this technique to determine
the effects of drugs on the oxygen tension in the subendocardial and the

subepicardial regions of the myocardium. This technique is based on the
fact that oxygen tension in the tissues reflects the balance between blood
flow and oxygen demand. The effects of drugs or physical alterations which
may increase or decrease metabolic demand or perfusion are reflected as
changes in the oxygen tension.

Oxygen tension is measured by small bare tip platinum–iridium electrodes polarographically, a technique that has been shown by Cater et al.
[91] to have good predictive validity. The electrodes are made from 0.18-
mm-diameter platinum–iridium wire insulated with Teflon. The insulation
is removed from the tip of each electrode for a distance of 0.2 to 0.3 mm
with the lead wire soldered at the opposite end. Each electrode is cali-
brated in vitro by exposure to different concentrations of oxygen dissolved
in saline. After calibration two matched electrodes are cemented together
with tips 6 mm apart. The circuit of Winbury et al. [26] for measuring
oxygen tension can register changes of less than 1 mmHg.

Drug effects on intramyocardial oxygen tension are usually examined
in anesthetized dogs. A left thoracotomy is performed and the pericardium
incised and sutured to the chest wall to form a cradle allowing free access
to the left side of the heart. A segment of the anterior descending branch
of the left coronary artery is isolated for placement of a ligature in order
to produce ischemia and placement of an electromagnetic flow probe for
monitoring. The double electrode is then pushed into the myocardium in
the area supplied by the left anterior descending coronary artery. Care
must be given during electrode placement to avoid high readings indicative
of bleeding which requires reinsertions. Inserted at the usual 3- and 9-mm
depths Winbury et al. [26] found an average epicardial/endocardial oxygen
tension ratio of 1.66. When the left anterior descending coronary artery
was occluded these investigators found a rapid fall in the subendocardial
oxygen tension although the subepicardial oxygen tension did not always
decline. On release of the occlusion there was rapid return to the oxygen
tension to control level, supporting the validity of the technique.

With this technique Winbury et al. [26] found that intravenous nitroglycerin, 0.005 to 0.02 mg/kg, increased subendocardial oxygen tension
approximately 40% over control values whereas subepicardial oxygen tension was not increased. Similar results were obtained with pentaerythritol
trinitrate [47]. In contrast, intravenous dipyridamole 0.25 mg/kg produced
a reduction in subendocardial oxygen tension in over 60% of the animals, in
spite of a twofold increase in total coronary flow.

D. Critique of Methods

We have selected for presentation and analysis three animal models for the
detection of antianginal activity. They were selected from a long list of
available models for their ability to differentiate between dipyridamole, a
drug that most feel is relatively ineffective clinically, and nitroglycerin, a

universally accepted antianginal. As such, we believe their predictive validity is high.

Nevertheless, the methods are not without disadvantages, including (a) the requirement for sophisticated instrumentation, (b) long-term treatment of animals, (c) low compound testing capacity, and (d) relatively high cost of compound evaluation. Because of these disadvantages, a rapid, low-cost screening procedure should be selected prior to testing with one or more of these methods.

IV. OUTLOOK FOR THE FUTURE

Epidemiological, clinical, and experimental data in man and animals indicate that the major risk factors responsible for coronary heart disease are hypercholesterolemia, cigarette smoking, and hypertension [92]. Studies in New York, Los Angeles, and Helsinki [93-95] have shown that ingestion of diets low in saturated fat and cholesterol results in a lower incidence of coronary heart disease than ingestion of high-fat-content diets. Despite the relatively small groups involved in these studies and the high dropout rates, it is clear that dietary modification (i.e., primary prevention) can lower the incidence of coronary heart disease and angina pectoris.

Elimination of cigarette smoking has also reduced the incidence of coronary heart disease. Two large studies [96,97] designed to examine mortality as a function of smoking history revealed that coronary heart disease mortalities of former cigarette smokers were significantly lower than those of individuals currently smoking. This suggests that the incidence of coronary heart disease can be reduced by cessation of cigarette smoking and that the beneficial effect is independent of serum cholesterol or blood pressure values [92].

Hypertension, another major risk factor responsible for coronary heart disease, was controlled in a recent study [98] by drug therapy. This procedure reduced the incidence of congestive heart failure and stroke although reduction of severe coronary atherosclerosis was less remarkable. Thus reduction of dietary intake of saturated fats and cholesterol, elimination of cigarette smoking, and control of hypertension will probably reduce the incidence of atherosclerotic disease. The Inter-Society Commission for Heart Disease Resources has recommended this approach in a recent report [92].

Reversal of coronary heart disease or inhibition of its progress has been attempted by the use of the lipid-lowering drug, clofibrate. Cohn et al. [99] in a double blind study compared clofibrate 2 g daily to placebo in a group of patients with well-established coronary artery disease. At the end of 1 year the patients were restudied by selective coronary angiography. The clofibrate group showed progressive narrowing of the coronary arteries not significantly different from the placebo group. Other studies involving clofibrate provide no convincing evidence that it will help patients with coronary artery disease [100].

On the other hand, the possiblity of developing better drugs to alleviate the frequency and severity of angina pectoris appears good. At present, nitroglycerin administered sublingually remains the drug of choice for the relief or prevention of anginal attacks. Unfortunately, its maximum duration of action is approximately 60 min. Although attempts have been made to synthesize organic nitrates with a more prolonged action the clinical results with these have been below expectations. Recently, the antianginal effect of nitroglycerin has been extended by combining it with an ointment base. This preparation, which depends on cutaneous absorption of nitroglycerin, has been shown to increase the exercise capacity of angina patients for at least 3 hr [101]. Chronic use of the ointment did not reduce the effect of sublingual nitroglycerin or the ointment. These results are encouraging but additional studies are required to examine possible tolerance development and toxicity.

Continued development of drugs that possess the clinical advantages of a nitroglycerin-propranolol combination but without the undesirable side effects seems appropriate. Such a pharmacological profile has been reported for perhexiline [73], and could represent a lead for the development of newer antianginal agents with improved safety and efficacy.

ACKNOWLEDGMENTS

The authors thank Mrs. Joan S. Gardner and Mrs. Susan L. Zehnder for valuable assistance in literature searches and Mrs. Betty L. Fitzgerald for excellent secretarial assistance.

REFERENCES

1. W. Heberden, Med. Trans. Roy. Coll. Physicians 2, 59 (1772).

2. C. K. Friedberg, Circulation 46, 1037 (1972).

3. T. Killip, in Textbook of Medicine (P. B. Beeson and W. McDermott, eds.), Saunders, Philadelphia, 1971, p. 1016.

4. R. E. Goldstein, D. R. Redwood, D. R. Rosing, G. D. Beiser, and S. E. Epstein, Circulation 44, 90 (1971).

5. K. Kitamura, C. R. Jorgensen, F. L. Gobel, H. Taylor, and Y. Wang, Am. J. Cardiol. 26, 643 (1970).

6. S. E. Epstein, M. Stampfer, G. D. Beiser, R. E. Goldstein, and E. Braunwald, N. Engl. J. Med. 280, 7 (1969).

7. A. Ansari and G. E. Burch, Arch. Intern. Med. 123, 371 (1969).

8. A. F. Ax, Psychosom. Med. 15, 433 (1953).

9. R. E. Goldstein and S. E. Epstein, Prog. Cardiovasc. Dis. 14, 360 (1972).

10. J. R. Nowlin, W. G. Troyer, W. S. Collins, G. Silverman, C. R. Nichols, H. D. McIntosh, E. H. Esters, Jr., and M. D. Bogdonoff, Ann. Intern. Med. 63, 1040 (1967).

11. W. S. Aronow, M. A. Kaplan, and D. Jacob, Ann. Intern. Med. 69, 529 (1968).

12. D. T. Watts, Ann. N.Y. Acad. Sci. 90, 74 (1960).

13. J. H. Burn, Ann. N.Y. Acad. Sci. 90, 81 (1960).

14. W. S. Aronow and A. J. Swanson, Ann. Intern. Med. 71, 599 (1969).

15. W. S. Aronow and A. J. Swanson, Ann. Intern. Med. 70, 1227 (1969).

16. W. B. Kannel and M. Feinleib, Am. J. Cardiol. 29, 154 (1972).

17. T. J. Reeves, A. Oberman, W. B. Jones, and L. T. Sheffield, Am. J. Cardiol. 33, 423 (1974).

18. W. Murrell, Lancet 1, 80 (1879).

19. H. E. Essex, R. G. Wegria, J. F. Herrick, E. J. Baldes, and F. C. Mann, Am. Heart J. 19, 554 (1940).

20. R. G. Wegria, H. E. Essex, J. F. Herrick, and F. C. Mann, Am. Heart J. 20, 557 (1940).

21. K. I. Melville, R. A. Gillis, and P. Sekelj, Can. J. Physiol. Pharmacol. 43, 9 (1965).

22. J. K. Vyden, M. Carvalho, E. Boszormenyi, T. Lang, H. Bernstein, and E. Corday, Am. J. Cardiol. 25, 53 (1970).

23. R. A. Gillis and K. I. Melville, Am. J. Cardiol. 28, 38 (1971).

24. W. M. Fam and M. McGregor, Circ. Res. 15, 355 (1964).

25. L. Bernstein, G. C. Freisinger, R. P. Lichtlen, and R. S. Ross, Circulation 33, 107 (1966).

26. M. M. Winbury, B. B. Howe, and H. R. Weiss, J. Pharmacol. Exp. Ther. 176, 184 (1971).

27. R. Forman, E. S. Kirk, M. J. Downey, and E. H. Sonnenblick, J. Clin. Invest. 52, 905 (1973).

28. R. Gorlin, N. Brachfeld, C. McLeod, and P. Bopp, Circulation 19, 705 (1959).

120 J. M. STUMP AND V. G. VERNIER

29. R. J. Bing, C. Cowan, D. Bottcher, G. Corsini, and C. G. Daniels, JAMA 205, 277 (1968).

30. C. Cowan, P. V. M. Duran, G. Corsini, N. Goldschlager, and R. J. Bing, Am. J. Cardiol. 24, 154 (1969).

31. P. F. Cohn and R. Gorlin, Med. Clin North Am. 58, 407 (1974).

32. L. D. Horwitz, R. Gorlin, W. J. Taylor, and H. G. Kemp, J. Clin. Invest. 50, 1578 (1971).

33. S. B. Knoebel, P. L. McHenry, A. J. Bonner, and J. F. Phillips, Circulation 47, 690 (1973).

34. W. Ganz and H. S. Marcus, Circulation 46, 880 (1972).

35. R. E. Goldstein, E. B. Stinson, J. L. Scherer, R. P. Seningen, T. M. Grehl, and S. E. Epstein, Circulation 49, 298 (1974).

36. H. B. Barner, G. C. Kaiser, and V. L. Willman, Am. Heart J. 88, 13 (1974).

37. J. C. Greenfield, J. C. Rembert, W. G. Young, Jr., H. N. Oldham, Jr., J. A. Alexander, and D. C. Sabisten, Jr., J. Clin. Invest. 51, 2724 (1972).

38. D. T. Mason and E. Braunwald, Circulation 32, 755 (1965).

39. G. W. Burggraf and J. O. Parker, Circulation 49, 136 (1974).

40. A. N. DeMaria, L. A. Vismara, K. Auditore, E. A. Amsterdam, R. Zelis, and D. T. Mason, Am. J. Med. 57, 754 (1974).

41. H. I. Russek, Am. J. Med. Sci. 252, 9 (1966).

42. R. E. Goldstein, D. R. Rosing, D. R. Redwood, G. D. Beiser, and S. E. Epstein, Circulation 43, 629 (1971).

43. A. P. Klaus, B. L. Zaret, B. L. Pitt, and R. S. Ross, Circulation 48, 519 (1973).

44. D. Brunner, N. Meshulam, and F. Zerieker, Chest 66, 282 (1974).

45. T. Winsor and C. S. Scott, Am. Heart J. 49, 414 (1955).

46. M. M. Winbury, in Problems in Laboratory Evaluation of Antianginal Agents (M. Winbury, ed.), North-Holland Publ., Amsterdam, 1967, p. 26.

47. H. R. Weiss and M. M. Winbury, Microvasc. Res. 4, 273 (1972).

48. H. A. Dewar, A. R. Horler, and D. J. Newell, Br. Heart J. 21, 315 (1959).

49. S. Oram and E. Sowton, Br. Med. J. 2, 1745 (1961).

50. G. R. Dagenais, R. E. Mason, G. C. Freisinger, C. Wender, and R. S. Ross, Johns Hopkins Med. J. 125, 301 (1969).

51. W. Evans and C. Hoyle, Q. J. Med. 2, 311 (1933).

52. S. L. Cole, H. Kaye, and G. C. Griffith, Am. J. Cardiol. 11, 639 (1963).

53. G. R. Dagenais, B. L. Pitt, R. E. Mason, G. C. Freisinger, and R. S. Ross, Am. J. Cardiol. 25, 90 (1970).

54. J. E. F. Riseman, G. E. Altman, and S. Koretsky, Circulation 17, 22 (1958).

55. S. A. Stephen, Am. J. Cardiol. 18, 463 (1966).

56. E. A. Amsterdam, R. Gorlin, and S. Wolfson, JAMA 210, 103 (1969).

57. D. J. Battock, H. Alvarez, and C. A. Chidsey, Circulation 39, 157 (1969).

58. M. M. Winbury, B. B. Howe, and M. A. Hefner, J. Pharmacol. Exp. Ther. 168, 70 (1969).

59. R. Charlier, in Antianginal Drugs, Springer-Verlag, New York, 1971, p. 188.

60. J. Grayson, M. Irvine, and J. R. Parratt, Cardiovasc. Res. 5, 41 (1971).

61. J. R. Parratt, I. McA. Ledingham, and C. S. McArdle, Cardiovasc. Res. 7, 401 (1973).

62. J. H. Maassen, Med. Klin. 58, 1269 (1963).

63. U. Storck, Med. Welt. 52, 2926 (1965).

64. H. Bell, D. L. Azarnoff, and M. Dunn, Clin. Pharmacol. Ther. 9, 40 (1968).

65. N. Conway, G. D. Gupta, and E. Sowton, Acta Cardiol. 23, 434 (1968).

66. H. Hunscha, M. Kaltenback, and W. Schellhorn, Therapiewoche 16, 1153 (1966).

67. R. J. Bing, S. R. Bender, M. I. Dunn, G. A. Fry, W. M. Fuller, S. C. K. Liu, H. S. Miller, J. W. Moses, L. W. Ritzmann, J. P. Segal, G. I. Shugoll, H. Fillmanns, and A. Wallace, Clin. Pharmacol. Ther. 16, 4 (1974).

68. W. J. Hudak, R. E. Lewis, R. W. Lucas, and W. J. Kuhn, Postgrad. Med. J. 49, 16 (1973).

69. G. Klassen, F. Sestier, A. L'Abbate, and D. Zborowska-Sluis, Am. J. Cardiol. 35, 149 (1975).

70. J. Morledge, Postgrad. Med. J. 49, 64 (1973).

71. A. Cherchi, M. Bina, R. Fonzo, and M. Raffo, Postgrad. Med. J. 49, 67 (1973).

72. J. Martins de Olivera, S. F. Loyola, and J. L. Da Cunha Chaves, Postgrad. Med. J. 49, 84 (1973).

73. C. J. Pepine, S. J. Schang, and C. R. Bemiller, Am. J. Cardiol. 33, 806 (1974).

74. R. Kadatz, Arzneim. Forsch. 9, 39 (1959).

75. G. Grabner, F. Kaindl, and O. Kraupp, Arzneim. Forsch. 9, 45 (1959).

76. T. Hockers and G. Bogelmann, Arzneim. Forsch. 9, 47 (1959).

77. W. M. Fam and M. McGregor, Circ. Res. 22, 649 (1968).

78. D. Kinsella, W. Troup, and M. McGregor, Am. Heart J. 63, 146 (1962).

79. L. A. Soloff, J. L. Gimenez, and W. L. Winters, Am. J. Med. Sci. 243, 783 (1962).

80. A. C. DeGraff and A. F. Lyon, Am. Heart J. 65, 423 (1963).

81. M. T. Newhouse and M. McGregor, Am. J. Cardiol. 16, 234 (1965).

82. M. C. Igloe, J. Am. Geriat. Soc. 18, 233 (1970).

83. R. Lofontant, H. Feinberg, and L. N. Katz, Circulation 22, 774 (1960).

84. H. J. Bartelstone, B. J. Scherlag, P. F. Cranefield, and B. F. Hoffman, Bull. N.Y. Acad. Med. 42, 951 (1966).

85. W. M. Fam and M. McGregor, in Problems in Laboratory Evaluation of Antianginal Agents (M. Winbury, ed.), North-Holland Publ., Amsterdam, 1967, p. 17.

86. A. Vineberg, B. Mahanti, and J. Litvak, Surgery 47, 765 (1960).

87. A. A. Kattus and D. E. Gregg, Circ. Res. 7, 628 (1959).

88. R. J. Lee and S. H. Baky, J. Pharmacol. Exp. Ther. 184, 205 (1973).

89. R. P. Gruber and J. J. Amato, Lab. Anim. Care 20, 741 (1970).

90. M. M. Winbury, J. K. Wolf, and M. T. I. Cronin, Am. J. Physiol. 200, 642 (1961).

91. D. B. Cater, I. A. Silver, and G. M. Wilson, Proc. Roy. Soc. Ser. B, Biol. Sci. 151, 256 (1960).

92. Inter-Society Commission for Heart Disease Resources: Primary Prevention of the Atherosclerotic Diseases, Circulation 42, A-55 (1970).

93. O. Turpeinen, M. Miettinen, M. J. Karvonen, P. Roine, M. Pekkarinen, E. J. Lehtosuo, and P. Alivirta, Am. J. Clin. Nutr. 21, 255 (1968).

94. S. H. Rinzler, Bull. N.Y. Acad. Med. 44, 936 (1968).

95. S. Dayton, M. L. Pearce, S. Hoshimoto, W. J. Dixon, and U. Tomiyasu, Circulation 40, Suppl. 2 (1969).

96. H. A. Kahn, in Epidemiological Approaches to the Study of Cancer and Other Diseases (W. Haenszel, ed.), National Cancer Institute Monograph, 1966, p. 1.

97. J. Stamler, Bull. N.Y. Acad. Med. 44, 1476 (1968).

98. Veterans Administration Cooperative Study Group on Antihypertensive Agents, Effects of Treatment on Morbidity in Hypertension. II. Results in Patients with Diastolic Blood Pressure Averaging 90 through 114 mmHg. JAMA 213, 1143 (1970).

99. K. Cohn, F. J. Sakai, and M. F. Langston, Jr., Am. Heart J. 89, 591 (1975).

100. P. M. S. Gillam, Am. Heart J. 87, 1 (1974).

101. N. Reichek, R. E. Goldstein, D. R. Redwood, and S. E. Epstein, Circulation 50, 348 (1974).

Chapter 5

ANTIARRHYTHMICS

John R. Cummings

Ayerst Research Laboratories
Montreal, Quebec, Canada

125

I. INTRODUCTION

Following a cursory computerized search of the recent literature on cardiac arrhythmias and antiarrhythmic drugs it became abundantly clear that a complete survey of the total, or even of the most important, findings in this field was outside the scope of this chapter. The intent of the present work then shifted to a more realistic approach, namely, to offer a personal view on how industry, both pharmaceutical and medical electronics, attempts to recognize, invent, develop, and eventually market drugs and devices for the management of various kinds of cardiac irregularities. Although serendipity has played a major role in the discovery of antiarrhythmic drugs in the past and the present, more rational concepts based on a better understanding of the pathogenesis and pathophysiology of cardiac rhythm disturbances and the relationship between drug activity and chemical structure hold out a promise for future advancements.

This chapter describes various studies on the genesis of cardiac arrhythmias, on the development of experimental arrhythmic models and their usefulness in studying antiarrhythmic drugs, and on selective structure-activity relationships. Pacemakers and defibrillators for the management of certain arrhythmias are also briefly considered.

II. HISTORICAL SYNOPSIS

In this modern era of new pharmaceuticals, it is noteworthy that two antiarrhythmic drugs widely used today, quinidine and digitalis, have a history dating back more than 200 years. Quinidine is one of the natural alkaloids found in cinchona bark; the latter was recognized in 1749 by Jean Baptiste de Senac [1] to have therapeutic value in the management of cardiac irregularities. This observation was apparently forgotten by the medical profession in the following years until the turn of the twentieth century when Wenckebach [2] published his findings on the value of quinine alkaloids in certain arrhythmias. A few years later Frey [3] studied quinine, cinchonine, and quinidine in patients with atrial fibrillation and found the latter to be particularly efficacious. In succeeding decades more and more investigators became aware of the antiarrhythmic efficacy of quinidine and, thus, the use of the drug became permanently established.

The recognition by Withering [4] that digitalis was the active ingredient in the Shropshire Lady's brew is a better known historical event than the early work with quinidine. Although Withering's observations were primarily limited to the diuretic action of digitalis in dropsy, he speculated that the drug had antiarrhythmic properties ("a power over the motion of the heart to a degree yet unobserved by any other medicine"). At the close of the nineteenth century and the start of the twentieth, Mackenzie [5] showed that digitalis could produce heart block in the presence of atrial fibrillation, and both he and later Lewis [6] gave great importance to the slowing effect of digitalis as being primarily responsible for clinical efficacy in heart failure.

The ability of muscles to respond to repeated electrical stimuli has been known, albeit poorly, since Galvani's study on frog skeletal muscle [7]. In 1871 Bowditch reported that the frog heart did not respond like skeletal muscle to trains of electrical stimuli, i.e., there was not always a 1:1 ratio between the number of shocks and the number of contractions [8a]. Using a similar technique, Marey concluded that the heart was refractory during the initial moments of systole [8a]. Rothberger and Winterburg [9] produced arrhythmia and ventricular fibrillation with faradic current. Wiggers [10] in the 1930s demonstrated in animals many of the physiological results of electrical stimulation of the heart. A thorough review of the problem as understood at that time was provided by Wiggers and Wegria [11]: for example, that the heart is most vulnerable to electrically induced ventricular fibrillation in the last part of systole.

Zoll [12] showed that closed-chest cardiac pacing was clinically beneficial. A few years later Furman and Robinson [13] demonstrated the feasibility of stimulating the canine and human right ventricular endocardium with a transvenously inserted electrode.

In this brief historical synopsis it is well to remember that each generation of cardiovascular pharmacologists, physiologists, and physicians working in the area of antiarrhythmic drug research is dependent on the techniques available to him at that time. As newer and improved cardiovascular methodology developed (e.g., in electrocardiography, intracellular microelectrode measurements, cardiac catheterization, hemodynamic recording systems, biochemical techniques), the cardiovascular actions of digitalis, quinidine, and a host of new antiarrhythmic drugs have become better known. Most likely the elaboration of further techniques will result in a clarification of our understanding of antiarrhythmic drugs or devices and of the etiology of cardiac irregularities, especially at the cellular and intercellular levels.

III. CARDIAC EXCITABILITY
      AND RHYTHM DISTURBANCES

Both cardiac electrophysiological abnormalities associated with arrhythmias and the mode of action of antiarrhythmic drugs can be characterized by studying the four basic properties of the heart, namely, automaticity, excitability, refractoriness, and conductivity. With the exception of certain parasystolic rhythms, nearly all arrhythmias are due either to enhanced automatic impulse formation (e.g., in the area of an infarction, after the administration of an overdose of digitalis) or to reentry (e.g., sinus node-atrial reentry, intraatrial reentry, intraventricular reentry), or to a

128   J. R. CUMMINGS

combination of both. The former mechanism is caused by an increase in
automaticity resulting in an occasional or repetitive discharge of an ectopic
focus. The latter mechanism is due to changes in excitability, refractoriness, and conductivity. Although the evidence is circumstantial rather
than definitive, both increased automaticity and reentry undoubtedly can
occur in man during periods of arrhythmia [14].

Automatic cells are found in the sinoauricular node, the His-Purkinje
system, the atrioventricular node, and some parts of the atrial tracts.
The normal mechanism of automaticity resides in an important feature of
the pacemaker action potential, namely, spontaneous slow diastolic depo-
larization (phase 4) of the resting membrane to the threshold level. Abnormal mechanisms which increase automaticity include myocardial injury,
ischemia, local changes in potassium and calcium concentrations, and local
alterations in pO_2, pCO_2, and pH [15,16].

After it has sequentially activated the atria and ventricles, the conducted impulse is normally extinguished since it is surrounded by tissue
which has just been excited and now is refractory. The concept of reentry
requires that under abnormal conditions the impulse persists long enough
that it can reenter and reexcite adjacent nonrefractory tissue, i.e., a one-
way block. This, in turn, implies that the impulse within the conducting
pathway is blocked, that conduction over an alternate path is slowed, and
that activation beyond the block is delayed.

In a biological system such as the heart it seems most likely that conductivity recovers nonsymmetrically. Propagation of an impulse unidirec-
tionally, therefore, is quite possible. For a self-sustained reentry circuit
to develop in the atrium as in atrial flutter, one of the bands of atrial conducting tissue must have a conduction defect at a critical moment. Investigators have grappled with the problem of the etiology and perpetuation of
atrial flutter in different ways. Wiener and Rosenblueth [17], for example,
developed a mathematical model to explain propagation of impulses in a
matrix which, like the atrium, is perforated by obstacles. This matrix
model could account for the maintenance of flutter. Using a computer
model, Moe et al. [18] showed that when they simulated fibrillation and then
created obstacles of suitable dimensions, a rhythmic reentry flutter developed. In this model no single ectopic impulse resulted in flutter without
a prior period of fibrillation.

In experimental flutter, anything that reduces the duration of the refractory period normally accelerates the flutter, and anything that prolongs
the refractory period reduces the frequency. As mentioned in subsequent
sections, the former relates to the action of digitalis [19] and the latter to
the action of quinidine [20] in the treatment of atrial flutter. The duration
of the refractory period interrelates with conduction velocity. Prolongation
of the refractory period results in a slowing of conduction.

In isolated rabbit atrioventricular nodal preparations, reentry leading to self-sustained supraventricular tachycardia has been demonstrated by several investigators [21-23]. This type of reentry activity has also been shown to occur clinically [24]. In the latter study it was demonstrated that in patients with occasional supraventricular tachycardia, it was possible to trigger identical arrhythmic episodes by premature electrical stimulation of the atrium. These investigators also terminated spontaneously occurring supraventricular tachycardia with a properly timed single stimulus applied to the atrium.

A combination of increased automaticity and reentry is implicated in the development and maintenance of ventricular arrhythmias. A few decades ago it appeared that the former mechanism was the only operative one in this irregularity, e.g., Prinzmetal's high-speed cinematographic studies of fibrillating ventricles [25] which showed no evidence of reentry. The concept of enhanced automaticity in the etiology of ventricular arrhythmias implies that there is rapid firing of impulses in one or more ectopic foci. It is supported, in part, on the assumption that the propagation of an impulse over an alternate pathway in the ventricles could not be slow enough to allow for reentry and reexcitation. More recently, however, Wit et al. [26] have reported relatively slow conduction velocities (< 50 mm/sec) in isolated Purkinje tissue. In addition, Sasyniuk and Mendez [27] recorded refractory periods of less than 40 msec in similar preparations. Reentry was demonstrated by both groups of investigators within loops only a few millimeters in circumference.

A newer approach in investigating cardiac electrophysiological mechanisms underlying ventricular arrhythmias has been to study the membrane responsiveness and refractory period of Purkinje fibers which were obtained from both infarcted and normal canine endocardium. With this in vitro method, the animal was sacrificed and portions of infarcted and noninfarcted tissue were removed 24 hr after coronary artery occlusion (i.e., at a time when the dog had developed sustained, multifocal ventricular extrasystoles). The action potentials of normal and ischemic Purkinje fibers were then examined [28-31]. Infarction enhanced automaticity and the development of reentry and, thereby, reexcitation. Moreover, antiarrhythmic agents affected cells in the infarcted zone differently from that recorded in noninfarcted Purkinje fibers [32,33]. For example, lidocaine caused a greater reduction in the membrane responsiveness of Purkinje fibers in the infarcted area as compared to the normal area. As a result, conduction was slowed more markedly through the infarcted zone than in the noninfarcted zone. Lidocaine shortened the action potential duration to a lesser degree in infarcted cells than in normal cells. And finally, lidocaine suppressed pacemaker activity in the infarcted area but not in the normal area [32].

IV. EXPERIMENTAL ARRHYTHMIA MODELS FOR
    DISCOVERING ANTIARRHYTHMIC DRUGS

In most pharmaceutical companies a sequential approach is employed to
find and evaluate compounds of value in the management of cardiac irregularities. The initial screen usually provides the pharmacologist with an
opportunity to test hundreds of compounds yearly if desired. Subsequent
tests in different arrhythmia model systems permit the recognition of agents
with the desired antiarrhythmic activity and an assessment of untoward actions which might limit or prevent clinical usage.

Although the carryover to the clinic occasionally has been poor in the
past [34,35] the concept of using several animal model systems to develop
an antiarrhythmic drug profile is undoubtedly valid. The problem is how to
make maximum use of meaningful methods in the proper sequence. In dis-
cussing various experimental arrhythmias, a modification of the outline
developed by Szekeres and Papp [36a] is followed.

A. Production of Arrhythmias
    by Electrical Stimulation

1. Fibrillation threshold:
    single pulse technique

An adequate square wave single shock applied during the vulnerable period
produces ventricular fibrillation, and weaker shocks evoke extrasystoles
whereas even strong shocks applied to the heart after complete recovery of
its excitability will cause only ectopic beats. Although several investigators
have used the single shock method for studying the ventricular fibrillation
threshold of antiarrhythmic drugs [37] the procedure has certain drawbacks.
If the electrical stimulus is to reach the heart in the vulnerable period,
artificial driving must be applied with the exclusion of the sinus impulse,
and a second extra stimulus must be delivered at a certain interval following the driving stimulus to measure the vulnerable period. In determining
the fibrillation threshold, the extra single stimuli are used to scan the vulnerable period of the cardiac cycle. Moreover, the production of ventricular fibrillation by a single shock requires a relatively strong stimulus
which may injure the cardiac tissue if applied too frequently. VanTyn and
McLean [38], for example, recommended that an interval equal to 10 to 15
contractions should elapse between the first and second extra stimuli.

2. Fibrillation threshold:
    multiple pulse technique

Most investigators studying antiarrhythmic drugs prefer to measure the
ventricular fibrillation threshold by applying a gated train of pulses to the
myocardium during the vulnerable period of the cardiac cycle [39,40].

With the serial shock method, rapid stimuli (10-60 Hz) are applied to the right ventricle and the strength of the current is gradually increased. As a consequence, a response can be elicited in the relative refractory phase; the number of responses per unit time increases up to a point where the heart can no longer follow the stimulus. The maximum frequency is determined by the effective refractory period. At this time, ventricular flutter is present and the minimum current intensity required to produce the arrhythmia (i.e., flutter threshold) is constant and reproducible. If the current intensity is increased still further, ventricular fibrillation develops since some of the stimuli fall within the vulnerable period of the cardiac cycle. Because of summation, the ventricular fibrillation threshold determined in this manner will be lower than that obtained with the single shock method. Using trains of pulses, the effects of antiarrhythmic drugs, e.g., lidocaine [39] and digitalis [40], on the ventricular fibrillation threshold have been studied.

3. Auricular flutter and fibrillation

The injury-stimulation method of Rosenblueth and Garcia-Ramos [41] for producing a long-lasting atrial flutter or fibrillation has been used by investigators in the development of an antiarrhythmic drug profile [34]. With this procedure a portion of the intervena caval bridge of the right atrium of an anesthetized dog is crushed with a hemostat followed by electrical stimulation of the atrium. In order to avoid thoracotomy, Ellis [42] modified this method whereby the atrium of a dog was stimulated by means of a stimulator connected to a transvenous catheter electrode placed on the atrial endocardium. The resulting atrial arrhythmia was used for screening compounds for antiarrhythmic activity. Another modification was described by Szekeres and Papp [36b], namely, epicardial electrodes were attached to the right atrium and right ventricle of an anesthetized dog, and atrial fibrillation and ventricular tachycardia were produced alternately. The potency and duration of action of antiarrhythmic drugs for correcting these two types of arrhythmias were then determined.

B. Quinidinelike Electrophysiological
     Alternations

1. In vitro procedures

In screening for antiarrhythmic drugs, automaticity, excitability, refractoriness, and conductivity are often measured directly or indirectly. Compounds which have some or all of the actions of quinidine (e.g., decrease in excitability, prolongation of the effective refractory period, inhibition of the pacemaker center, slowing of conduction) are considered to be of potential value as antiarrhythmic drugs. Either the method of Dawes [43] or, as mentioned subsequently, one of the modifications of this model provides a simple, indirect approach to the problem; that is, isolated rabbit atria are stimulated at increasing frequencies until the tissue can no longer follow with a 1:1 stimulus-response ratio. Measurements of the maximum driving rate are made before and after the test compound is placed in the tissue bath. A quinidinelike action is indicated by a decrease in the highest driving frequency, i.e., indirect evidence that the drug prolongs the effective refractory period. An improvement in the in vitro model has been described by Szekeres and Vaughan Williams [44] and Papp and Vaughan Williams [45]. Using isolated rabbit or guinea pig atria, the amplitude of the intracellular action potential, its rate of rise, the force of contraction, conduction velocity, and the atrial flutter and fibrillation thresholds were directly recorded. With this technique, various antiarrhythmic drugs have been examined by these authors, for example, quinidine, procainamide, propranolol, and practolol. Recently, Wang and Maxwell [46] modified the technique so that comparisons could be made between electrophysiological effects of bretylium on isolated heart tissue of normal and immunosympathectomized rats.

2. In vivo procedures

In addition to isolated cardiac tissue assays, numerous investigators have examined the quinidinelike electrophysiological effects of various antiarrhythmic drugs in intact animals [8b,36c,47,48]. Damato and associates [49] have extended these studies to man using the technique of premature atrial stimulation and His bundle recordings for studies on atrial refractoriness. In these investigations, a tripolar electrode catheter was positioned under fluoroscopic visualization across the tricuspid valve in order to record atrioventricular nodal, His bundle, and right bundle branch potentials. For premature stimulation, a bipolar electrode catheter was placed against the lateral wall of the right atrium. With this procedure, the investigators have studied a variety of antiarrhythmic drugs administered to patients in clinically effective dosages, e.g., the effect of propranolol on cardiac conduction [50].

C. Production of Arrhythmias
    with Chemical Substances
    Applied Locally or Parenterally

1. Local administration

The local application of the arrhythmogenic agent, aconitine, on the heart was described by Scherf [51]. Using dogs, aconitine was applied to the right atrium in the form of a soaked cotton pledget or subepicardially which resulted in a sustained atrial flutter or fibrillation. Moe and Abildskov [52] found that the aconitine-induced atrial flutter could be converted to fibrillation by stimulating the vagi, and under in vitro conditions, Yelnosky and Clark [53] showed that acetylcholine could antagonize the effect of aconitine in isolated rabbit hearts. More recently, Hashimoto and Moe [54] found that pacemaker activity in specialized atrial fibers is suppressed by acetylcholine. The procedure used to induce an atrial tachysystole has a marked effect on the kind of antiarrhythmic activity observed. Mendez and Kabela [55], for example, demonstrated that potassium can terminate the arrhythmia caused by aconitine without altering the arrhythmia due to injury and stimulation-induced reentry, whereas the antiarrhythmic agent clemizole has the opposite action. This is an interesting model because it allows the investigator the opportunity to determine drug activity in terms of both reentry and automaticity. A long-lasting atrial flutter may also be evoked by applying delphinine [56], methacholine [57], or veratrine [58] onto the atrium. An improved method for administering constant concentrations of aconitine to a restricted area of the atrium (the "cup technique") was described by Nakayama et al. [59].

2. Parenteral administration

In addition to local application, experimental cardiac irregularities can be produced by intravenous or intraarterial administration of a variety of arrhythmogenic agents. Both Szekeres [60] and Fekete and Boisy [61] evoked a relatively prolonged atrial and/or ventricular arrhythmia in rats by intravenous injections of aconitine. The former group used this procedure to test a series of compounds for their ability to convert the aconitine-induced arrhythmia to normal sinus rhythm whereas the latter were interested in finding agents which prevented the appearance of the irregularity.
   Investigators have also used intravenous administrations of cardiac glycosides at toxic dosages to evoke arrhythmias in various laboratory species. Clark and Cummings [62] found that intravenous administration of large doses of ouabain to dogs caused a prolonged ventricular tachycardia which usually progressed to ventricular fibrillation. Procainamide showed antiarrhythmic activity against the ventricular tachycardia (i.e., a reversion to normal sinus beats) but not against the development of ventricular fibrillation; ambonestyl had the opposite effect; and quinidine was antiarrhythmic using both criteria. A similar procedure was employed by Lucchesi and Shivak [63] and Sekiya and Vaughan Williams [64]; namely, after pretreatment with the test compound the amount of ouabain or acetylstrophanthidin required to induce arrhythmias was recorded and compared with the vehicle control. Another modification is the measurement of the amount of acetylstrophanthidin necessary to cause nodal arrhythmia in isolated rabbit hearts before and after the introduction of the antiarrhythmic test compound [65]. Recently Laddu et al. [66] described the use of an infusion of the cardiac glycoside, thevetin, into guinea pigs for screening antiarrhythmic agents. Although the effect of the test compound on ventricular

arrhythmia and/or cardiac arrest was also noted, the endpoint in this model was taken as the time required for the disappearance of the P wave. With this test, various clinically useful antiarrhythmic or antifibrillatory drugs were effective, e.g., bretylium, diphenylhydantoin, lidocaine, propranolol, and quinidine.

A number of other classes of drugs and chemicals have been used to produce experimental arrhythmias. For instance, intracoronary injections of the sclerosing agent tetrafluorohexachlorobutane to dogs and baboons caused a ventricular arrhythmia which could be modified by various antiarrhythmic drugs [67,68]. Recently a new antiarrhythmic benzylamine derivative was discovered using this procedure [69].

D. Production of Arrhythmias by a Combination
    of Drugs Plus "Sensitizing" Agents

That an anesthetic such as chloroform may "sensitize" the hearts of dogs to the administration of an adrenergic drug was appreciated years ago by Levy [70]. Later, cyclopropane replaced chloroform in this type of investigation, and epinephrine was either injected into the dog in a fixed dose [71] or slowly infused at a standard rate (1 μg/kg/ml/20 sec) until multiple ventricular extrasystoles developed [72]. More recently, halothane has been substituted for cyclopropane [73]. In mice, chloroform alone can evoke arrhythmias including ventricular fibrillation without the concomitant administration of exogenous sympathomimetics. This model has been used by several investigators to search for antiarrhythmic drugs [34,74,75]. Although the method has a number of inherent problems (e.g., the separation of mortality due to anoxia versus mortality due to fibrillation), the use of the mouse has obvious advantages in screening.

Agents other than general anesthetics have also been used to "sensitize" the heart. Thus, amarin, which slows conduction, coupled with epinephrine, which increases ventricular automaticity, produced a long-lasting ventricular arrhythmia [8c,76]. Leveque developed a method wherein insulin and glucose were used to sensitize the hearts of dogs to the arrythmogenic action of acetylcholine. This procedure was employed to demonstrate the antiarrhythmic action of guanethidine [77] and bretylium [78].

E. Arrhythmias Caused by Coronary Ligation

A two-stage ligation of the left anterior descending coronary artery of the dog, as described by Harris [79], provides a useful preparation with a predictable, long-lasting ventricular tachycardia. The technique of coronary ligation has been used by numerous investigators evaluating antiarrhythmic drugs because of its similarity to myocardial infarction occurring in man.

The persistence of the arrhythmia permits repeated injections of the test
compound and thus an assessment of duration of antiarrhythmic activity.
The use of a conscious animal allows for an evaluation of certain untoward
actions, for example, CNS stimulation [39, 62, 80]. Within 5 to 7 hr after
complete coronary artery occlusion, premature ventricular beats appear
and then increase in frequency until there exists a relatively high rate,
multifocal ventricular tachycardia. The assessment of antiarrhythmic
activity of the test compound is measured approximately 10 to 36 hr post-
occlusion. By the third or fourth day after ligation, the ventricular ectopic
rhythm spontaneously reverts to normal sinus rhythm. Notwithstanding,
the infarcted myocardium is unusually sensitive at this time to epinephrine,
vasopressin, nicotine, and other arrhythmic agents, and this fact allows
the investigator to use another model for assessing antiarrhythmic activity
[62, 81-83]. Another variation in the coronary ligation preparation was
introduced by Varma and Melville [84], namely, a combination of hypothermia with one-stage coronary ligation. The resultant ventricular fibrillation
in 100% of the control dogs was used as a basis for assessing the activity
of various antiarrhythmic drugs.

F. Arrhythmias Caused by Hypothermia

In dogs subjected to hypothermia (25°C), temporary occlusion of the venous
supply to the heart and an incision of the right ventricle caused ventricular
fibrillation [85]. Using this model, Covino et al. [86] found that procainamide and diphenylhydantoin had little or no antiarrhythmic effect. In this
model, Angelakos and Hegnauer [87] found that quinidine afforded protection
against ventricular fibrillation, procainamide increased the incidence of
fibrillation, ambonestyl had weak antiarrhythmic activity, and antazoline
and methapyrilene had the most antiarrhythmic activity. Using an isolated
cat heart preparation [88], Szekeres and Papp [36d] examined the effect of
quinidine, procaine, and papaverine on the auricular and ventricular fibrillation threshold to electrical stimulation at normal body temperature and
at 26°C. They found that cooling influences the effect of the antiarrhythmic
drugs. For example, procaine increased the auricular threshold for fibrillation at 38°C more than at 26°C; at 38°C, papaverine was more effective
against ventricular fibrillation than quinidine and procaine; and during hypothermia procaine was more active than papaverine.

V. STRUCTURE-ACTIVITY RELATIONSHIPS

As previously mentioned, the empiric approach in which large numbers of
compounds are screened in a battery of procedures has often resulted in the

discovery of antiarrhythmic agents. More recently the search for new
drugs has also been guided by a more rational approach founded on an ap-
preciation of the biochemical and electrophysiological abnormalities under-
lining the disorder. Regardless of how an active antiarrhythmic lead is
discovered, medicinal chemists and pharmacologists working in a pharmaceutical house normally prepare and test a number of chemical analogs and
homologs. The intent is to find compounds with more efficacy, greater
potency, less toxicity, prolonged or shorter duration of action, and so on.
Despite the fact that efforts to relate antiarrhythmic activity to a single
common structure have failed (which is hardly surprising in view of the
diverse etiologies involved), it is often possible to demonstrate a relationship between structure and activity within certain series of compounds.
For the purpose of illustration, two chemically and pharmacologically different types of antiarrhythmic agents are considered briefly.

A. β-Adrenergic Blocking Agents

The structure of the first recognized β-receptor antagonist, dichloroiso-
proterenol [DCl (1)] is closely related to the β-adrenergic agonist, isoproterenol (2). Under proper experimental conditions, DCl protects against
arrhythmias induced by electrical stimulation plus norepinephrine infusion
[89] and by arrhythmogenic doses of cardiac glycosides [65, 82]. However,
DCl also has intrinsic β-adrenergic stimulating actions and, as a consequence, it has no clinical usefulness.

(1)

(2)

Structural analogs of DCl were then synthetized, and these included the substituted phenethylamines, pronethalol (3) and sotalol (4). Pronethalol represented the first "specific" β-adrenergic blocking agent, i.e., it lacked β-adrenergic agonist activity. Because of this it showed (along with

(3)

(4)

structurally related compounds) a number of pharmacologic advantages over DCl. Both pronethalol and sotalol were found to have antiarrhythmic activity. Results supporting this property of pronethalol came from experiments in which toxic doses of cardiac glycosides were employed [64,90]; results with sotalol included studies in which arrhythmias were induced in dogs by injections of methylchloroform [91,92]. At β-blocking dosages, sotalol has only a narrow antiarrhythmic profile; e.g., it was nearly inactive in correcting cardiac irregularities caused by infusing toxic amounts of ouabain or by coronary artery ligation [93-95]. However, much higher doses of sotalol did afford protection against ouabain-induced arrhythmias [95].

In an effort to develop more efficacious and less toxic compounds, it was found that insertion of an $-OCH_2-$ bridge between the aromatic and the aliphatic side chain resulted in increased β-adrenergic blocking activity. The antiarrhythmic effects of propranolol (5) have been studied more extensively than any other β-blocker. At doses causing β-adrenergic blockade but little or no quinidinelike activity, propranolol blocked the cardiac effects of catecholamines and of sympathetic nerve stimulation in experimental animals [96]. However, the well-established effectiveness of propranolol in blocking arrhythmias caused by ouabain [64,97] seems to be associated with the drug's quinidinelike action. This is based on the findings that

(5)

d-propranolol (which has essentially no β-blocking action) is as effective in blocking digitalis toxicity as the l-isomer; that the β-blocking activity of l-propranolol is evident at lower doses than is the antiarrhythmic action; and that more selective β-adrenergic blockers often fail to prevent digitalis cardiac toxicity [93,98,99]. Notwithstanding, more recent investigations indicate that blockade of β-adrenergic receptors does play a role in propranolol's protective effect against digitalis-induced arrhythmias [96]. Moreover, studies in man on propranolol have failed to reveal any significant effect on conduction or refractoriness in the His-Purkinje system [50, 100]. These and related findings led Sasyniuk and Ogilvie [33] to conclude that the use of the term "quinidinelike" in reference to propranolol's antiarrhythmic action is a misnomer. A number of analogs of propranolol have been found to have varying degrees of antiarrhythmic activity. These include the following: alprenolol (6) [101-103], oxprenolol (7) [104], pindolol (8) [105-107], and practolol (9) [45,108].

(6)

(7)

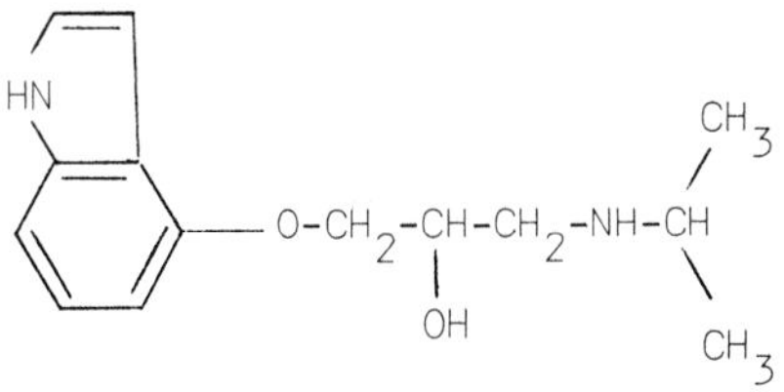

(8)

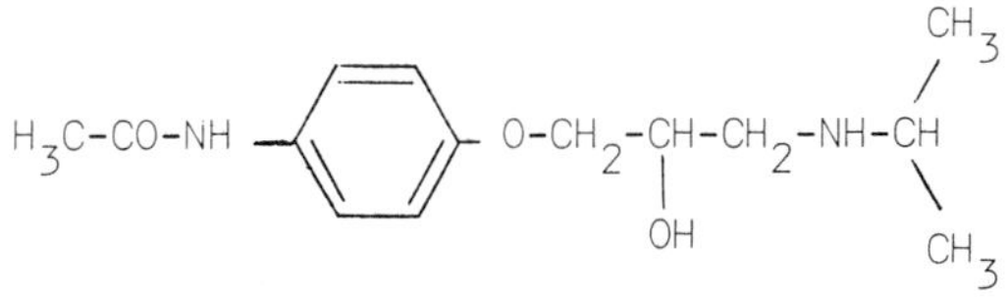

(9)

When the isopropylamine group was replaced by the tertiary butyl group, β-adrenergic activity increased severalfold. Bunolol (10) is a representative member of this group [109]. However, bunolol is less active as an antiarrhythmic than propranolol [110]. Besides, at the present state

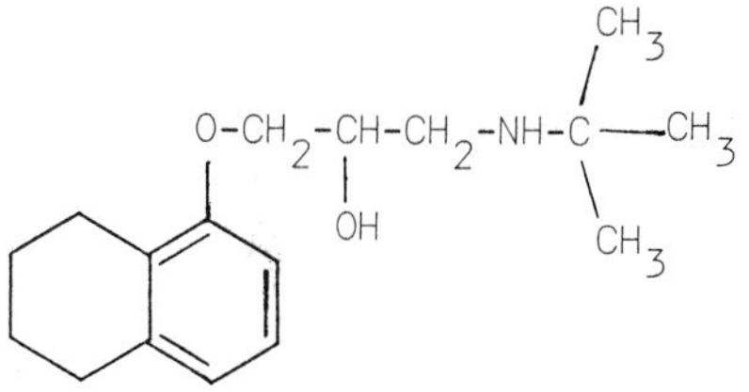

(10)

of the art, greater β-adrenolytic potency is only of secondary importance. What is of prime interest today is the discovery of less toxic compounds with selective pharmacologic properties, e.g., relatively safe compounds which affect only the β_1 receptors of the heart without inhibiting the β_2 receptors of the bronchi and the blood vessels. Practolol (9) was the first clinically useful "cardioselective" β_1-blocking agent [111]. For example, VanDurme et al. [112] found that practolol corrected supraventricular tachyarrhythmias in patients who could not tolerate propranolol because of its bronchoconstrictor effects. Bunitrolol (11) is a more potent β-adrenergic

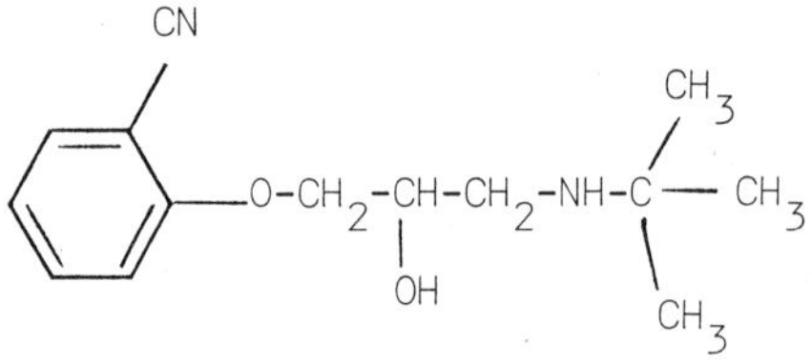

CN

—O-CH$_2$-CH-CH$_2$-NH-C — CH$_3$

OH

CH$_3$ / CH$_3$ \ CH$_3$

(11)

blocking agent which also has "cardioselective" and antiarrhythmic activities [113]. As in the case with practolol, bunitrolol has been successfully employed as an antiarrhythmic in patients who suffer from bronchial asthma [114].

Finally, recent studies on the quarternary derivative of propranolol, UM-272 (12), serve as a reminder that β-adrenolytic activity per se is not a requisite for the prevention or reversion of cardiac arrhythmias [115]. Like d-propranolol, UM-272 is devoid of β-adrenergic receptor blocking activity. However, unlike d-propranolol, UM-272 lacked local anesthetic activity. The latter finding is in agreement with the results of others which suggest that a local anesthetic effect is not necessary for antiarrhythmic activity [116,117].

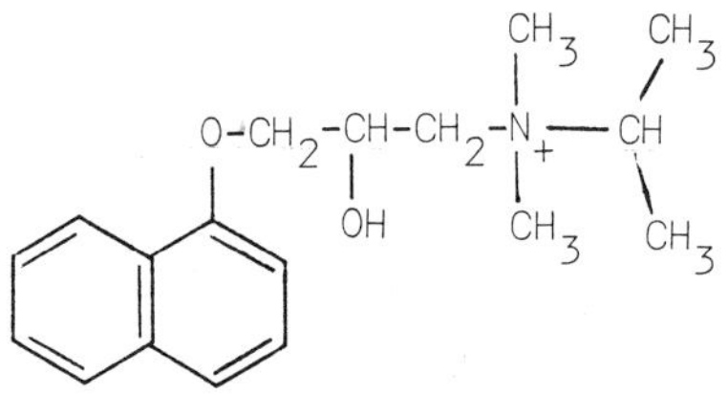

O-CH$_2$-CH-CH$_2$-N$^+$— CH

OH

CH$_3$ CH$_3$ / CH$_3$ \ CH$_3$

(12)

B. Digitalis and Allied Cardiac Glycosides

Because of its vagal-mediated and direct effects on ectopic atrial pacemakers and atrioventricular conduction, digitalis has a long-established clinical usefulness in the treatment of various cardiac arrhythmias, e.g., atrial premature beats, supraventricular tachycardia, atrial fibrillation, atrial flutter, and tachyarrhythmias associated with the Wolff-Parkinson-White syndrome [118]. Notwithstanding, excessive doses of digitalis glycosides and their aglycones often result in undesirable and sometimes lethal arrhythmias, a situation which led Lown et al. [119] to jest sadly: "It may be said that lanatoside is now replacing homicide as a leading cause of death."

Naturally occurring digitalis agents have a steroid nucleus attached to the β-carbon atom of an α,β-unsaturated lactone. Digitoxigenin (13) serves as an example. In an effort to reduce the incidence of serious intolerance to digitalis, a variety of compounds extracted from natural sources

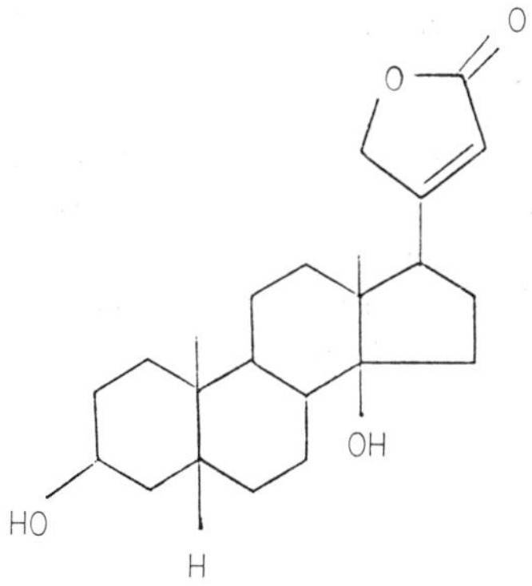

(13)

and semisynthetic cardiac glycosides and aglycones have been prepared over the years. Numerous investigators have reviewed the extensive literature on the botanical sources and major chemical components of this series of compounds [120-124]. Unfortunately, most studies have been limited to measurements of lethal doses in laboratory animals or to in vitro experiments with little or no attention directed to quantitative differences in the inotropic and arrhythmogenic actions of these compounds. Recently, though, a new semisynthetic cardenolide, actodigin (14), has been examined which

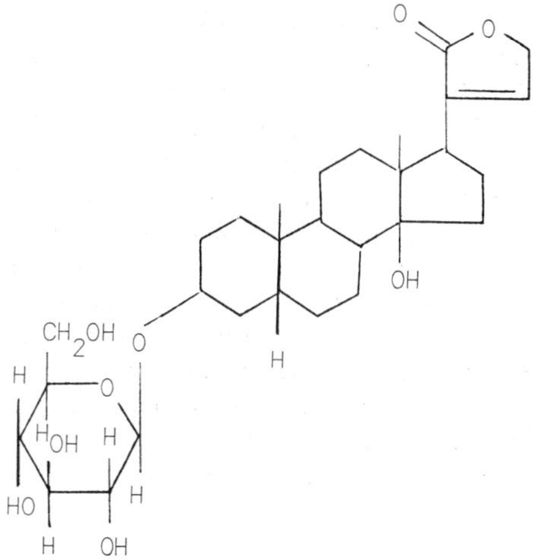

(14)

has an ultrashort cardiotonic onset and duration of action in dogs [125,126] and a therapeutically useful effect in patients with atrial arrhythmias [127]. This drug was chosen from a series of compounds in which the steroid nucleus is attached α to the carboxyl function in the lactone (15) rather than β to the carboxyl function (16) as in the natural glycosides. The structure of actodigin is the same as that of digitoxin except for the sugar moiety (a monoglucose rather than a tridigitoxose) and the aforementioned attachment of the steroid nucleus to the α-carbon of the lactone. The synthesis of actodigin and other semisynthetic cardenolides and related compounds has been described by Ferland et al. [128], Deghenghi [129], and Ferland [130]. On the basis of a variety of in vitro and in vivo pharmacologic experiments, actodigin appears to be significantly less arrhythmogenic than equiinotropic concentrations or doses of ouabain, acetylstrophanthidin, digitoxin, and other digitalis glycosides [125,126,131,132].

(15)   (16)

VI.   IMPLANTABLE PACEMAKERS
AND DEFIBRILLATORS

Within the last decade the use of cardiac pacemakers has evolved into the principal means of managing patients with Adams-Stokes seizures, other acute or chronic bradycardia, some types of supraventricular tachycardia with or without the Wolff-Parkinson-White syndrome, and ventricular arrhythmias unresponsive to antiarrhythmic drug therapy [133-136]. The growing importance of cardiac pacing is indicated by its increasing usage. Parsonnet [137] reported that over 70,000 patients throughout the world have pacemakers implanted, and that 15,000 are inserted yearly in North America. A more recent and generous estimate is that there are 100,000 pacemakers in patients in the United States alone [138].

The development of newer and better fixed-rate and demand pacemakers by the medical electronic industry in many ways resembles the development of newer and better antiarrhythmic drugs by the pharmaceutical industry. Thus, efficacy is normally established in laboratory animals and confirmed in patients with cardiac irregularities; research is directed toward improving the product by correcting or minimizing existing untoward effects; and so on. Although not routinely established as with new antiarrhythmic drugs, chronic toxicologic and efficacy studies in one or more animal species are sometimes undertaken with new models of pacemakers, e.g., investigations in sheep and large dogs over a 4 to 20-month period on the effect of fixed-rate and ventricular synchronous pacers with regard to pulse threshold, repetition rate, pulse wave shape, ECG, and gross and histopathology [139]. Advances in the search for improved pacemakers include the development of pulse generators with greater reliability, longevity, and smaller size; the development of electrodes which can be implanted in the atrium or ventricle and are more fracture-proof and less likely to cause exit block; the development of more sophisticated electronic circuitry (e.g., ventricular-inhibited pacers); and improved protection of the pulse generator from moisture by better hermetical sealing [134, 140,141].

Implanted standby defibrillators represent an intriguing approach to the problem of sudden death in patients with coronary heart disease. Studies conducted by Mirowski et al. [142-144] in dogs and in man have shown that this device can reverse ventricular fibrillation at relatively low sources of energy. In this defibrillation system, the catheter electrodes were put into position transvenously. The distal electrode was wedged into the apex of the right ventricle and the proximal one was located in the superior vena cava. Changes in blood pressure indicative of either ventricular fibrillation or successful defibrillation served as the trigger for the device. The implanted countershock pulse generator was capable of delivering 5 to 20 W/sec of energy at variable pulse widths. At the present time, however, a number of technical and nontechnical problems must be overcome before implanted standby defibrillators become a widely acceptable means of preventing fatal ventricular fibrillation in patients with heart disease [145].

VII. INTRODUCTION OF ANTIARRHYTHMIC DRUGS
      INTO CLINICAL PRACTICE

When the pharmacologic data on a new antiarrhythmic agent appear sufficiently promising, a decision to proceed toward a clinical trial is normally made. The sometimes rickety bridge between a lead compound and a marketed drug has been described in several recent reviews [146-150]. An affirmative decision to try to cross this bridge usually signals the participation of scientists in allied disciplines in the pharmaceutical house whose organic chemists and pharmacologists discovered the drug. For example, the chemist in the pilot plant assumes the responsibility for producing bulk quantities of acceptable purity, particle size, and cost; the pharmaceutical chemist and biochemist study the drug from the standpoint of stability,

formulation, metabolism, and in vitro and in vivo pharmacokinetics; and
the toxicologist assesses the acute and chronic toxicity of pyramiding pharmacologically excessive doses in two or more species of laboratory animals.
    In these preclinical phases of new drug development, emphasis is
placed on the outcome of the toxicologic investigation. Acute toxicity consists of the administration of single, increasingly larger dosages to different
species. Toxic signs occurring in the animals, the time in which they
appear, and the median lethal dose (LD50) are recorded. The length and
design of the subacute and chronic toxicity studies depend on various factors,
e.g., the intended route, frequency, and duration of administration to humans; the way the drug is metabolized in different species; and compliance
with regulatory guidelines. Before a drug can be marketed, chronic toxicity
studies must be conducted in two or more species for at least 12 months in
a nonrodent and at least 18 months in a rodent. However, in the beginning,
shorter term toxicity studies normally suffice for a cautious clinical trial
conducted by a qualified clinical pharmacologist in subjects or patients who
have given their informed consent. Included in the chronic toxicity study
are measurements at regular intervals of food consumption, body weight,
electrocardiogram, urinalysis, and hematological, renal, and hepatic function tests. At predetermined times, the animals are sacrificed and gross
and histopathological examinations are made. Potential carcinogenic and
teratological effects are also assessed under appropriate experimental conditions. In all of these chronic toxicity studies, three dose levels are normally used, namely, a low nontoxic dose which is greater than the amount
evoking a pharmacologic response and two to five times more than the
expected human dose, a high dose large enough to cause toxicity upon repeated administration, and an intermediate dose.
    Clinical investigations of a new antiarrhythmic drug are controlled by
laws administered by governmental regulatory agencies, e.g., the United
States Federal Food, Drug and Cosmetic Act of 1938 and the subsequent
Kefauver-Harris Amendments of 1962. The regulations and schedules which
must be followed in the United States, the composition of an IND (Notice of
Clinical Investigational Exemption for a New Drug), an NDA (New Drug
Application), and related matters, have been reviewed by Abrams [146].
Additional information on the intent, interpretation, and enforcement of
these regulations and those of other countries may be found in the Federal
Register [151], the FDA Papers [152], the Ethical Guidelines for Clinical
Investigators of the AMA [153], and the Declaration of Helsinki of the World
Medical Association [154].

VIII. OUTLINES FOR ANTIARRHYTHMIC
       DRUG PROGRAMS

In the search for clinically useful, novel antiarrhythmic drugs, there is no
one "correct" sequence for screening and no one "ideal" drug. All the

methods and treatments reviewed have deficiencies and limitations, and these should be recognized and weighed by the investigator working in this field. Some suggested outlines on methodologies which have appeared in the literature are as follows:

Search and Development of Antiarrhythmic Drugs

OUTLINE 1 [34]

I. Initial Step

    A. Determine maximum tolerated dose in normal, unanesthetized dogs

II. Step 2

    A. Measure antiarrhythmic effect at maximum tolerated dose

        1. Conscious dogs with multifocal ventricular arrhythmias the day after coronary ligation

III. Step 3

    A. Determine activity against atrial irregularities of those compounds with antiarrhythmic effects in Step 2 at doses <21 mg/kg, i.v.

        1. Arrhythmias produced in open-chest dogs by aconitine or crush + stimulation

IV. Step 4

    A. Same as in Step 3 with compounds active at doses >21 mg/kg, i.v.

OUTLINE 2 [42]

I. Initial Step

    A. Measure the maximum driving rate of isolated guinea pig atria

        1. Provides an estimate of the effect of compounds on the refractory period

II. Step 2

    A. Measure the effect on the duration of a dog's P wave of those compounds which lengthen the interval between stimuli (Step 1)

        1. Provides an estimate of the effect of compounds on conduction velocity

III. Step 3

    A. Determine activity of those compounds which slow conduction
(Step 2) against atrial arrhythmias induced by a transvenous electrode placed in the right atrium of dogs

OUTLINE 3 [155]

  I. Initial Step

    A. Implant either a 25-mg pellet of DCA subcutaneously into rats
and/or guinea pigs or a 10-mg pellet into mice. Exchange tap
water for 1% saline as the drinking fluid.

  II. Step 2

    A. In control experiments, inject dl-isoproterenol, 150 μg/kg, s.c.,
17 to 23 days later. Record ECG evidence of cardiac irregularities.

    B. Regarding antiarrhythmic screening, inject the test compound
subcutaneously 10 min before the administration of isoproterenol
and determine if the typical ventricular arrhythmias (including
VF) are prevented

OUTLINE 4 [36e]

  I. Initial Step

    A. Determine antiarrhythmic activity against atrial and ventricular
arrhythmias induced in rats by intravenous administration of
aconitine (40 μg/kg)

      1. Anesthetized rats (1 g/kg urethane, i.p.)

  II. Step 2

    A. Determine antiarrhythmic activity against electrically induced
atrial fibrillation and ventricular arrhythmias in anesthetized dogs

      1. Arrhythmias produced by means of electrodes attached to the
epicardial surface of the right atrium and ventricle. Following
placement, pneumothorax reduced and spontaneous respiration
restored

      2. Atrium and ventricle stimulated alternately

III. Step 3

    A. Determine antiarrhythmic activity against ventricular arrhythmias
induced in conscious rabbits by barium chloride

      1. Long-lasting cardiac irregularity caused by $BaCl_2$, 4 mg/kg, i.v.

ACKNOWLEDGMENT

The help of Dr. G. Beaulieu in the preparation of this manuscript is gratefully acknowledged.

REFERENCES

1. F. A. Williams and T. E. Keys, Mayo Clin. Proc. 17, 294 (1942).

2. K. F. Wenckebach, Die unregelmässige Herztätigkeit und ihre klinische
   Bedeutung, W. Engelman, Leipzig, 1914.

3. W. Frey, Wien. Klin. Wochenschr. 55, 849 (1918).

4. W. Withering, An Account of the Foxglove, M. Swinney, Birmingham,
   1785.

5. J. Mackenzie, Br. Med. J. 1, 587 (1905).

6. T. Lewis, Br. Med. J. 2, 621 (1919).

7. R. M. Green, English translation of L. Galvani's De viribus electrici-
   tatis in motu commentarius, Elizabeth Licht, Cambridge, Mass., 1953.

8. C. McC. Brooks, B. F. Hoffman, E. E. Suckling, and E. Orias,
   Excitability of the Heart, Grune & Stratton, New York, 1955: (a) p. 1;
   (b) p. 243; (c) p. 260.

9. C. J. Rothberger and H. Winterburg, Pfluegers Arch. Ges. Physiol.
   160, 42 (1914).

10. C. J. Wiggers, Am. J. Physiol. 20, 399 (1940).

11. C. J. Wiggers and R. Wegria, Am. J. Physiol. 131, 296 (1940).

12. R. M. Zoll, N. Engl. J. Med. 247, 768 (1952).

13. S. Furman and G. Robinson, Surg. Forum 9, 245 (1958).

14. G. K. Moe, Rev. Physiol. Biochem. Pharmacol. 72, 56 (1975).

15. B. F. Hoffman and P. F. Cranefield, Electrophysiology of the Heart,
    McGraw-Hill, New York, 1960, p. 323.

16. A. S. Harris, Am. Heart J. 71, 797 (1966).

17. N. Wiener and A. Rosenblueth, Arch. Inst. Cardiol. (Mexico) 16, 205
    (1946).

18. G. K. Moe, W. C. Rheinboldt, and J. A. Abildskov, Am. Heart J. 67,
    200 (1964).

19. A. Farah and T. A. Loomis, Circulation 2, 742 (1950).

20. B. B. Brown and G. H. Acheson, Circulation 6, 529 (1952).

21. C. Mendez and G. K. Moe, Circ. Res. 19, 378 (1966).

22. M. J. Janse, F. J. L. vanChappelle, G. E. Freud, and D. Durrer, Circ. Res. 28, 403 (1971).

23. A. L. Wit, B. N. Goldreyer, and A. N. Damato, Circulation 43, 862 (1971).

24. J. T. Bigger, Jr. and B. N. Goldreyer, Circulation 42, 673 (1970).

25. M. Prinzmetal, Circulation 7, 607 (1953).

26. A. L. Wit, B. F. Hoffman, and P. F. Cranefield, Circ. Res. 30, 1 (1972).

27. B. Sasyniuk and C. Mendez, Circ. Res. 28, 3 (1971).

28. P. L. Friedman, J. R. Stewart, J. J. Fenoglio, Jr., and A. L. Wit, Circ. Res. 33, 597 (1973).

29. P. L. Friedman, J. R. Stewart, and A. L. Wit, Circ. Res. 33, 612 (1973).

30. R. Lazzara, N. El-Sherif, and B. J. Scherlag, Circ. Res. 33, 722 (1973).

31. B. I. Sasyniuk and T. Kus, Pharmacologist 15, 178 (1973).

32. B. I. Sasyniuk and T. Kus, Fed. Proc. 33, 476 (1974).

33. B. I. Sasyniuk and R. I. Ogilvie, Annu. Rev. Pharmacol. 15, 131 (1975).

34. M. M. Winbury, Ann. N.Y. Acad. Sci. 64, 564 (1956).

35. L. L. Terry, Ann. N.Y. Acad. Sci. 64, 574 (1956).

36. L. Szekeres and J. Gy. Papp, Experimental Cardiac Arrhythmias and Antiarrhythmic Drugs, Akademiai Kiado, Budapest, 1971: (a) p. 25; (b) p. 62; (c) p. 59; (d) p. 146; (e) p. 58.

37. R. Wegria and N. D. Nickerson, Am. Heart J. 25, 56 (1943).

38. R. A. VanTyn and L. D. McLean, Am. J. Physiol. 201, 457 (1961).

39. F. J. Kniffen, T. E. Lomas, N. L. Nobel-Allen, and B. R. Lucchesi, Circulation 49, 264 (1974).

40. A. George, J. F. Spear, and E. N. Moore, Circulation 50, 353 (1974).

41. A. Rosenblueth and J. Garcia Ramos, Am. Heart J. 33, 677 (1947).

42. C. H. Ellis, Ann. N.Y. Acad. Sci. 64, 552 (1956).

43. G. S. Dawes, Br. J. Pharmacol. 1, 90 (1946).

44. L. Szekeres and E. M. Vaughan Williams, J. Physiol. (London) 160, 470 (1962).

45. J. Gy. Papp and E. M. Vaughan Williams, Br. J. Pharmacol. 37, 380 (1969).

46. C. M. Wang and R. A. Maxwell, Pharmacologist 16, 267 (1974).

47. C. Steiner, A. L. Wit, and A. N. Damato, Circ. Res. 24, 167 (1969).

48. I. Barr, T. W. Smith, M. D. Klein, F. Hagemeijer, and B. Lown, J. Pharmacol. Exp. Ther. 180, 710 (1972).

49. A. N. Damato, S. H. Lau, R. D. Patton, C. Steiner, and W. D. Berkowitz, Circulation 40, 71 (1969).

50. W. D. Berkowitz, A. L. Wit, S. H. Lare, C. Steiner, and A. N. Damato, Circulation 40, 855 (1969).

51. D. Scherf, Proc. Soc. Exp. Biol. 64, 233 (1947).

52. G. K. Moe and J. A. Abildskov, Am. Heart J. 58, 59 (1959).

53. J. Yelnosky and B. B. Clark, Br. J. Pharmacol. 15, 448 (1960).

54. K. Hashimoto and G. K. Moe, Circ. Res. 32, 618 (1973).

55. R. Mendez and E. Kabela, Annual Review of Pharmacology (H. W. Elliott, ed.), Palo Alto, 1970, p. 293.

56. D. Scherf, S. Blumenfeld, and M. Gildiz, Cardiologia (Basel) 43, 133 (1963).

57. L. H. Nahum and H. E. Hoff, Am. J. Physiol. 129, 428 (1940).

58. D. Scherf and F. B. Chick, Am. Heart J. 42, 212 (1951).

59. K. Nakayama, T. Oshima, S. Kumakura, and K. Hashimoto, Eur. J. Pharmacol. 14, 9 (1971).

60. L. Szekeres, Proc. 2nd Hungarian Conf. Therap. Pharmacol. Res. Akademiai Kiado, 1964, p. 165.

61. M. Fekete and J. Boisy, Med. Exp. (Basel) 10, 93 (1964).

62. B. B. Clark and J. R. Cummings, Ann. N.Y. Acad. Sci. 64, 543 (1956).

63. B. R. Lucchesi and R. Shivak, J. Pharmacol. Exp. Ther. 143, 366 (1964).

64. A. Sekiya and E. M. Vaughan Williams, Br. J. Pharmacol. 21, 462 (1963).

65. B. R. Lucchesi and H. F. Hardman, J. Pharmacol. Exp. Ther. 132, 372 (1961).

66. A. R. Laddu, P. Scully, M. J. Fahrenbach, and R. Z. Gussin, 26th Int. Congr. Physiol. Sci. (New Delhi) 11, 32 (1974).

150

J. R. CUMMINGS

67. E. T. Angelakos and M. L. Torchiana, Cardiac Arrhythmias (L. Dreifus and W. Likoff, eds.), Grune & Stratton, New York, 1973, p. 505.

68. M. L. Torchiana and C. A. Stone, Pharmacologist 12, 304 (1970).

69. M. L. Torchiana, C. A. Stone, H. C. Wenger, R. Evans, B. Lagerquist, and T. O'Mallery, J. Pharmacol. Exp. Ther. 194, 415 (1975).

70. A. G. Levy, Heart 4, 319 (1913).

71. W. J. Meek, H. R. Hathaway, and O. S. Orth, J. Pharmacol. Exp. Ther. 61, 299 (1937).

72. J. R. Cummings and H. W. Hays, Anesthesiology 17, 314 (1956).

73. R. L. Katz, R. S. Matteo, and E. M. Papper, Anesthesiology 23, 597 (1962).

74. J. W. Lawson, J. Pharmacol. Exp. Ther. 160, 22 (1968).

75. M. Hirata, Y. Oku, and K. Kikuchi, J. Takeda Res. Lab. 30, 589 (1971).

76. F. H. Smirk, J. Nolla-Panades, and T. Wallis, Am. J. Cardiol. 14, 79 (1964).

77. P. E. Leveque, Arch. Int. Pharmacodyn. Ther. 149, 297 (1964).

78. P. E. Leveque, Nature 207, 203 (1965).

79. A. S. Harris, Circulation 1, 1318 (1950).

80. M. M. Winbury and M. L. Hemmer, J. Pharmacol. Exp. Ther. 113, 402 (1955).

81. H. M. Mailing and N. C. Moran, Circ. Res. 5, 409 (1957).

82. N. C. Moran, J. I. Moore, H. K. Holcomb, and G. Mushet, J. Pharmacol. Exp. Ther. 136, 327 (1962).

83. T. Balzas, S. Ohtake, J. R. Cummings, and J. F. Nobel-Allen, Toxicol. Appl. Pharmacol. 15, 189 (1969).

84. D. R. Varma and K. I. Melville, Can. J. Biochem. 41, 511 (1963).

85. B. G. Covino and A. H. Hegnauer, Surgery 40, 475 (1956).

86. B. G. Covino, R. Wright, and D. A. Charleson, Am. J. Physiol. 181, 54 (1955).

87. E. T. Angelakos and A. H. Hegnauer, J. Pharmacol. Exp. Ther. 127, 137 (1960).

88. L. Szekeres, J. Mehes, and J. Gy. Papp, Br. J. Pharmacol. 17, 167 (1961).

89. J. L. Gilbert, G. G. Lange, and C. McC. Brooks, Circ. Res. 7, 417 (1959).

90. B. Levitt, S. J. Ehrreich, and J. Roberts, Pharmacologist 6, 166 (1964).

91. H. C. Stanton, T. Kirchgessner, and K. Parmenter, J. Pharmacol. Exp. Ther. 149, 174 (1965).

92. P. Somani, J. G. Fleming, G. K. Chan, and B. K. B. Lum, J. Pharmacol. Exp. Ther. 151, 32 (1966).

93. P. Somani and B. K. B. Lum, J. Pharmacol. Exp. Ther. 147, 194 (1965).

94. J. R. Schmid and C. Hanna, J. Pharmacol. Exp. Ther. 156, 331 (1967).

95. G. J. Kelliher and J. Roberts, Am. Heart J. 87, 458 (1974).

96. C. Raper and J. Wale, Eur. J. Pharmacol. 4, 1 (1968).

97. B. N. Benfey and D. R. Varma, Br. J. Pharmacol. 26, 3 (1966).

98. B. R. Lucchesi, L. S. Whitsit, and N. L. Brown, Can. J. Physiol. Pharmacol. 44, 543 (1966).

99. B. J. Koerpel and L. D. Davis, Circ. Res. 30, 681 (1972).

100. S. F. Seides, M. E. Josephson, W. P. Batsford, G. M. Weisfogel, S. H. Lau, and A. N. Damato, Circulation 48 (Suppl. IV), IV-7 (1973).

101. J. Proctor and A. J. Wasserman, Fed. Proc. 26, 401 (1967).

102. B. R. Madan and R. S. Gupta, Arch. Int. Pharmacodyn. 178, 43 (1969).

103. B. N. Singh and E. M. Vaughan Williams, Br. J. Pharmacol. 38, 749 (1970).

104. E. M. Vaughan Williams and J. Gy. Papp, Postgrad. Med. J. 46, Suppl. 22 (1970).

105. K. Saameli, Helv. Physiol. Pharmacol. Acta 25, CR-432 (1967).

106. J. F. Giudicelli, H. Schmitt, and J. R. Boissier, J. Pharmacol. Exp. Ther. 168, 116 (1969).

107. G. E. Moore and S. R. O'Donnel, J. Pharm. Pharmacol. 22, 180 (1970).

108. A. R. Laddu and P. Somani, J. Toxicol. Appl. Pharmacol. 15, 287 (1969).

109. R. D. Robson and H. R. Kaplan, J. Pharmacol. Exp. Ther. 175, 157 (1970).

110. H. R. Kaplan and R. D. Robson, J. Pharmacol. Exp. Ther. 175, 168 (1970).

111. D. Dunlop and R. G. Shanks, Br. J. Pharmacol. 32, 201 (1968).

112. J. P. VanDurme, L. Bossaert, P. Verneire, and R. Pannier, Am. Heart J. 86, 284 (1973).

113. T. Baum, G. Rowles, and A. T. Shropshire, J. Pharmacol. Exp. Ther. 176, 350 (1971).

114. H. W. VonKlempt and F. Bender, Arzneim. Forsch. 23, 1064 (1973).

115. D. P. Schuster, B. R. Lucchesi, N. L. Nobel-Allen, M. N. Mimnaugh, R. E. Counsell, and F. J. Kniffen, J. Pharmacol. Exp. Ther. 184, 213 (1973).

116. V. Lanzoni and B. B. Clark, Circ. Res. 3, 335 (1955).

117. I. M. Glynn and A. E. Warner, Br. J. Pharmacol. 44, 271 (1972).

118. E. O. Theilen, D. L. Warkentin, and L. E. January, Prog. Cardiovasc. Dis. 7, 261 (1964).

119. B. Lown, F. Hagemeijer, I. Barr, and M. Klin, Basic and Clinical Pharmacology of Digitalis (B. H. Marks and A. M. Weissler, eds.), Thomas, Springfield, Illinois, 1972, p. 299.

120. K. K. Chen and R. C. Anderson, J. Pharmacol. Exp. Ther. 90, 271 (1947).

121. L. F. Fieser and M. Fieser, Steroids, Van Nostrand-Reinhold, Princeton, New Jersey, 1959, p. 727.

122. G. K. Moe and A. E. Farah, Pharmacological Basis of Therapeutics (L. S. Goodman and A. Gilman, eds.), 4th ed., Macmillan, New York, 1970, p. 678.

123. R. Thomas, J. Boutagy, and A. Gelbart, J. Pharmacol. Exp. Ther. 191, 219 (1974).

124. R. Thomas, J. Boutagy, and A. Gelbart, J. Pharm. Sci. 63, 1649 (1974).

125. G. Beaulieu, I. Vavra, and J. R. Cummings, Pharmacologist 16, 245 (1974).

126. R. Mendez, G. Pastelin, and E. Kabela, J. Pharmacol. Exp. Ther. 188, 189 (1974).

127. R. Bojorges, M. Cardenas, G. Pastelin, and R. Mendez, Arch. Inst. Cardiol. (Mexico) 44, 615 (1974).

128. J. M. Ferland, Y. Lefebvre, R. Deghenghi, and K. Wiesner, Tetrahedron Lett. 30, 3617 (1966).

129. R. Deghenghi, Pure Appl. Chem. 21, 153 (1970).

130. J. M. Ferland, Can. J. Chem. 52, 1652 (1974).

131. G. Pastelin and R. Mendez, Eur. J. Pharmacol. 19, 291 (1972).

132. J. I. Gliklich, R. Gaffney, M. R. Rosen, and B. J. Hoffman, Eur. J. Clin. Pharmacol. 32, 1 (1975).

133. H. B. Burchall, D. C. Connolly, and F. H. Ellis, Am. J. Med. 37, 764 (1964).

134. S. Furman and D. J. W. Escher, Principals and Techniques of Cardiac Pacing, Harper & Row, New York, 1970, p. 183.

135. A. J. Moss and R. J. Rivers, Circulation 50, 942 (1974).

136. R. A. Johnson, A. M. Hutter, R. W. Desanctis, P. M. Yurchak, R. C. Leinbach, and J. W. Harthorne, Ann. Intern. Med. 80, 380 (1974).

137. V. Parsonnet, Chest 61, 165 (1972).

138. W. H. Fleming and J. C. Toler, Circulation 50, 111, 226 (1974).

139. J. R. Cummings, R. Gelok, J. L. Grace, and A. J. Salkind, J. Thorac. Cardiovasc. Surg. 66, 645 (1973).

140. K. E. Wright and H. D. McIntosh, Circulation 47, 1108 (1973).

141. D. J. W. Escher, Circulation 47, 1119 (1973).

142. M. Mirowski, M. M. Mower, W. S. Staewen, B. Tabatzik, and A. I. Mendleloff, Arch. Intern. Med. 126, 158 (1970).

143. M. Mirowski, M. M. Mower, W. S. Staewen, R. H. Denniston, and A. I. Mendleloff, Arch. Intern. Med. 129, 773 (1972).

144. M. Mirowski, M. M. Mower, V. L. Gott, and R. K. Brawley, Circulation 47, 79 (1973).

145. B. Lown and P. Axelrod, Circulation 46, 637 (1972).

146. W. B. Abrams, Anesthesiology 35, 176 (1971).

147. L. Lasagna, Am. J. Med. Sci. 263, 8 (1972).

148. M. Tishler, Clin. Pharmacol. Ther. 14, 479 (1973).

149. P. deHaen, Clin. Pharmacol. Ther. 16, 413 (1974).

150. C. J. Cavallito, Drug Develop. Comm. 1, 259 (1975).

151. Federal Register, May 8, 1970; Nov. 19, 1976.

152. W. J. Gyarfas and A. Welch, F.D.A. Papers 3, 27 (1969).

153. Human Experimentation, Code of Ethics of the World Medical Association, Br. Med. J. 2, 177 (1964).

154. AMA Endorsed Declaration of Helsinki, JAMA 197(3), 18; (11), 31 (1966).

155. G. Guideri, M. Barletta, R. Chou, M. Green, and D. Lehr, Recent Advances in Studies on Cardiac Structure and Metabolism (P.-E. Roy and G. Rona, eds.), Vol. 10, Univ. Park Press, Baltimore, 1975, p. 661.

Chapter 6

MAJOR TRANQUILIZERS

William H. Funderburk and David N. Johnson

A. H. Robins Company
Richmond, Virginia

I. INTRODUCTION

Schizophrenia, one of the oldest disorders of the mind, has fascinated physicians and philosophers for hundreds of years. Although it is so widespread that everyone is familiar with the symptoms of this disorder, its diagnosis is not clearly defined, a situation that remains a source of embarrassment for psychiatrists. For years patients suffering from schizophrenia were managed only with custodial care until it was found that hot baths relaxed some disturbed patients, and subsequently such baths were used frequently for the unruly. Sedatives (paraldehyde, bromides, barbiturates, and others) were used to quiet the back wards of state hospitals but they were of no value in the treatment of the basic disorder.

In the 1930s, after centuries without real progress, there occurred certain events which appeared to herald the achievement of some success in the treatment of schizophrenia. After observing that an accidental overdose of insulin to a diabetic drug addict appeared to clear up the patient's confused mental state, Sakel [1] reported treating schizophrenia with insulin-induced hypoglycemic coma. This treatment was so difficult to manage and required so much nursing care that it was usually reserved for young and acutely ill patients. It did appear to be effective in some patients, many of whom were released from the hospitals, although eventually they did return for further treatment.

Meduna introduced a form of convulsive therapy produced by pentylenetetrazol in 1935, although camphor-induced convulsions had been used for the treatment of schizophrenia many years earlier. These chemically induced seizures were replaced with electroconvulsive therapy shortly after its introduction by Cerletti and Bini in 1938 [2]. So skillful were some in the use of this new therapy that straitjackets and padded cells could be abandoned in the management of patients.

Other forms of treatment were constantly being introduced, and each had their champions. Modified electrostimulation techniques were tried, both nonconvulsive [3] and electronarcosis [4]. In 1935, Fulton and Jacobsen [5] found that monkeys with frontal lobe extirpations appeared to suffer no impairment of memory or intelligence and remained calm when frustrated. Application of this finding to schizophrenic patients did not become popular until 1950 when Freeman and Watts [6] perfected the lobotomy technique.

Carbon dioxide therapy was actually used by Loevenhart et al. [7] before insulin coma was introduced. It is also of interest to note that this treatment was used after the discovery that sodium cyanide, which was first used to stimulate respiration in hypoventilated mental patients, was beneficial in the treatment of mental illness. Carbon dioxide was not extensively used until Meduna [8] gave it wide publicity in the early 1950s.

One after another these therapies were discarded as being of little value and only electroconvulsive and insulin therapy continued to be used throughout the years. During all the time that physical means of treating schizophrenia were being used, another school of psychiatrists was hard at work trying to treat this disorder with psychotherapy. Many claimed success but the populations in mental hospitals continued to rise.

By 1952 some advances had been made; the hospitals were quieter and the patients were more comfortable with their illness. Large research units were hard at work in an effort to learn how to treat schizophrenia and most felt a major breakthrough was imminent. In that year, on May 26, a paper was presented at the centenary meeting of the Societe Medico-Psychologique in Paris by Delay, Deniker, and Hard. It was entitled "The Therapeutic Use of a Phenothiazine with Selective Central Action (RP4560)." This drug, chlorpromazine, had been used by Laborit et al. [9] to help produce a kind of hibernation in high-risk surgery patients, and they encouraged Delay and his coworkers to try it in schizophrenic patients [10]. As with many new psychotherapeutic discoveries, serendipity played a major role in chlorpromazine's introduction into the field of mental disease.

About the same time, Bein [11] reported that reserpine, long used as a hypotensive agent, had sedative action, and a year later Kline [12] confirmed the tranquilizing effect of this drug.

Many other phenothiazines followed the introduction of chlorpromazine, and some appeared to be more efficacious. Certain types, or certain symptoms, of schizophrenia appeared to respond better to some of these drugs than to others. This concept was held for a long time by many investigators but Hollister and coworkers [13] have recently indicated that it is not experimentally supportable.

To date, hundreds of phenothiazine derivatives have been synthesized and tested in laboratory animals. Of these, well over 100 have reached the clinical phase of drug development and over 40 are currently available in the United States and Europe.

No new types of drugs for the treatment of schizophrenia were introduced until Divry and colleagues [14] found that a butyrophenone, haloperidol, was effective. Similar drugs were synthesized and trifluperidol was widely studied, but only haloperidol and the short-acting droperidol are available in this country at the present time. Others are being studied in the clinic and may be available soon. One, lenperone, appears somewhat less potent than haloperidol and may be less likely to produce extrapyramidal signs at therapeutic doses [15,16].

Chemical modifications of these available major tranquilizers have resulted in other clinically effective drugs. Chlorprothixene [17] and thiothixene [18], both 4-phenylbutylamines, have been available for a number of years and clopenthixol and flupenthixol are under clinical investigation. Newer still is the dihydroindolone, molindone [19], and the dibenzoheteroazepines, loxapine [20], metiapine [21], and clozapine [22]. Clozapine, in particular, is claimed to cause little or no extrapyramidal activity. The French compound, sulpiride, is currently undergoing clinical trials in this country and abroad [23].

Of particular interest in recent years is the introduction of long-acting major tranquilizers which provide a duration of action of from 1 to 8 weeks. Injectable fat-soluble decanoate and enanthate salts of fluphenazine [24] are available and the palmitic ester, pipothiazine palmitate [25], is under investigation. Also under clinical investigation is the orally active penfluridol which has elicited antischizophrenic effects for 1 week following a single dose [26].

In the United States, the phenothiazine class of major tranquilizers accounts for approximately 90% of the prescriptions written, and haloperidol and thiothixene or chlorprothixene are responsible for an additional 6 and 2%, respectively. The remaining prescriptions are for lithium carbonate which is not a major tranquilizer but is used in the treatment of mania.

The introduction of chemotherapy for schizophrenia has already been quite beneficial. In the years since chlorpromazine was introduced, hospital populations are down sharply, many patients have been helped to lead productive lives, and many millions of dollars have been saved. Yet, many patients do not respond to our best drugs, for we do not understand the etiology of the disorder. As Hollister [13] has said, we have many patients who are improved but still too few who are cured. Much progress has been made since 1952. Many investigators are still at work in large laboratories, and there is a feeling that a major breakthrough is not far off. Our attitude has not changed much in the intervening years.

II. METHODOLOGY

With the discovery that chlorpromazine was an effective major tranquilizer, pharmacologists began to study its actions in animals and a number of methods were quickly developed for the identification of other, similar drugs [27-29]. This was not difficult once the prototype became available. Each investigator had his favorite tests and perhaps most were good ones. With use, these tests were sifted and the better ones were used by more and more investigators. It was quickly realized that these methods would only identify similar drugs with the same type of actions, a fact that still holds. Pimozide, sulpiride, and clozapine have shown that the original methods must be altered and new ones sought.

There is still some disagreement on tests that must be carried out to evaluate major tranquilizers, but in general routine tests are well known. It is accepted by most investigators that major tranquilizers should have the following properties:

1. Inhibit amphetamine toxicity in grouped mice.

2. Suppress fighting behavior in mice.

3. Inhibit amphetamine- or apomorphine-induced stereotypic behavior.

4. Reduce apomorphine-induced emesis.

5. Suppress conditioned avoidance behavior.

6. Reduce exploratory behavior without undue sedation.

7. Induce a cataleptic state.

8. Induce palpebral ptosis.

9. Decrease body temperature.

10. Block norepinephrine lethality.

11. Induce dopaminergic receptor blockade.

12. Inhibit arousal.

13. Block self-stimulation in the reward area.

All drugs that satisfy these criteria are not major tranquilizers because many compounds have been studied in patients and found to be ineffective as antipsychotic agents. Ethomoxane, developed many years ago, is a notable example. This drug was a very potent inhibitor of conditioned avoidance behavior, and satisfied all criteria established at that time for a major tranquilizer. When evaluated in the clinic, however, it was found to have no antipsychotic activity. It is for this reason that several tests are usually used before such drugs are tested in man. These tests are also included in this discussion. Many tests other than those described herein have been developed and used in various laboratories from time to time, but they have not withstood the test of time or appear to add little, or nothing, to the more widely used procedures.

A. Suppression of d-Amphetamine Lethality

Gunn and Gurd [30] and Chance [31] pointed out a differential lethality of amphetamine in isolated and aggregated mice. More recently, Lasagna and McCann [32] and Burn and Hobbs [29] found that chlorpromazine and reserpine prevented amphetamine-induced lethality in the aggregated animals, whereas in isolated mice, the LD50 values of amphetamine were not altered by either of these major tranquilizers. Indeed, these observations so impressed Burn and Hobbs that they titled their paper "A Test for Tranquilizing Drugs."

Although major tranquilizers are screened in aggregated mice, other compounds which affect the sympathetic nervous system have also been reported to give positive results. Phenoxybenzamine [33], guanethidine [34], α-methyl dopa, and α-methyl-m-tyrosine [35] have all been reported to afford protection. Various other compounds have been tested with essentially negative results [36].

In this test, d-amphetamine was given in geometrically spaced doses to groups of 10 mice. Each group of animals was placed in a separate wire mesh cage (6 × 10 × 4 in.) which was elevated by 2-in. legs to allow free air circulation. Thus, each animal was afforded 6-in.^{2} of floor space.

The effects of d-amphetamine (5-44 mg/kg, i.p.) were readily visible. Physiological effects included salivation, pilo-erection, vocalization, and marked increases in aggressiveness and spontaneous motor activity. Within a few hours most animals lay exhausted in the cage, although aggressive interactions still occurred. Lethality usually occurred within 2 to 8 hr, although the animals were left undisturbed for 24 hr after amphetamine administration.

From these data, the LD90 was calculated using probit analysis [37]. In all subsequent studies, the LD90 dose (21 mg/kg, i.p.) was administered to groups of 10 mice at predetermined intervals after administration of the test compound. Positive controls, run at the same time, were given saline plus d-amphetamine at the LD90 level.

Protective ED50 values were calculated using the method of Litchfield and Wilcoxon [37] and defined as that dose which prevented 50% of the mice from succumbing to the effects of d-amphetamine.

Effects of a phenothiazine, butyrophenone, and diphenylbutyl-amine given 60 min prior to d-amphetamine are shown in Table 1. All major tranquilizers are active in this test in doses below those which produce marked motor impairment. Furthermore, the test does not give false positives for sedatives or antianxiety agents in reasonable doses.

Control of environmental factors is known to be an important consideration in conducting this experiment. Clark and coworkers [38] reported the effects of amphetamine on rectal temperatures in aggregated and isolated mice. In all studies it was observed that mice with body temperatures below 40°C survived and those with temperatures above 40.6°C usually succumbed. Experience has shown that ambient temperatures of 20 to 21°C, with a relative humidity of 70 to 80%, give consistent results.

TABLE 1 Protection of d-Amphetamine-Induced Lethality in Mice under Aggregated Conditions

Drug	Protective ED50 (95% confidence limits; mg/kg, i.p.)
Chlorpromazine	0.30 (0.16-0.48)
Haloperidol	0.10 (0.05-0.20)
Penfluridol	1.28 (0.90-1.91)
Pentobarbital	No protection up to 20 mg/kg, i.p.
Chlordiazepoxide	No protection up to 30 mg/kg, i.p.

Other environmental factors that have been reported to influence the LD50 of d-amphetamine in aggregated mice include noise [31] and light intensity [39]. In our studies, lights are left on the entire 24 hr after d-amphetamine administration and the animals are not subjected to loud or sudden noise.

B. Inhibition of Fighting Behavior

In 1959, Yen et al. [40] reported that major tranquilizers were capable of suppressing isolation-induced aggression in mice. Further studies by Janssen and coworkers [41] and Scriabine and Blake [42] improved on the methodology but large numbers of animals were still needed. DaVanzo and coauthors [43] added aversive stimuli to the period of isolation and found that the number of reliable fighters was markedly increased. Other differences in producing reliable fighters reported by the latter investigators were strain differences (C57 B1/10J mice were more sensitive than ICR-DUB mice), seasonal variations (fewer fighters in the summer months than during the rest of the year), and, of course, length of isolation.

Methods involved the isolating of mice for 21 days in 4 × 5 × 9-in. solid-walled cages such that the animals did not have visual contact with each other. After the 21-day period of isolation, the animals were individually exposed to several forms of aversive stimuli. They were gently prodded on the hindquarters with long forceps and their tails were pinched. After 5 min of aversive stimuli, a nonisolated "intruder" mouse was placed in the home cage of the isolated animal. The two mice were allowed to remain together for 5 min, or until the isolated animal attacked the intruder. Only animals which consistently attacked were used in subsequent drug studies.

For these studies, test compounds were administered in geometrically spaced doses to groups of five isolated mice, and the incidence of attack directed toward an intruder was determined at preselected intervals (0.5, 1, 2, and 4 hr) thereafter. Protective ED50 values were calculated and defined as the dose which blocked 50% of the isolated mice from attacking at the time of peak effect. Results from the studies of DaVanzo et al. [43] are shown in Table 2.

TABLE 2   Drug Effects on Isolation-Induced Aggression in Mice

Drug	Protective ED50 (mg/kg, i.p.)
Chlorpromazine	1.54
Fluphenazine	1.66
Reserpine	No protection in doses below those that produce neurotoxicity

While Yen and coworkers [40] claimed this test to be specific for major tranquilizers, DaVanzo reported various antidepressants, antihistamines,
anticonvulsants, analgesics, and autonomic agents to be effective. Barnett
et al. [44] also reported protection with anticholinergic agents, but suppression of isolation-induced aggression was not correlated with antihistamine
or antitetrabenazine activity.

C. Inhibition of Stereotypy

Amphetamine-induced stereotypy is believed to be due to central stimulation of dopamine receptors [45]. Although the precise anatomical areas are
unknown, most investigators feel that the nigrostriatal pathway is involved
[46]. Specific behavioral alterations produced by amphetamine are dose
related, but most investigators report continuous sniffing, licking, or biting,
with compulsive gnawing in rats. Cats make continuous head movements
as if looking around, whereas monkeys continuously repeat simple behavioral patterns [47].

      With the exception of reserpine [48], all major tranquilizers block
amphetamine-induced stereotypy in rats [49]. The methods reported by
Randrup and Munkvad [50] and Costall and Naylor [51] are frequently used.
In the latter technique, an arbitrary scoring system was adopted over a
30-sec observation period 0.25, 0.5, 1, 1.5, 2, 3, and 4 hr after administration of d- or l-amphetamine.

      In this method, a score of "zero" was assigned to drug-treated mice
whose behavior did not differ from that of saline-treated animals. Discontinuous sniffing with some locomotor activity in the animals resulted in a
score of 1; behavior consisting of continuous sniffing, some head movement,
and periodic locomotor activity was scored as 2. An animal with a stereotypic score of 3 appeared similar to an animal with a 2, but discontinuous
biting or chewing was also seen. Continuous gnawing, biting, or licking
with no locomotor activity resulted in a score of 4.

      Using this technique, minimal stereotypy (score = 1) was observed
after 1.25 mg/kg, i.p., of d-amphetamine with maximal stereotypy
(score = 4) observed after 5 mg/kg, i.p. Drug effects in reducing the
mean stereotypy score by 50% were determined when 5 mg/kg, i.p., of
d-amphetamine was given.

      In the method of Randrup and Munkvad [50] 3 mg/kg, s.c., of
d-amphetamine was used. Episodes of grooming behavior were counted,
in addition to stereotyped sniffing and locomotor activity. These authors
reported a marked increase in grooming behavior after perphenazine
(0.03 mg/kg, s.c.) plus d-amphetamine while the normal stereotyped behavioral patterns were abolished.

D. Blockade of Apomorphine-Induced Emesis

Since the realization that all major tranquilizers are potent antiemetic agents, various methods have been developed to determine this activity for unknown compounds. Most methodology is concerned with stimulating the chemoreceptive trigger zone [52] by pharmacological means and determining the incidence of vomiting. Most widely used of the pharmacologic agents is apomorphine, described in an early study by Chen and Ensor [53]. Other agents used include morphine [54], digitalis [55], emetine [56], and copper sulfate. Most studies are performed in dogs, although cats and monkeys have also been used.

"All or none" techniques were described by Niemegeers [57] for the effects of apomorphine in dogs. In this technique adult mongrel dogs, fasted for 12 to 18 hr, were fed a standard diet 1 to 2 hr prior to apomorphine administration (0.31 mg/kg, s.c.). The percentage of animals totally protected from vomiting was used to calculate the protective dose 50% (PD50) at preselected time intervals after administration of test compounds.

In other methods a quantal technique was employed whereby the dose necessary to suppress the number of episodes of vomiting by 50% was determined [58]. A minimum of three dogs was used at each of four or more geometrically spaced doses. Using the all-or-none method, the data listed in Table 3 were determined at the time of peak effect [59].

E. Inhibition of Conditioned Avoidance Behavior

One of the early findings for identifying major tranquilizers reported by Courvoisier and her coworkers [27] was that chlorpromazine suppressed avoidance response in rats but did not impair escape behavior.

TABLE 3 Antiapomorphine Activity in Dogs

Drug	Time of peak effect (hr)	ED50
Chlorpromazine	0.75	0.64 (mg/kg, s.c.)
Thioridazine	3	3.34 (mg/kg, s.c.)
Haloperidol	0.5	0.19 (μg/kg, s.c.)

TABLE 4   Drug Effects on Learned Behavior in Mice (N = 4)

Drug	Dose (mg/kg, i.p.)	Mean % correct avoidance response						
		0	15	30	60	90	120	180 (min)
Chlorpromazine	5	100	77	35	17	25	30	92
Haloperidol	1	93	83	34	15	13	20	5
Chlordiazepoxide	25	100	100	100	100	100	—	—
Pentobarbital	10	96	98	100	98	100	—	—

In contrast to the effects of major tranquilizers, sedative agents are not selective in that both avoidance and escape behavior are blocked. This effect occurs only at large doses which produce marked impairment of coordination and spontaneous motor activity.

Although most studies are performed in rodents because of the ease in handling and low cost of these animals, other studies have been performed in cats and dogs [60,61] and monkeys [62]. Methodology has been expanded to include shuttle box procedures [63], lever pressing methods [64], various types of discriminating behavior situations [65], and others.

One fairly simple conditioned avoidance apparatus which has been used successfully was reported by McKean and Pearl [66]. An electrically activated solenoid pushed a mouse off an elevated platform onto a grid floor. Five seconds later the grid became electrified (400 Hz, 1 mA, 0.4 msec pulse width) and the animal escaped the shock by climbing back onto the platform. Naive mice, placed in the apparatus for approximately 25 trials three or four times each day, quickly learned to escape the shock, and within 5 days were avoiding the shock 95 to 100% of the time. Effects of major tranquilizers in suppressing conditioned avoidance responding in mice are shown in Table 4 [67].

F.   Blockade of Exploratory Behavior

It is well known that major tranquilizers decrease exploratory behavior and locomotion in laboratory animals. The methods used to quantitate these data are concerned either with suppression of exploration in a novel environment or with blockade of locomotor activity. Janssen and coworkers [68] reported that haloperidol, in doses of 0.04 mg/kg, s.c., and higher, decreased exploratory behavior in rats; rearing and defecation were suppressed by 0.08 and 2.5 mg/kg, s.c., respectively. The technique involved placing a naive male Wistar rat (200–250 g) in the center of an "open field arena." Dimensions of the field were 100 cm in diameter and 50 cm high with the black floor equally divided into six sections by painted gray lines. The number of lines crossed (ambulation score) during a 3-min observation

TABLE 5   Drug Effects on Exploratory Behavior in Rats 30 min after Drug Administration

Drug	Dose (mg/kg, s.c.)	Mean score		
		Ambulation	Rearing	Defecation
Saline	—	26.7	5.8	1.4
Chlorpromazine	1.25	19.7	8.9	1.1
	2.5	14.5^a	5.0	0.95
	5	11.1^a	3.3^a	0.10^a
Haloperidol	0.02	22.6	6.3	1.2
	0.04	11.8^a	4.3	1.8
	0.08	8.7^a	2.3	1.6
	2.5	0.15^a	0.05^a	0.3^a

$^a p \leq 0.01$.

period was determined at 30-min intervals. In addition, the incidence of rearing during this time and the number of fecal boluses excreted were noted. Nonparametric statistical analyses of the mean numbers (five rats per dose level) are summarized in Table 5.

Tedeschi and coauthors [69] measured locomotion according to the method of Winter and Flataker [70] as modified by Cook et al. [28]. In this technique, mice were placed in individual photocell-counting chambers and the total number of counts recorded periodically. Using dose-response curves for drug-treated versus saline-treated mice, the dose which suppressed spontaneous motor activity (SMA) by 50% was determined. Tedeschi et al. [69] reported that chlorpromazine produced a significant decrease in SMA at 2.5 mg/kg, p.o., and trifluoperazine produced a similar effect at one-sixth the dose.

The distinguishing characteristic of the major tranquilizers, compared to sedative hypnotics, in suppression of locomotor activity is the relative lack of other behavioral signs at the dose which decreases SMA. That is, pentobarbital and phenobarbital produce decreased locomotor activity only at doses which produce obvious signs of neurotoxicity (ataxia, muscle weakness, etc.).

Other investigators have used more or less elaborate devices to measure locomotor activity. Boyd and Miller [71] used rats fasted for 3 days and measured activity wheel revolutions before and after chlorpromazine (0.5-2.5 mg/kg, p.o.). Marked suppression of running behavior was seen at all doses, with complete absence of activity at the highest dose tested.

Archer [72] studied the effects of chlorpromazine in a multiple T-maze and reported no effects at 0.5 mg/kg, s.c., but decreased running speed and, to a slight extent, less accuracy at higher doses.

G. Catalepsy

In the evaluation of new agents of potential utility for the treatment of psychoses and neuroses, the catalepsy test is used to determine the incidence of extrapyramidal side effects which might be expected in man. Some investigators believe this to be an indication of antipsychotic activity, speculating that the antipsychotic activity and extrapyramidal effects of these compounds are inseparable [73,74]. Others believe these properties are not necessarily interrelated [75].

The stages of catalepsy induced by phenothiazines were reported by Courvoisier and coworkers [76] with subsequent modifications suggested by Tedeschi and others [69]. The methods of Wirth et al. [77] and Janssen and coworkers [48] are other important contributions in this area.

In the method described by Wirth, one front foot of an adult rat is placed on a rubber stopper 3 cm high. Failure to correct the imposed posture within 10 sec is considered a positive cataleptic response and a score of 0.5 is assigned. After using both forepaws, the stopper is removed and each forepaw placed, in turn, on a 9-cm-high stopper. Failure to remove the paw from this stopper is assigned a score of 1. Using a scoring system for right and left forepaws, a catalepsy score of 0 (control rat) to 3 (maximal response) for each animal is obtained.

Catalepsy scores are determined at 0.5, 1, 1.5, 2, 3, and 6 hr after drug administration and ED50 values are calculated [37] and defined as the dose which produced one-half maximal response (mean score of 1.5). Using this method, the data given in Table 6 were determined [78].

H. Ptosis

Janssen [79] was among the first to recognize that major tranquilizers produce closure of the palpebral fissure (ptosis) in rats. Although the ptotic

TABLE 6   Calculated Cataleptic ED_{50} Values at Time of Peak Effect

Drug	ED50 (95% confidence limits; mg/kg, i.p.)
Haloperidol	5.1 (4.14-6.17)
Chlorpromazine	15.8 (12.6-19.7)

phenomena may be related to antipsychotic activity, a host of peripherally acting agents also produce this effect. The predominant peripheral mechanisms include sympathetic ganglionic blockade (hexamethonium), postganglionic, α-adrenergic blockade (phentolamine), and interference or depletion of sympathetic nerve transmitters (guanethidine, bretylium). Central mechanisms are less well understood but may be due to preganglionic inhibition of sympathetic outflow (chlorpromazine, reserpine).

Fujita and Tedeschi [80], using a technique which was an improvement of the method described by Janssen [79], reported that various centrally acting drugs produce ptosis in rats. In this procedure, the rat was given the test compound and left undisturbed for up to 4 hr. At predetermined intervals the degree of ptosis was determined before and 90 sec after exteroceptive stimulation. By briefly handling the animal, spontaneous ptosis was eliminated. Stimulation reversed the ptosis induced by centrally acting agents and this reversal continued for approximately 1 min. In contrast, peripheral agents which produced ptosis were generally nonreversible. The data in Table 7 show the relative potency of major tranquilizers in causing ptosis in rats [73].

I. Body Temperature

Courvoisier and her coworkers [27] reported that the subcutaneous administration of chlorpromazine lowered the body temperature of mice kept in an environment of 25° C. This effect has been noted for other major tranquilizers [81] and has been used extensively as a screening method.

Mice and rats are commonly used, although rabbits produce similar effects (see the review by Gordon [82]). Mice were used in the method of Lessin and Parkes [83], wherein each animal was individually housed and given free access to water. Chlorpromazine was given in geometrically spaced doses to groups of eight animals each, with control animals receiving an equal volume of saline. Rectal temperatures were ascertained at 0, 1,

TABLE 7   Effects of Drugs in Producing Ptosis in Rats

Drug	ED50 (mg/kg, p.o.)
Chlorpromazine	10.3
Haloperidol	0.5
Reserpine	0.5
Promazine	80.1

2, 3, 4, and 5 hr using an Ellab Model TE3 thermometer with the thermistor probe inserted 2 to 3 cm. Mean body temperatures were calculated and compared with the saline controls.

Results of chlorpromazine and reserpine on body temperature in mice are shown in Table 8 [83]. As pointed out by Lessin and Parkes [83] and emphasized by others [84], a number of other psychoactive agents lower body temperature in experimental animals. Bartholini et al. [84] reported a hypothermic effect in rats after diazepam administration which may have been related to the decrease in brain homovanillic acid (HVA) levels. However, HVA is increased after major tranquilizer administration and thus cannot be a contributing factor in the depression of body temperature.

J. Norepinephrine Antagonism

Prior to the suggestion that dopamine may be involved in the etiology of mental illness, it was believed that norepinephrine was somehow responsible for psychotic states. This was because of the peripheral α-adrenergic blocking effects which were seen after phenothiazine administration. Janssen et al. [48] reported that the results of this test correlate well with the action of various major tranquilizers in blocking norepinephrine-induced lethality in mice.

Rats were pretreated with test compound in geometrically spaced doses subcutaneously 1 hr prior to administration of a lethal dose (1.25 mg/kg, i.v.) of norepinephrine. The protective ED50 value was calculated by probit analysis [37] and compared with the protective ED50 value for the same test drug in blocking the compulsory gnawing or chewing movements induced by 10 mg/kg, i.v., of d-amphetamine.

The ratio (ED50, d-amphetamine test)/(ED50, norepinephrine test) was a measurement of the relative peripheral α-adrenergic blocking potency of the test compound. The effects of various butyrophenones and phenothiazines are shown in Table 9.

TABLE 8   Hypothermic Effects of Test Drugs in Mice

Drug	Dose (mg/kg, i.p.)	0	1	2	3	4	5 (hr)
		Mean rectal temperature (°C)					
Chlorpromazine	3	38.3	37.1	34.7	36.3	36.8	—
Chlorpromazine	5	38.3	32.3	28.7	28.3	29.1	29.7
Reserpine	1	38.2	37.7	37.1	—	35.3	—
Reserpine	1.5	38.2	37.7	35.9	—	32.4	—

TABLE 9   Relative Potency of Compounds

Drug	Protective ED50 (mg/kg, s.c.)		Ratio
	d-Amphetamine	Norepinephrine	
Haloperidol	0.03	2	1/70
Droperidol	0.03	0.1	1/3
Trifluoperazine	0.3	7	1/23
Chlorpromazine	1	0.5	2
Thioridazine	100	0.7	143
Promazine	30	0.7	43

Janssen concluded that the major tranquilizers fell into various groups, including

1. the haloperidol category (ratio = 1/3 to 1/100), which was practically devoid of peripheral adrenolytic effects at tranquilizing dose levels;

2. the chlorpromazine category (ratio = 2-6), which had moderate activity at tranquilizing dose levels;

3. the promazine category (ratio = 43-143), which exerted potent peripheral adrenolytic effects at tranquilizing doses.

Above this ratio, compounds did not possess major tranquilzing properties.

K. Caudate Mice

In 1966, Anden and coworkers [85] reported a method of unilateral lesioning of the corpus striatum in rats. This area, known to be rich in dopamine, is thought to be associated with the incidence of drug-induced catalepsy in animals and with the production of major tranquilizer-induced extrapyramidal side effects in man. Inhibition of dopamine in these rats is believed to produce postural asymmetries and pivoting toward the unoperated side (contralateral) and also to block body asymmetries and pivoting toward the operated side (ipsilateral) after treatment with apomorphine, a dopamine receptor stimulant [86]. Subsequent work by Ungerstedt [87] and Von Voigtlander and Moore [88] resulted in better techniques for lesioning of the striatum in rats using intracerebral administration of 6-hydroxydopamine in rats and mice.

Lotti [89] reported a simple technique for lesioning the caudate nuclei of mice by aspiration which did not require a stereotaxic apparatus, and hence a large number of animals could be prepared in 1 day. In this method, a 20-gauge hypodermic needle, filed to a 5-mm length, was placed through the skull two-thirds of the distance from the external auditory meatus to the corner of the eye and 1 mm lateral to the midline. Using a vacuum system, brain tissue was aspirated by rapidly raising and lowering the needle several times.

After 5 to 14 days recovery, each animal was given 2 mg/kg, i.p., of apomorphine and the presence or absence of body asymmetries and pivoting was determined during the next 30 min. In animals with successful unilateral lesions, apomorphine caused the mice to pivot continuously toward the side of the lesion and they could not be prodded to pivot in the other direction. In further drug studies, only those animals which pivoted consistently on each of three drug trials 1 day apart were used.

Major tranquilizers produced contralateral pivoting in mice with unilateral caudate lesions although the postural asymmetries were not as pronounced as those produced by dopamine stimulants. The endpoint for these studies may be either an all-or-none response or a quantal response. The data in Table 10 [67] were obtained by determining the number of animals with contralateral pivoting after major tranquilizer administration or the number of animals which did not show ipsilateral pivoting after administration of major tranquilizer plus apomorphine (2 mg/kg, i.p.).

Quantal data in rats have been determined by Ungerstedt and Arbuthnott [90] with 6-hydroxydopamine lesions in the nigrostriatal pathways, unilaterally. In this procedure, the rat, wearing a harness, was placed in a bowl and the number of pivots determined by a microswitch-counting device. The effects of d-amphetamine, a dopamine stimulant, were effectively abolished by the administration of haloperidol (1 mg/kg) or spiroperidol (0.1 mg/kg) within 30 min [87].

TABLE 10   Drug Effects on Pivoting in Mice with Unilateral Lesions of the Caudate Nuclei

Drug	ED50 (mg/kg, i.p.)	
	Contralateral pivoting	Blockade of apomorphine–induced ipsilateral pivoting
Chlorpromazine	1.3	4.1
Haloperidol	0.1	0.4

L. EEG Effects of Major Tranquilizers

A large number of publications have appeared concerning the effects of the
phenothiazines on spontaneous and evoked electrical activity from cortical
and subcortical areas in curarized or freely moving animals. Although
most work is done with cats, monkeys and rabbits are used in some laboratories. Early work with chlorpromazine was reported by Preston [91] who
proposed that the major site of action of this drug was in the amygdala.

The results of the studies of Killam and coworkers [92] on the limbic
pathways and on the reticular formation suggested that chlorpromazine
facilitated amygdaloid and hippocampal seizures, and to some extent suppressed cortical desynchronization induced by stimulation of the reticular
activating system. Ishikawa et al. [93] reported similar effects for chlorpromazine as well as reserpine using the hippocampal afterdischarge
technique.

Effects of the butyrophenones have not been studied as extensively,
yet Itil and Fink [94] stated that haloperidol produced EEG effects in man
similar to those produced by the phenothiazines. Janssen [95] believes
that the more potent tranquilizers, such as haloperidol, act primarily on
only a few highly localized centers of the midbrain whereas chlorpromazine
acts on a larger group of midbrain structures. Johnson and coworkers [15],
however, found that haloperidol but not chlorpromazine blocks afterdischarges in the amygdala and hippocampus.

Techniques for recording electrical activity from the cortex and from
subcortical areas of acutely prepared cats have been described in detail
by Oliver and Funderburk [96].

1. Spontaneous cortical activity

Adult mongrel cats (2.5-3.2 kg) of both sexes were anesthetized with ether,
and cannulae were inserted in the trachea for artificial ventilation and in a
femoral artery and a cephalic vein for blood pressure recording and drug
administration, respectively. The animal was placed in a stereotaxic
apparatus and stainless steel screws (0.25 in.) were placed bilaterally in
the exposed calvarium so that their tips rested on the dura over the sigmoid,
suprasylvian, and posterior lateral gyri. A screw of the same type was
placed in the bone over a frontal sinus and served as a common electrode.
Prior to removal of the anesthetic the cat was given 1 mg/kg, i.v., of
tubocurarine and artificial ventilation was instituted (10 ml air/kg every
3 sec). Wound edges and pressure points were infiltrated with procaine.
The animal was placed in a dimly lit, sound-attenuated, electrically shielded
cage in order to minimize the effects of external stimuli (noise, drafts, etc.).

After sufficient time for the effects of the anesthetic to dissipate
(minimum of 1 hr), monopolar tracings of spontaneous cortical activity

were recorded, along with arterial blood pressure and EKG (lead II) on an
EEG polygraph.

In most instances, EEG activity was recorded for 2 or 3 min every 10
min. When cumulative effects of increasing doses of a test compound were
desired, the drug was given in doses of 0.5, 1, 3, 5, 10, and 20 mg/kg,
i.v., at 20-min intervals.

Computer analysis of the EEG has been gaining popularity in recent
years. This method of automated EEG analysis consists of digitizing the
analog EEG signal and processing it on a digital computer. Several methods of numerical analyses have been developed for use on a digital computer.
Power spectrum analysis has been used by Schallek et al. [97] to investigate drug effects on the EEG. This technique transforms an EEG recording
into a single graph with power plotted against frequency [97,98]. Walter
[99] described several mathematical operations which can be performed on
the EEG tracing with a computer including the autospectrogram or power
spectrum analysis used by Schallek.

In power spectrum analysis, the phenothiazines produce an increase
in total power and the dominant frequency shifts to the slow components [98].
The butyrophenones have not been investigated as extensively in the power
spectral techniques, but subjective inspection of the records suggests that
the results are similar to those of the phenothiazines.

2. Cortical afterdischarge

After preparing the animal for recording cortical potentials, an additional
pair of electrodes approximately 1 mm apart was placed over the right
frontal area.

Stimulation of this area was accomplished using Grass equipment
(Model S4-E stimulator; Model SIU5 stimulus isolation unit; Model CCU1A
constant current unit) and the duration of stimulation was controlled by a
Hunter timer (Model 111B). The cortex was stimulated for 5 sec every 10
min with 60 Hz, 1-msec-duration pulses, and the intensity of stimulation
increased stepwise (beginning at 0.5 mA) until an afterdischarge of 5 to 10
sec was recorded on each of five consecutive trials. Drug administration
and recording techniques were as described previously.

3. Hippocampal afterdischarge

The cat was prepared as described previously for recording cortical activity except that a bur hole was drilled in the calvarium over the left suprasylvian gyrus. Stainless steel coaxial electrodes (David Kopf, Model NEX-
100) were stereotaxically implanted in the ventral hippocampus (F = 9.0 mm,
L = 7.0 mm, V = -6.0 mm) using the maps of Jasper and Ajmone Marsan
[100]. Using stimulating equipment already described, evoked responses

from the hippocampus (and occasionally from the cortex) were obtained with the following parameters of stimulation: 100 Hz, 5 msec pulse width for 5 sec every 10 min. The intensity of stimulation was adjusted so that the duration of hippocampal afterdischarge was consistently between 5 and 15 sec on each of five control trials. Changes in the duration of the after-discharges after drug administration or in the intensity of stimulation to produce a similar duration were determined.

4. Reticular activation

For this procedure, coaxial electrodes were implanted in the mesencephalic portion of the reticular activating system (F = 4.0 mm, L = 3.5 mm, V = 1.5 mm) using the atlas of Jasper and Ajmone Marsan [100]. Cortical electrodes were placed as described previously. Stimulation equipment and parameters were identical to those used for hippocampal afterdischarges. The intensity of stimulation was increased stepwise (beginning at 0.1 mA) until cortical desynchronization resulted, and outlasted the stimulation by at least 20 sec. Of utmost importance in this technique is to provide a quiet, isolated environment for the preparation to allow the normal slowing of the cortical waves to occur. Drug effects on the duration of the desynchroniza-tion are determined.

5. Thalamic recruitment

After preparing the cat with cortical electrodes as described previously, coaxial electrodes were placed in the nucleus reuniens near the middle of the thalamus (F = 11.0 mm, L = 0.5 mm, V = 0 mm) using the atlas of Jas-per and Ajmone Marsan [100]. Frequencies of 8 to 14 Hz and 1 msec pulse width were used every 10 min at threshold and supramaximal intensity of stimulation. Threshold was defined as the minimum stimulus intensity which resulted in recruiting responses from the cortex. With increasing intensities of stimulation, recruitment improved and then plateaued at the supramaximal intensity. Compounds are given as described previously, with changes in recruitment noted at both threshold and supramaximal inten-sities at 10-min intervals.

Using the procedures already described, certain characteristic changes were seen with chlorpromazine and haloperidol as indicated in Table 11 [15].

Following experiments in which subcortical electrodes were used, the animals were anesthetized and the site of the electrode was marked by passing a 3-mA direct current for 30 sec through the animal using the elec-trode as the anode and attaching the cathode to the body of the animal. This deposited iron in the brain and the Prussian blue technique was used to detect the iron [101]. This was done by perfusing the animal with a saturated solu-tion of potassium ferricyanide in 10% formaldehyde. The brain was removed

TABLE 11   Comparative Effects of Chlorpromazine and Haloperidol on
EEGs in Cats

	Chlorpromazine	Haloperidol
Spontaneous cortical activity	Depressed with convulsive-type discharges beginning in limbic system (amygdala) and spreading to cortex	Same
Cortical afterdischarge	Prolonged	Suppressed
Hippocampal afterdischarge	Prolonged	Suppressed
Reticular activation	Blocked	Blocked
Thalamic recruitment	Biphasic; improved with low doses, decreased with high doses	Same

and stored in formaldehyde. After 3 or 4 days the brain was sectioned to
verify electrode placement.

M. Self-Stimulation

Blockade of self-stimulation in laboratory animals by specific chemical entities has been used by some investigators as a useful tool in the study of
major tranquilizers. The pharmacology of this system was reviewed by
Stein [102], and more recently by Wauquier et al. [103-106].
        In general, parenteral administration of drugs with central adrenergic
effects will facilitate or suppress this type of behavior with the degree of
effect apparently related to the degree of adrenergic manipulation. Thus,
drugs which deplete brain monoamines (α-methyl-p-tyrosine) or which suppress adrenergic transmission (chlorpromazine, haloperidol) suppress
self-stimulation whereas central administration of norepinephrine facilitates
such behavior [107]. In contrast to the effects of major tranquilizers, pentobarbital and meprobamate are without effect in these procedures [108].
        The method of Olds and Olds [108] was used to implant a pair of silver
wires, 0.01 in. in diameter and insulated except for the cross section of
the tips, in the lateral hypothalamus of male albino rats (300-400 g). The
methodology for the standardization of the stereotaxic coordinates was
described by Olds and Olds [109], with the placement of the electrodes
described as 3 to 4 mm posterior, 1 mm lateral, and 8 mm deep in relation
to the bregma.

After sufficient time for recovery from surgery, the animals were trained to bar press for hypothalamic stimulation (60 Hz sine wave at an intensity of 40-60 μA for 250 msec).

Chlorpromazine, in doses of 1, 1.5, and 2 mg/kg, i.p., suppressed self-stimulation patterns in each of five implanted rats in a dose-dependent manner. Other psychoactive drugs tested were d-amphetamine (3 mg/kg, i.p.), meprobamate (100 mg/kg, i.p.), and LSD (0.20 mg/kg, i.p.), all of which were without consistent effect in altering response rates.

In contrast to these results, Van Rossum et al. [110] reported that self-stimulation was blocked by classes of drugs other than major tranquilizers. They reported that there was no striking correlation of inhibition of self-stimulation with tranquilizing activity, but rather with sleep-inducing activity.

III. SPECIFICITY OF ACTION

How sensitive and selective are these tests, and are all of them necessary? All of these tests are probably not needed, but they all add something to the profile of activity of any new major tranquilizer. Many of these tests are not specific for the action of major tranquilizers but, on the other hand, no single test will identify a major tranquilizer. In addition, some of these tests, if not most of them, are probably based on side effects of such drugs and are not related to their antipsychotic action.

The fighting mice test has been shown to be a nonspecific test for major tranquilizers since a large number of experimental compounds devoid of antipsychotic activity act positively in this test. In fact, Vinař and Kršiak [111] found no statistically significant correlations in tests using mice, and concluded that mice are not a good model for drugs to be used in man. Nevertheless, the antipsychotic phenothiazines and butyrophenones block fighting behavior in mice.

Inhibition of stereotyped movements and the hyperactivity produced by d-amphetamine are properties of major tranquilizers. These are very useful test procedures since they are sensitive and rather selective. However, there are some compounds that inhibit amphetamine that do not have antipsychotic activity. Phenothiazines and butyrophenones are potent antagonists of apomorphine-induced stereotyped behavior in rats and emesis in dogs but the latter is not specific since many drugs (antiemetics) block the effects of apomorphine in dogs but have no antipsychotic action.

All of the older major tranquilizers, at least, produce catalepsy if given in high enough doses, but there are drugs that produce this phenomenon which are not major tranquilizers, e.g., bulbocapnine. This is probably more closely correlated with the side effect, Parkinsonism, than to the antipsychotic actions of the drugs.

Blockade of exploratory behavior by major tranquilizers is said to be a sensitive and selective test [112]. Sedative drugs such as barbiturates and others will block this behavior, but major tranquilizers do this without producing sedation. Ptosis is produced by the well-known major tranquilizers. In order to be meaningful, the ptosis must be reversible when the animal is handled since the use of sedatives and adrenolytics produces ptosis that is not readily reversed. This test may also be associated with the extrapyramidal side effect because rats in which the caudate nucleus has been removed do not respond with ptosis when treated with major tranquilizers [110].

"Caudate mice" are used to evaluate dopamine blockade at the level of the caudate nucleus. All the major tranquilizers used in this test cause pivoting away from the lesion and block ipsilateral pivoting produced by apomorphine. This is a relatively new test, especially for use with major tranquilizers, and until recently was thought to be selective. However, this test too is probably related more to extrapyramidal side effects than to antipsychotic activity. In recent experiments, Muller and Seeman [113] found evidence that this model is not specific for drugs that directly block dopamine, and thus the results should be evaluated with caution.

Conditioned avoidance behavior is undoubtedly the most widely used test for major tranquilizers. The type of conditioned behavior does not appear to be of any significance since all types are blocked by major tranquilizers. It is unfortunate that several experimental compounds block this behavior but do not possess antipsychotic action.

The older major tranquilizers inhibit intracranial self-stimulation in the reward areas but this is not specific for this group of drugs since it appears to be correlated with sleep-inducing drugs [110].

Major tranquilizers cause a decrease in body temperature and all protect against epinephrine and norepinephrine toxicity; the latter is probably due to α-adrenergic receptor blockade. Neither of these tests can be considered very selective for major tranquilizers.

Inhibition of EEG arousal due to stimulation of the ascending activating system cannot be said to be a specific effect of major tranquilizers. However, most tranquilizers do cause somnolence in animals and man, and this test will so indicate. Somnolence is also suggested by slowing of the spontaneous cortical activity.

For years, cortical and hippocampal afterdischarges were used by the authors to identify major tranquilizers. It was believed that any drug with sedative action that prolonged these afterdischarges was likely to be a major tranquilizer and should be studied further for this type of activity. This test appeared to be very selective for phenothiazines and reserpine. When butyrophenones were encountered, however, the test was found to be nonspecific since these drugs blocked both afterdischarges rather than prolonged them. This was the first laboratory test to show qualitative differences between the butyrophenones and the phenothiazines.

Although many of these methods cannot be considered specific for identifying major tranquilizers, the group taken as a whole establishes quite well the profile of activity of proven major tranquilizers.

IV. THE ROLE OF DOPAMINE

In recent years neurochemists have been actively studying the effects of major tranquilizers on cerebral catecholamine metabolism. Attention has been focused mainly on dopamine content and turnover in specific areas. It has been shown that major tranquilizers markedly increase the turnover rate of dopamine, mainly in, but not limited to, the caudate nucleus. This appears to be a characteristic common to all the major tranquilizers studied and could well become a method for evaluating such drugs.

This finding, along with many other similar observations, has attracted the attention of pharmacologists and other neuroscientists to dopamine as playing a major role in the etiology of schizophrenia and in the mechanism of action of major tranquilizers. It has been established that in patients with Parkinson's disease, a deficiency of dopamine exists in the extrapyramidal system and that major tranquilizers produce extrapyramidal signs as side effects.

There is abundant evidence that major tranquilizers block the action of dopamine or, in the case of reserpine, deplete dopamine. This amine is not generally found throughout the brain but is localized in rather precise areas. It has been found in the medulla, corpus striatum, some areas of the limbic system, the olfactory tubercle, nucleus accumbens, and the cortex [114]. It is intriguing to assume that major tranquilizers block the emetic effect of apomorphine in the medulla, produce extrapyramidal signs by blocking dopamine receptors in the corpus striatum, and exert their antipsychotic effect in the limbic system or elsewhere. The latter has been suggested by Andén [115]. We have very specific antiemetic drugs (e.g., diphenidol), compounds that produce catalepsy but are not antipsychotic agents (e.g., bulbocapnine), and major tranquilizers that have both effects in addition to their antipsychotic action, suggesting that there may well be more than one type of dopamine receptor such as are known to exist for adrenergic receptors.

From the dopamine-blocking action of major tranquilizers it is fascinating to assume overactivity of dopamine synthesis or diminished metabolism of this catecholamine as the basis for schizophrenia. But there is a great deal of evidence against such a hypothesis. The disorder is not frequently cured completely by the administration of these drugs. Snyder and his coworkers [116] pointed out that the prevention by physostigmine of the psychosis-worsening action of methylphenidate [117] suggests a balance between catecholamines and acetylcholine in modulating psychotic symptoms. Matthysse [114] also finds fault with the dopamine mechanism, since cerebrospinal fluid homovanillic acid concentrations in schizophrenics appear to be within normal limits. Persson and Roos [118] reported no significant abnormality in CSF homovanillic acid in chronic schizophrenics, an observation confirmed by Rimon et al. [119].

If tranquilizers have but one action, at therapeutic antischizophrenic doses they should all produce the same degree of extrapyramidal signs. But it is well known that these drugs differ markedly in producing extrapyramidal effects. Haloperidol, trifluoperazine, and perphenazine produce more such signs than does chlorpromazine. Thioridazine produces fewer signs and clozapine produces the lowest incidence of extrapyramidal signs. Snyder et al. [120] have shown that such differences can be explained by the differences in the degree of anticholinergic actions of these drugs. These authors suggest that by blocking cholinergic receptors, the tranquilizers might antagonize their own tendency to elicit extrapyramidal signs produced by dopamine receptor blockade. They studied the affinity of the drugs for central muscarinic cholinergic receptors and showed that the incidence of extrapyramidal signs produced by the drugs was inversely related to their antimuscarinic activity. Thus, they found that haloperidol had the lowest and clozapine had by far the highest affinity for muscarinic receptors, and the other drugs fell in between as predicted.

Snyder and his coworkers [120] extended this study to show that relative affinities are the same in the corpus striatum as in whole brain of rats, a finding that is applicable to primates. They also found the same relative affinities of clozapine, chlorpromazine, and trifluoperazine in the guinea pig ileum, making it possible to investigate this property by conventional pharmacological techniques. Using techniques similar to those used originally by Snyder et al. [120] to study the affinities of tranquilizers for central muscarinic receptors, Miller and Hiley [121] came to the same conclusions.

Separation of anticholinergic activity from the antipsychotic activity requires the relative affinities for the dopamine and muscarinic cholinergic receptors to differ. Miller and Iversen [122] determined the inhibition of several of these drugs on striatal dopamine-sensitive adenyl cyclase and showed that blockade of dopamine receptors does not correlate at all with the affinities for muscarinic receptors.

In another effort to study the separation of extrapyramidal signs and antipsychotic effects of major tranquilizers, Bunney and Aghajanian [123] recorded the firing rates of dopaminergic cells that project to the limbic system (grouping A10) and dopaminergic cells in the substantia nigra that project to the corpus striatum (grouping A9). These investigators found that the drugs most prone to produce extrapyramidal effects increased the firing rate of A9 neurons as much as 100% above baseline. Those drugs with a low incidence of extrapyramidal side effects (thioridazine and clozapine) did not increase A9 cell firing rate. The authors showed that antipsychotic drugs reversed d-amphetamine-induced depression of A9 and A10 cells. Mepazine, a phenothiazine with little antipsychotic action but one that produces extrapyramidal signs, was found to reverse d-amphetamine-induced depression of A9 cells but had no effect on A10 cells. Bunney and Aghajanian suggest that reversal of d-amphetamine-induced depression of A10 cells correlates best with the antipsychotic properties of the drugs. By testing the ability of a potential tranquilizer to reverse the depressed A10 cells and to increase the firing rate of A9 cells above baseline, it may be possible to predict whether such a drug will have antipsychotic properties and a high or low incidence of extrapyramidal side effects.

V. FUTURE AREAS OF RESEARCH

There is no assurance that schizophrenia is a single entity. As Kety [124] pointed out, it may be that the term schizophrenia has been applied to a diffuse segment of a continuum of social maladaptation. Thus, it may be proven that some patients suffer from overactivity of the dopaminergic system whereas others suffer from metabolic lesions that produce psychotogenic substances, and, of course, there may be other causes of schizophrenia that we have not yet conceived. Until the etiology of the mental disorder has been elucidated, it will be very difficult to develop significant new drugs that will be more beneficial than those currently available. To assume that any one of the current theories is correct would be foolhardy since this would tend to polarize our attention perhaps on the wrong mechanism of action of the major tranquilizers.

We need to know the etiology of schizophrenia before going further in the development of new specific drugs since it is impossible to develop such drugs without first knowing what action is needed. The current major tranquilizers have helped tremendously in the control of patients with schizophrenia but there are too few patients who are cured. We have an abundance of hypotheses and each of them should receive sufficient attention for purposes of rejection or acceptance.

Until we know the cause or causes of schizophrenia, we must continue in our present mode of study hoping that the right drug will be found. In this quest we have only serendipity to guide us. This may not be all bad because we have been guided in this way since 1933 when hypoglycemic treatments were discovered quite fortuitously by Sakel. We do need to remain alert to be able to recognize important leads when they appear.

Until the shining light appears, pharmacologists should busy themselves studying the leads we now have, and develop methods to show how new drugs, such as sulpiride, act. We also have several leads for agents that have a much longer duration of action, such as penfluridol, fluspirilene, and the decanoate and enanthate salts of fluspirilene. Continued efforts should be made in this direction, for a truly long-acting drug would be of great value in reducing hospital nursing care and especially in treating newly released outpatients. With such methods of treatment, the psychiatrist could be assured of the continued treatment of patients, although seeing them infrequently.

Neurochemists should study mechanisms of action of both new and old drugs with their specialized techniques, because this is probably the way that advances will be made in the near future. This is undoubtedly true for the elucidation of both the etiology of schizophrenia and the mechanism of action of new major tranquilizers. The chemists will probably also play an ever increasing role in the development of new drugs, and it is entirely within the realm of reality that such drugs will be screened in vitro without the use of animal models.

REFERENCES

1. M. Sakel, Wien. Klin. Wochenschr. 46, 1372 (1933).

2. U. Cerletti and L. Bini, Arch. Gen. Neurol. Psichiatria. Psicoanal. 19, 266 (1938).

3. A. Sweel, North Carolina Med. N. 15, 246 (1954).

4. O. V. Kerbikov, Lancet 1, 744 (1955).

5. J. F. Fulton and C. F. Jacobsen, Adv. Mod. Biol. (Moscow) 4, 113 (1935).

6. W. Freeman and J. W. Watts, Psychosurgery in the Treatment of Mental Disorders and Intractable Pain, 2nd ed., Thomas, Springfield, Illinois, 1950.

7. A. S. Loevenhart, W. F. Lorenz, and R. M. Waters, JAMA 92, 880 (1929).

8. L. J. Meduna, Carbon Dioxide Therapy, Thomas, Springfield, Illinois, 1950.

9. H. Laborit, P. Huguenard, and R. Alluaume, Presse Med. 60, 206 (1952).

10. J. Delay, P. Deniker, and J. M. Hard, Ann. Med. Psychol. 110, 267 (1952).

11. H. J. Bein, Experientia 9, 107 (1953).

12. N. S. Kline, Ann. N.Y. Acad. Sci. 59, 107 (1954).

13. L. E. Hollister, in The Phenothiazines and Structurally Related Drugs (I. S. Forrest, C. J. Carr, and E. Usdin, eds.), Raven Press, New York, 1974, pp. 667–673.

14. P. Divry, J. Bobon, and J. Collard, Acta Neurol. Belg. 58, 878 (1958).

15. D. N. Johnson, W. H. Funderburk, and J. W. Ward, Arch. Int. Pharmacodyn. Ther. 194, 197 (1971).

16. G. M. Simpson and V. Varga, Curr. Ther. Res. 16, 477 (1974).

17. I. Møller Nielsen and K. Neuhold, Acta Pharmacol. Toxicol. 15, 335 (1959).

18. A. A. Sugarman, H. Stohlberg, and J. Herrmann, Curr. Ther. Res. 7, 310 (1965).

19. F. J. Ayd, Dis. Nerv. Syst. 35, 447 (1974).

20. R. M. Steinbook, B. J. Goldstein, B. Brauzer, S. S. Moreno, and A. F. Jacobson, Curr. Ther. Res. 15, 1 (1973).

21. M. Kramer, B. Blackwell, T. Roth, and M. Wray, Curr. Ther. Res. 15, 465 (1973).

22. G. M. Simpson and E. Varga, Psychopharmacol. Bull. 11, 14 (1975).

23. M. Toru, Y. Shimazono, M. Miyasaka, T. Kokubo, Y. Mori, and T. Nasu, J. Clin. Pharmacol. 12, 221 (1972).

24. A. J. Sanseigne, H. L. Yale, S. M. Hess, J. C. Burke, and Z. P. Horovitz, Agressologie 9, 309 (1968).

25. D. M. Gallant, Psychopharmacol. Bull. 11, 11 (1975).

26. A. Jus, R. Pineau, K. Jus, A. Villeneuve, J. Gautier, P. Pires, A. Drolet, M. Cote, and R. Villeneuve, Curr. Ther. Res. 16, 1041 (1974).

27. S. Courvoisier, F. Fournel, R. Ducrot, M. Kolsky, and P. Koetschet, Arch. Int. Pharmacodyn. Ther. 92, 305 (1953).

28. L. Cook, E. Weidley, E. F. Morris, and P. A. Mattis, J. Pharmacol. Exp. Ther. 113, 11 (1955).

29. J. H. Burn and R. Hobbs, Arch. Int. Pharmacodyn. Ther. 113, 290 (1958).

30. J. A. Gunn and M. R. Gurd, J. Physiol. (London) 97, 453 (1940).

31. M. R. A. Chance, J. Pharmacol. Exp. Ther. 97, 214 (1946).

32. L. Lasagna and W. P. McCann, Science 125, 1241 (1957).

33. D. R. Maxwell, in Proc. 1st Int. Congr. Neuropharmacology (P. B. Bradley, P. Deniker, and C. Radovco-Thomas, eds.), Elsevier, Amsterdam, 1959, p. 365.

34. J. Cohen and H. Lal, Pharmacologist 5, 261 (1963).

35. H. Lal, S. Ginocchio, and A. Shefner, Life Sci. 3, 190 (1963).

36. J. F. Gardocki, M. E. Schuler, and L. Goldstein, Toxicol. Appl. Pharmacol. 9, 536 (1966).

37. J. T. Litchfield, Jr. and F. Wilcoxon, J. Pharmacol. Exp. Ther. 96, 99 (1949).

38. W. C. Clark, H. J. Blackman, and J. E. Preston, Arch. Int. Pharmacodyn. Ther. 170, 350 (1967).

39. J. M. Littleton, Acta Pharmacol. Toxicol. 34, 92 (1974).

40. C. Y. Yen, R. L. Stanger, and N. Millman, Arch. Int. Pharmacodyn. Ther. 123, 179 (1959).

41. P. A. J. Janssen, A. H. Jageneau, and C. J. E. Niemegeers, J. Pharmacol. Exp. Ther. 129, 471 (1960).

42. A. Scriabine and M. Blake, Psychopharmacologia 3, 224 (1962).

43. J. P. DaVanzo, M. Daugherty, R. Ruckart, and L. Kang, Psychopharmacologia 9, 210 (1966).

44. A. Barnett, J. B. Molick, and R. I. Taber, Psychopharmacologia 19, 359 (1971).

45. J. Scheel-Krüger and A. Randrup, Acta Pharmacol. Toxicol. 25, 61 (1967).

46. A. Randrup and I. Munkvad, in International Symposium on Amphetamines and Related Compounds (E. Costa and S. Garattini, eds.), Raven Press, New York, 1970, p. 695.

47. I. Munkvad, in Modern Problems of Pharmacopsychiatry, Vol. 5, The Neuroleptics (D. B. Bobon, P. A. J. Janssen, and J. Bobon, eds.), Karger, Basel, 1970, p. 44.

48. P. A. J. Janssen, C. J. E. Niemegeers, and K. H. L. Schellekens, Arzneim. Forsch. 15, 104 (1965).

49. A. Randrup, in Modern Problems of Pharmacopsychiatry, Vol. 5, The Neuroleptics (D. B. Bobon, P. A. J. Janssen, and J. Bobon, eds.), Karger, Basel, 1970, p. 60.

50. A. Randrup and I. Munkvad, Psychopharmacologia 7, 416 (1965).

51. B. Costall and R. J. Naylor, Eur. J. Pharmacol. 25, 121 (1974).

52. S. C. Wang and H. L. Borison, Arch. Neurol. Psychiatry 63, 928 (1950).

53. G. Chen and C. R. Ensor, J. Pharmacol. Exp. Ther. 98, 245 (1950).

54. V. V. Glaviano and S. C. Wang, J. Pharmacol. Exp. Ther. 114, 358 (1955).

55. M. T. Peng and S. C. Wang, Proc. Soc. Exp. Biol. Med. 110, 211 (1962).

56. H. L. Borison, J. Physiol. 147, 172 (1959).

57. C. J. E. Niemegeers, Pharmacology 6, 353 (1971).

58. C. A. Leonard, T. Fujita, D. H. Tedeschi, C. L. Zirkle, and E. J. Fellows, J. Pharmacol. Exp. Ther. 154, 339 (1966).

59. P. A. J. Janssen, C. J. E. Niemegeers, and K. H. L. Schellekens, Arzneim. Forsch. 15, 1196 (1965).

60. E. F. Domino, A. J. Karoly, and E. L. Walker, J. Pharmacol. Exp. Ther. 141, 92 (1963).

61. A. Wikler, Am. J. Psychiatry 105, 329 (1948).

62. M. Sidman, Psychopharmacologia 1, 1 (1959).

63. R. Ader and D. W. Clink, J. Pharmacol. Exp. Ther. 121, 144 (1957).

64. M. D. Aceto, V. D. Lynch, and R. K. Thoms, J. Pharm. Sci. 50, 823 (1961).

65. M. Sidman, Science 118, 157 (1953).

66. D. B. McKean and J. Pearl, Physiol. Behav. 3, 795 (1968).

67. D. N. Johnson, W. H. Funderburk, and J. W. Ward, Arch. Int. Pharmacodyn. Ther. 211, 326 (1974).

68. P. A. J. Janssen, A. H. M. Jageneau, and K. H. L. Schellekens, Psychopharmacologia 1, 389 (1960).

69. D. H. Tedeschi, R. E. Tedeschi, L. Cook, P. A. Mattis, and E. J. Fellows, Arch. Int. Pharmacodyn. Ther. 122, 129 (1959).

70. C. A. Winter and L. Flataker, J. Pharmacol. Exp. Ther. 103, 93 (1951).

71. E. M. Boyd and O. K. Miller, Fed. Proc. 13, 338 (1954).

72. J. D. Archer, Fed. Proc. 13, 332 (1954).

73. D. H. Tedeschi, in The Present Status of Psychotropic Drugs (A. Corletti and F. J. Bové, eds.), Excerpta Medica Foundation, Amsterdam, 1969, pp. 145-153.

74. L. Julou, in Modern Problems of Pharmacopsychiatry, Vol. 5, The Neuroleptics (D. P. Bobon, P. A. J. Janssen, and J. Bobon, eds.), Karger, Basel, 1970, pp. 50-54.

75. B. Costall and R. J. Naylor, Psychopharmacologia 32, 161 (1973).

76. S. Courvoisier, R. Ducrot, and L. Julou, in Psychotropic Drugs (S. Garattini and V. Ghetti, eds.), Elsevier, Amsterdam, 1957, pp. 375-377.

77. W. Wirth, R. Gosswald, U. Horlein, K. H. Risse, and H. Kreiskott, Arch. Int. Pharmacodyn. Ther. 115, 1 (1958).

78. D. N. Johnson, unpublished work, 1974.

79. P. A. J. Janssen, Arzneim. Forsch. 11, 932 (1961).

80. T. Fujita and D. H. Tedeschi, Pharmacologist 7, 155 (1965).

81. E. A. Swinyard, H. H. Wolf, G. B. Fink, and L. S. Goodman, J. Pharmacol. Exp. Ther. 126, 312 (1959).

82. M. Gordon, in Psychopharmacological Agents, Vol. 2, Academic Press, New York, 1967, p. 68.

83. A. W. Lessin and M. W. Parkes, Br. J. Pharmacol. 12, 245 (1957).

84. G. Bartholini, H. Keller, L. Pieri, and A. Pletscher, in The Benzodiazepines (S. Garattini, E. Mussini, and L. O. Randall, eds.), Raven Press, New York, 1973, pp. 235-240.

85. N.-E. Andén, A. Dahlstrom, K. Fuxe, and K. Larsson, Acta Pharmacol. Toxicol. 24, 263 (1966).

86. N.-E. Andén, A. Rubenson, K. Fuxe, and T. Hökfelt, J. Pharm. Pharmacol. 19, 627 (1967).

87. U. Ungerstedt, Acta Physiol. Scand. Suppl. 367, 49 (1971).

88. R. F. Von Voigtlander and K. E. Moore, Neuropharmacology 12, 451 (1971).

89. V. J. Lotti, Life Sci. 10, 781 (1971).

90. V. Ungerstedt and G. Arbuthnott, Brain Res. 24, 485 (1970).

91. J. B. Preston, J. Pharmacol. Exp. Ther. 118, 100 (1956).

92. E. K. Killam, K. F. Killam, and T. Shaw, Ann. N.Y. Acad. Sci. 66, 784 (1957).

93. I. Ishikawa, Y. Sadanaga, S. Katsuta, J.-I. Ishiyama, and T. Kobayashi, in Progress in Brain Research (T. Tokizane and J. P. Schadé, eds.), Part B, Vol. 21B, Elsevier, Amsterdam, 1966, pp. 40-53.

94. T. Itil and M. Fink, Dis. Nerv. Syst. 30, 524 (1969).

95. P. A. J. Janssen, Symposium Internazionale sull' Haloperidol e Triperidol, Instituto Luso Farmaco d'Italia, Milano, 1962.

96. K. L. Oliver and W. H. Funderburk, EEG Clin. Neurophysiol. 19, 501 (1965).

97. W. Schallek, T. Lewinson, and J. Thomas, Int. J. Neuropharmacol. 6, 253 (1967).

98. W. Schallek, T. Lewinson, and J. Thomas, Int. J. Neuropharmacol. 7, 37 (1968).

99. D. O. Walter, Exp. Neurol. 8, 155 (1963).

100. H. H. Jasper and C. Ajmone Marsan, A Stereotaxic Atlas of the Diencephalon of the Cat, Natl. Res. Council Canada, Ottawa, 1954.

101. W. H. Marshall, Stain Technol. 15, 133 (1940).

102. L. Stein, in Antidepressant Drugs (S. Garattini and M. N. G. Dukes, eds.), Excerpta Medica Foundation, Amsterdam, 1967, pp. 130-140.

103. A. Wauquier, C. J. E. Niemegeers, and H. A. Geivers, Psychopharmacologia 23, 238 (1972).

104. A. Wauquier and C. J. E. Niemegeers, Psychopharmacologia 27, 191 (1972).

105. A. Wauquier and C. J. E. Niemegeers, Psychopharmacologia 30, 163 (1973).

106. A. Wauquier and C. J. E. Niemegeers, Psychopharmacologia 34, 265 (1974).

107. C. D. Wise and L. Stein, Science 163, 299 (1969).

108. M. E. Olds and J. Olds, Int. J. Neuropharmacol. 2, 309 (1964).

109. M. E. Olds and J. Olds, J. Comp. Neurol. 120, 259 (1963).

110. J. M. Van Rossum, P. A. J. Janssen, J. R. Boissier, L. Julou, D. M. Loew, I. Møller Nielsen, I. Munkvad, A. Randrup, G. Stille, and G. H. Tedeschi, in Modern Problems of Pharmacopsychiatry, Vol. 5, The Neuroleptics (D. P. Bobon, P. A. J. Janssen, and J. Bobon, eds.), Karger, Basel, 1970, pp. 23-32.

111. O. Vinař and M. Kršiak, in Phenothiazines and Structurally Related Drugs (I. S. Forrest, C. J. Carr, and E. Usdin, eds.), Raven Press, New York, 1974, pp. 675-683.

112. D. M. Loew, in Modern Problems of Pharmacopsychiatry, Vol. 5, The Neuroleptics (D. P. Bobon, P. A. J. Janssen, and J. Bobon, eds.), Karger, Basel, 1970, pp. 47-50.

113. P. Muller and P. Seeman, J. Pharm. Pharmacol. 26, 981 (1974).

114. S. Matthysse, Fed. Proc. 32, 200 (1973).

115. N.-E. Andén, J. Pharm. Pharmacol. 24, 905 (1972).

116. S. H. Snyder, S. P. Banerjee, H. I. Yamamura, and D. Greenberg, Science 184, 1243 (1974).

186   W. H. FUNDERBURK AND D. N. JOHNSON

117. J. M. Davis and D. Janowsky, in Frontiers in Catecholamine Research (E. Usdin and S. H. Snyder, eds.), Pergamon Press, New York, 1974, p. 977.

118. T. Persson and B. E. Roos, Br. J. Psychiatry 115, 95 (1969).

119. R. Rimon, B. E. Roos, V. Rakkolainen, and Y. Alanen, J. Psychosom. Res. 15, 375 (1971).

120. S. Snyder, D. Greenberg, and H. I. Yamamura, Arch. Gen. Psychiatry 31, 58 (1974).

121. R. J. Miller and C. R. Hiley, Nature 248, 596 (1974).

122. R. J. Miller and L. L. Iversen, quoted in reference 121.

123. B. S. Bunney and G. K. Aghajanian, Psychopharmacol. Bull. 10, 17 (1974).

124. S. S. Kety, N. Engl. J. Med. 276, 325 (1967).

Chapter 7

MINOR TRANQUILIZERS

Allan D. Rudzik

The Upjohn Company
Kalamazoo, Michigan

I. INTRODUCTION

The finding of the broad pharmacological and clinical activity of the benzodiazepine derivatives, chlordiazepoxide [1] and diazepam [2], has markedly
increased the interest of both medicinal chemists and biologists in the investigation of the pharmacological properties of the minor tranquilizing
agents. The mechanism of the anxiolytic action of minor tranquilizers is

difficult to characterize because of the diversity of activities produced by these agents. Compounds of this type possess sedative-hypnotic, muscle relaxant, and anticonvulsant activity, antiaggressive or taming behavior, marked activity in operant behavior procedures, and effects on food intake. All these effects have been used to assess the minor tranquilizing activity of new compounds.

Of more importance to the industrial pharmacologist has been the attempt to find animal test systems which best correlate with anxiolytic activity in humans since this is the most important indication for the clinical usage of these agents. Also of importance to the medicinal chemist and pharmacologist has been the attempt to discover compounds in which anxiolytic activity is separated from sedative activity. Since sedation is the major clinical side effect seen with these agents, compounds with high anxiolytic but low sedative potential would possess marked clinical utility.

To establish a logical testing and evaluation sequence, this chapter is subdivided into several sections, each of which analyzes a particular pharmacological activity. The methodology cited primarily involves small animal systems, but large animal systems are included where available.

II. CHEMISTRY

Figure 1 shows the chemical structures of various benzodiazepine derivatives. Most of the compounds listed are available to the practicing clinician. Two of the compounds (triazolam and alprazolam) are new chemical entities and are undergoing clinical study.

III. PHARMACOLOGICAL ACTIVITIES

A. Assessment of Gross Behavior

Initial evaluation of potential minor tranquilizing agents usually involves an analysis of their effects on the gross behavior of laboratory animals. Initial testing in mice can be followed by more elaborate testing in cats or dogs. Irwin [3] has developed a gross behavioral assessment procedure in mice which is widely used. In this study, he evaluated a number of sedative-hypnotic and minor tranquilizing agents such as alcohol, chloral hydrate, glutethimide, pentobarbital, phenobarbital, meprobamate, and the benzodiazepines, chlordiazepoxide, oxazepam, and diazepam. Special emphasis was given to the differences in activity of sedative-hypnotics and minor tranquilizers.

Compounds were administered to groups of mice, six per dose level, and changes of function were rated on a 0 to 8 scale. Functional changes observed were impaired gait (as ataxia and limb weakness); impaired righting (failure of animals to land on all fours when somersaulted into the air);

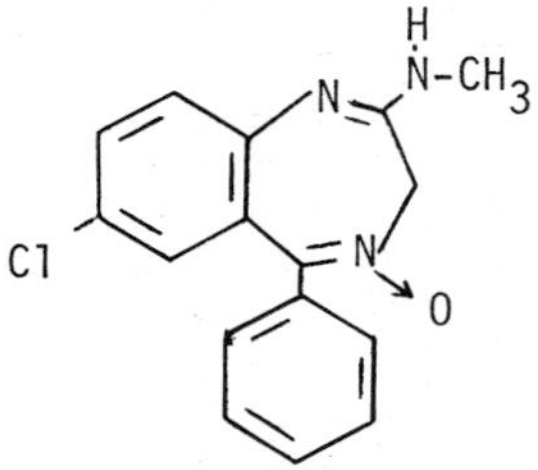

Chlordiazepoxide

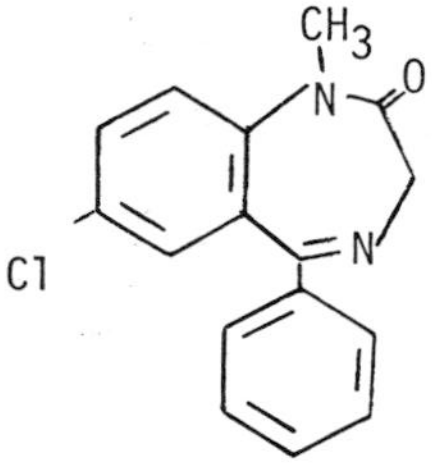

Diazepam

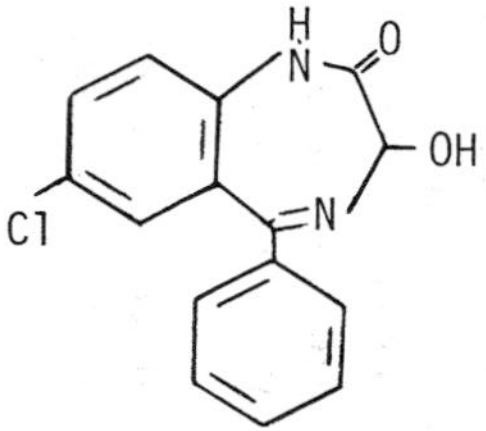

Oxazepam

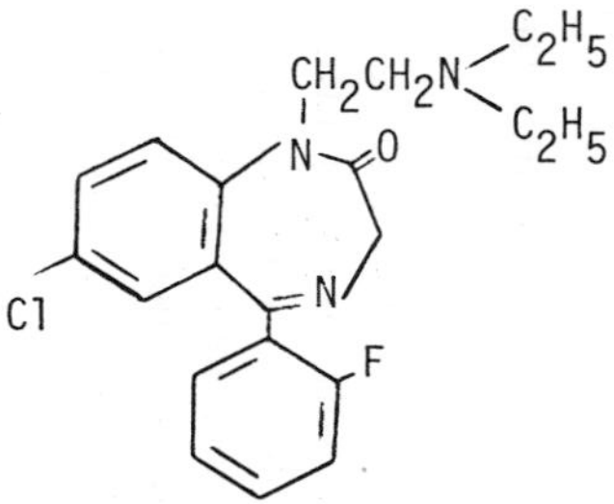

Flurazepam

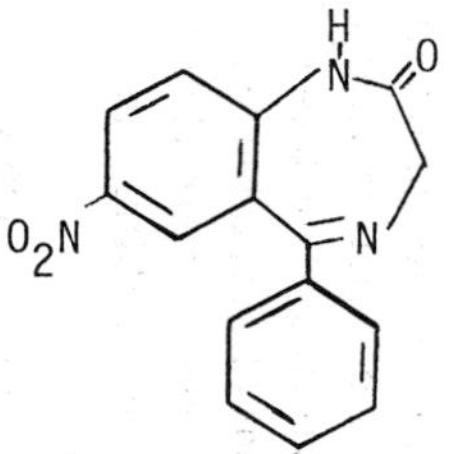

Nitrazepam

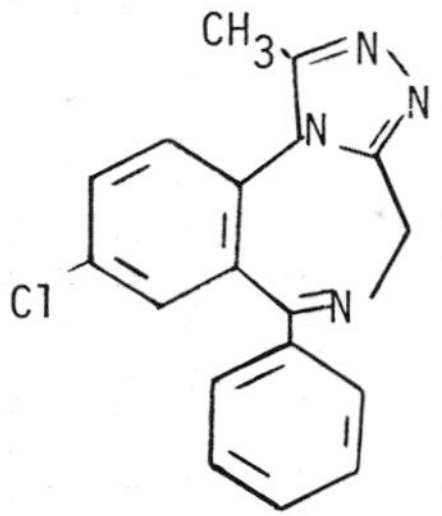

Alprazolam

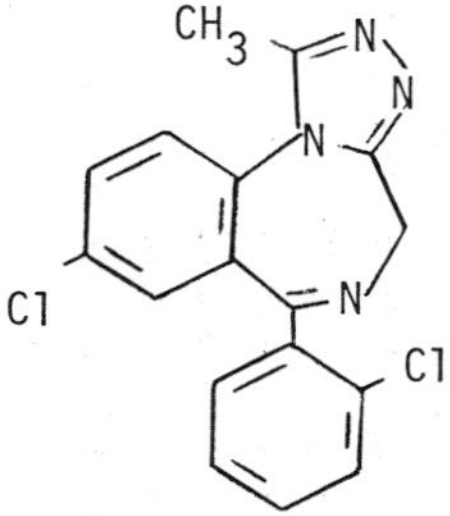

Triazolam

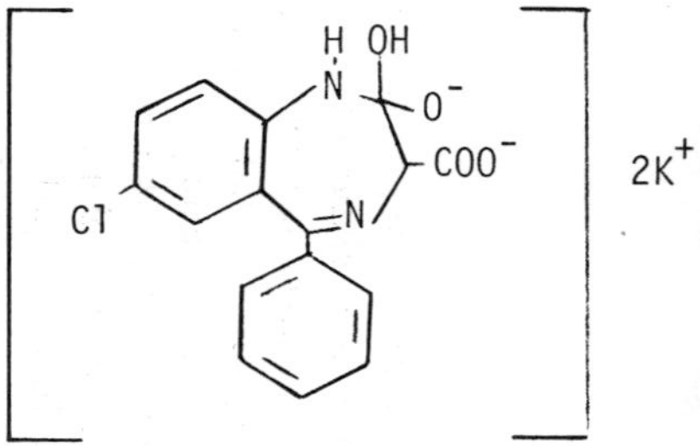

Clorazepate Dipotassium

FIGURE 1. Structures of various standard benzodiazepines.

muscle tone reduction; sensoromotor responses (pinna, corneal, and toe-pinch reactions); irritability avoidance (finger withdrawal, provoked biting, provoked freezing, and grasp responses); locomotor activity (measured immediately after transfer to a new environment); finger approach (approach behavior on presentation of an extended index finger); and reduced behavioral arousal (relaxed dulled appearance of animals immediately after transfer to a new environment).

The minor tranquilizers, oxazepam and diazepam, caused impairment of gait and righting reflex. They also selectively reduced muscle tone whereas the sedative-hypnotics were without effect until gait impairing doses were administered, and then pentobarbital actually increased muscle tone. Sensoromotor responses were increased by both sedative-hypnotics (with the exception of chloral hydrate and glutethimide) and minor tranquilizers, occurring over a wide dose range in the benzodiazepine group. A reduction in levels of behavioral arousal occurred with all compounds, probably reflecting their sedative action.

In these gross behavioral tests, dose-response curves for the benzodiazepines tend to be flatter than those of sedative-hypnotics and meprobamate.

Norton and De Beer [4] and Irwin [3] have developed systematic observational procedures for cats. Sedative-hypnotics (chloral hydrate, pentobarbital, and phenobarbital) decrease wakefulness in cats at about twice their neurotoxic dose levels whereas the benzodiazepines increase wakefulness at minimal neurotoxic doses.

B. Hypnotic Activity

The hypnotic activity of minor tranquilizing agents is generally evaluated by measuring the compound's effect on simple covert or overt assays in the rodent or by neurophysiological measurements of sleep stages. The pertinent methodology has recently been reviewed by Straw [5].

In rodents, the simple test systems commonly used measure sleeping time [7], loss of righting reflex [8], potentiation of known CNS depressants such as pentobarbital, alcohol, or chlorprothixene [8], or gross behavioral changes [3]. But there are inherent limitations in these systems. Minor tranquilizing agents generally do not produce loss of righting reflex in the mouse nor does potentiation of known CNS depressants such as alcohol or the barbiturates correlate well with clinical efficacy. Furthermore, the assessment of gross behavior, although useful, is only semiquantitative. Table 1 shows comparative data on the potentiation of the CNS depressants ethanol, pentobarbital, and chlorprothixene by standard benzodiazepine compounds.

Perhaps more appropriate for the evaluation of hypnotic activity are the neurophysiological techniques used to measure drug effects on sleep stages of cats or monkeys. Minor tranquilizing agents are active in these tests [8].

TABLE 1   Potentiation of Depressants

Compound	ED50 (mg/kg, i.p.) to potentiate		
	Ethanol	Pentobarbital	Chlorprothixene
Chlordiazepoxide	11	14	6.3
Diazepam	0.9	5.0	2.3
Nitrazepam	—	0.5	0.7
Flurazepam	1.3	4.5	—
Alprazolam	0.16	0.45	0.16
Triazolam	0.6	2.0	0.3

The benzodiazepines have also been evaluated in rhesus monkeys using specific electroencephalographic procedures [5]. Several of these derivatives shared a common effect in the 7.5 to 15, 15 to 25, 25 to 35, and 35 to 100 Hz bands of the rhesus monkey EEG, but differed qualitatively in the 0 to 7.5 Hz band. Those clinically effective anxiolytics with relatively little sedative effect (e.g., diazepam and ketazolam) had no effect or a decrease in this band in the doses studied. In contrast, flurazepam and triazolam, which are effective as hypnotics, produce significant increases in this band. The usefulness of this technique in predicting the clinical utility of drugs remains to be proven.

C. Muscle Relaxant Activity

Minor tranquilizing agents have been found to be effective in treating various forms of muscle spasms, and their pharmacological [6] and clinical [9] activities have been reviewed.

The methodologies used to evaluate muscle relaxant activity in animals involve either simple test systems such as antagonism of strychnine lethality [10], traction response [10], inclined screen [3], or gross observation of muscle tone in rodents [3,11], or complex (and possibly more precise) neurophysiological methods in decerebrate or high spinal cats [12].

Minor tranquilizers antagonize strychnine lethality and inhibit the traction response. The approximate potency of a series of benzodiazepine derivatives was the same in both test systems, the newer triazolobenzodiazepines being approximately 20 times more active than the standard, diazepam [10]. Table 2 shows comparative data on the antagonism of strychnine lethality, traction response, and spinal reflexes in the cat for various standard benzodiazepine compounds.

Gross observation of behavior in rodents or in cats has also been a reliable method of evaluating muscle relaxant activity [11]. Muscle

192

A. D. RUDZIK

TABLE 2   Muscle Relaxant Activity

Compound	Antistrychnine ED50 (mg/kg, i.p., mouse)	Traction ED50 (mg/kg, i.p., mouse)	Spinal reflexes potency ratio (decerebrate cat, i.v.)
Chlordiazepoxide	63	11	0.1
Diazepam	8.0	7.0	1
Nitrazepam	3.6	1.2	—
Flurazepam	22	9.0	0.2
Alprazolam	0.3	0.6	6
Triazolam	0.2	0.6	11

relaxant activity in cats is measured by determining the minimum dose of
test agent which causes the cats to hang relaxed when suspended by the
scruff of the neck. The muscle relaxant doses obtained in these experiments agree closely with the clinical data previously published by Zbinden
and Randall [12]. Neurophysiological techniques have shown that diazepam
is a potent depressant of both patellar and linguomandibular reflexes in the
intact cat [13]. In the high spinal cat only the linguomandibular reflexes
were depressed. Small doses of diazepam also abolished the rigidity of the
midcollicular decerebrate cat. Evidence exists for both a brain stem
reticular and a spinal cord site for the action of diazepam on motor systems.

D. Anticonvulsant Activity

One of the most sensitive measures of minor tranquilizer activity in mice
is the antagonism of convulsions, especially those induced by chemical
agents such as pentylenetetrazol [7,8,10,14], nicotine [10], bemegride [10],
and 3-mercaptopropionic acid [15]. The minor tranquilizing agents are
somewhat less active against both minimal and maximal electroshock
seizures.
      Antipentylenetetrazol activity in mice has long been considered an
indicator of potential antiepileptic (petit mal) activity in man. In recent
years, a positive correlation has been established between the clinical
sedative and/or anxiolytic activity of various benzodiazepines and antipentylenetetrazol activity in animals [12]. Chen and Bohner [16] interpret pentylenetetrazol antagonism as a measure of sedation in mice. Antagonism of
pentylenetetrazol can also be assessed in rats [10], rabbits [17], and cats [18].

Initial evaluation of anticonvulsant activity is usually made in groups of male mice. Convulsants such as pentylenetetrazol (85 mg/kg, s.c.) and bemegride (40 mg/kg, s.c.) are administered 30 min after test compounds and evaluations are made 15 min later. Thiosemicarbazide (20 mg/kg, i.p.) is administered simultaneously with test compounds and evaluated 4 hr later. Table 3 shows comparative data for the effect of various standard compounds on the convulsions produced by pentylenetetrazol, nicotine, thiosemicarbazide, and electroshock in mice and pentylenetetrazol convulsions in rats and cats.

3-Mercaptopropionic acid produces a convulsive syndrome in mice characterized by running, tonic extensor, and lethality phases [15]. The tonic extensor phase of the convulsion is antagonized by both major and minor tranquilizing agents, antidepressants, and anticonvulsants. Antagonism of the running phase is more difficult and only certain benzodiazepine derivatives (chlordiazepoxide and the triazolobenzodiazepines) are active in this regard. Antagonism of 3-mercaptopropionic acid convulsions should be a part of the initial evaluation of any compound thought to have minor tranquilizing activity.

The neuropharmacological approach to anticonvulsant testing is based on electrical stimulation of specific brain areas believed to be involved in different forms of epilepsy. Repetitive stimulation of these areas induces afterdischarges in the EEG which resemble the seizure discharges seen in clinical epilepsy.

In immobilized cats, Schallek and Kuehn [19] found that chlordiazepoxide caused decreased duration of afterdischarge in the septum and hippocampus and decreased amplitude of afterdischarge in the amygdala. Other studies in cats by Requin et al. [20] showed that chlordiazepoxide and diazepam depressed afterdischarge in the amygdala.

In the freely moving cat, stimulation of the amygdala or hippocampus induces staring, dilatation of the pupils, facial twitching, and drooling, behavior resembling that seen during psychomotor seizures in man. Chlordiazepoxide increases the threshold for these behavioral manifestations of afterdischarge in the amygdala [21].

E. Antiaggression and Taming Activity

Another characteristic activity of minor tranquilizing agents in animals is their ability to reduce aggressive behavior in mice and rats [12, 22] and to tame vicious monkeys and zoo animals [23]. Aggressive behavior can be induced in mice by prolonged isolation [22] or electroshock [10, 24] and in rats by electroshock [24] or midbrain lesions [24]. The benzodiazepines reduce aggressive behavior produced by electroshock in both mice and rats at relatively low doses whereas amobarbital is inactive and only high doses of meprobamate are effective in this type of aggressive behavior [24]. The benzodiazepines are also extremely effective in reducing aggressive behavior

TABLE 3   Anticonvulsant Activity

	Chlordiazepoxide	Diazepam	Nitrazepam	Flurzepam	Alprazolam	Triazolam
Antagonism in mice of:						
Pentylenetetrazol	3.1	0.8	0.4	0.7	0.2	0.04
Nicotine	1.0	0.28	0.09	0.2	0.02	0.01
Thiosemicarbazide	4.0	0.7	0.3	0.8	0.2	0.03
Electroshock	40	20	32	50	25	23
Antagonism in rats of:						
Pentylenetetrazol	4.0	1.4	1.2	—	0.3	0.2
Antagonism[a] in cats of:						
Pentylenetetrazol	0.25	1.0	2	—	5	12

[a]Expressed as potency ratio compared to diazepam (diazepam = 1); all other values in mg/kg, i.p.

in rats induced by lesions in the midbrain [24]. But differences in potency are evident within this class of tranquilizers when electroshock-induced aggression is compared with midbrain lesion aggression.

Rhesus monkeys are known to be spontaneously aggressive, retreating and/or launching an attack at the approach of an observer [24]. After chlordiazepoxide, they walk without any noticeable motor deficit, take food, sit peacefully in their cages, and allow an observer to reach in and touch them. Chlordiazepoxide is also effective in reducing the aggressive behavior in monkeys elicited by electrical stimulation of Forel's field or by radio stimulation of specific brain structures [25].

The taming effect of the minor tranquilizing agents while prominent in animals is more difficult to elaborate in humans and, in fact, much controversy exists as to whether the benzodiazepines increase or decrease aggressive behavior in man.

Table 4 shows comparative data for various standard benzodiazepine compounds in antagonizing foot-shock-induced aggressive behavior in mice and taming effects in monkeys.

F. Activity in Behavioral Procedures

The activity of the benzodiazepines in many operant behavioral procedures has been reviewed by Zbinden and Randall [12] and by Randall and Schallek [14]. In this section only those procedures are discussed which appear to be specific for minor tranquilizing agents.

Geller and Seifter [26] have developed a method for inducing and quantifying automated conflict behavior in laboratory animals. This conflict behavior procedure is sensitive to the actions of a number of CNS depressants [27]. Since meprobamate and chlordiazepoxide, anxiolytic agents of

TABLE 4   Antiaggressive Behavior

Compound	Foot-shock-induced aggression, mouse (ED50 mg/kg, i.p.)	Taming effect, monkey (effective dose, p.o.)
Chlordiazepoxide	7.0	3-10
Diazepam	1.8	3-10
Nitrazepam	1.3	10
Flurazepam	2.1	10
Alprazolam	0.13	0.3
Triazolam	0.3	0.3

known clinical utility, were effective in attenuating the conflict behavior, the method was suggested as a preclinical evaluator of this class of compounds [28].

The rat conflict procedure appears to be a useful laboratory technique for identifying psychopharmacological agents such as chlordiazepoxide and other minor tranquilizers. In addition, the potency of various compounds in this system corresponds to their clinical potency [29,30]. Table 5 shows comparative data for various standard benzodiazepine compounds in the rat conflict procedure.

Several other procedures seem to be predictive of anxiolytic activity. For example, Vogel et al. [31] have developed a simple conflict test in which thirsty naive rats are periodically administered shocks for licking water. Results from this test indicate that benzodiazepines, meprobamate, and pentobarbital but not d-amphetamine sulfate, magnesium pemoline, or scopolamine increase punished responding.

In a continuous avoidance procedure, animals were trained to postpone an electric foot shock by pressing a lever at a regular rate and to terminate a shock by pressing a second lever in the case of avoidance failure [12]. Some depressant drugs lower the rate of lever pressing, increase the number of shocks received, and cause failure of lever pressing to terminate shock. The continuous avoidance procedure distinguishes tranquilizing agents of the benzodiazepine type from sedative-hypnotics but fails to differentiate between benzodiazepines and phenothiazine neuroleptics.

G. Effect on Food Intake

Randall et al. [1] found that chlordiazepoxide increased the food intake of starved rats by some 20 to 60%. Amphetamine caused an inhibition of food intake under these conditions. Similarly in chronic experiments, chlordiazepoxide administered in the diet increased food intake and enhanced growth in rats.

TABLE 5 Effects on Operant Behavior

Compound	Conflict behavioral technique in rats (effective dose mg/kg, p.o.)
Chlordiazepoxide	5-10
Diazepam	5-10
Flurazepam	10-20
Alprazolam	2
Triazolam	0.25

Hanson and Stone [32] related the food intake of starved rats to the
anxiolytic effects of chlordiazepoxide. Low doses of chlordiazepoxide increased food intake whereas high sedative doses decreased food intake.
Major tranquilizing agents and amphetamine only decreased food intake.

Poschel [33] devised a simple and specific screen for benzodiazepinelike drugs based on their ability to increase food intake. Naive, nonhungry,
nonthirsty rats tested with benzodiazepines ingested inordinate amounts of
a sweetened milk solution when given their first opportunity to drink the
solution. Among a number of other drugs tested only phenobarbital induced
a similar, although clearly weaker effect. This method provides a simple,
rapid, sensitive, and specific test for benzodiazepinelike drugs. The effects
of the drugs were interpreted as overcoming a rat's natural aversion to an
unfamiliar food substance without at the same time greatly sedating the
animal.

H. Biochemical Activity

A biochemical mechanism which explains the anxiolytic action of minor
tranquilizing agents has not been established. Many studies have attempted
to relate the behavioral effects of these agents to the metabolism of biogenic
amines. Taylor and Laverty [34] have found that minor tranquilizing agents
such as chlordiazepoxide, diazepam, and nitrazepam decrease the turnover
of both norepinephrine in the thalamus-midbrain, cortex, and cerebellum,
and dopamine in the striatum. These compounds also antagonized the increased catecholamine turnover in the same regions due to electro-foot-
shock stress.

Additional studies by the same investigators [35] showed that electroshock stress reduced the endogenous levels of norepinephrine and of [^{3}H]nor-
epinephrine after intraventricular administration of [^{3}H]dopamine. Minor
tranquilizing agents such as chlordiazepoxide, diazepam, and nitrazepam
maintained the levels of norepinephrine and [^{3}H]norepinephrine formed
from [^{3}H]dopamine at values above the stress-induced depleted levels. The
effect was greater in the cortex, cerebellum, and thalamus-hypothalamus-
midbrain regions than in the brain stem. Thus the effects on dopamine
metabolism were greater in those regions in which the benzodiazepines prevented the increase in catecholamine turnover induced by stress.

Rat brain levels of serotonin and its primary metabolite 5-hydroxyin-
doleacetic acid were not significantly changed by chlordiazepoxide or diazepam [36]. Chase et al. [37] found that diazepam did not influence the uptake
of radioactive serotonin in rat brain. However, diazepam caused increased
retention of serotonin in brain after intraventricular administration of radioactive serotonin and a marked elevation of 5-hydroxyindoleacetic acid.
These effects of diazepam were interpreted as indicating a decreased metabolism of serotonin and a decreased transport of its metabolite.

Minor tranquilizing agents appear to effect only the turnover of catecholamines and histamine and not the endogenous levels of these biogenic
amines. Other CNS drugs such as the phenothiazines, tricyclic antidepressants, and amphetamines modify endogenous levels, metabolism, and
reuptake mechanisms of biogenic amines in the brain.

The most prominent biochemical changes that occur with minor tranquilizers relate to their effect on stress-induced increases in plasma corticoids. One result of psychic stress is an increase in plasma corticoids
[38,39]. For example, plasma corticoids have been shown to increase in
animals which are transferred from a home cage to an experimental cage.
This phenomenon has been used to evaluate the anxiolytic activity of a
series of minor tranquilizing agents [40,41]. Minor tranquilizers were
found to be specific inhibitors of the elevation of plasma corticoids in rats
subjected to mild stress. Other psychoactive compounds such as chlorpromazine, imipramine, protriptyline, amitriptyline, and morphine were
not active. Thus, this test system appears to be specific for minor tranquilizing agents, and the rank order of potencies for these agents was found
to correspond to their clinical rank order.

IV. FUTURE RESEARCH

Minor tranquilizing agents at present have certain deficiencies and future
research in this area should attempt to develop compounds which will reduce anxiety or tension without producing excessive drowsiness or decreased
performance. New compounds should not impair discrimination, memory,
or learning.

Future research will require a more concerted effort to discover the
mechanism(s) and site(s) of action of the minor tranquilizers in animals
and man. Research should be most fruitful in neuropharmacology to eluci-
date the mechanism of action of drugs on the limbic system and in psychopharmacology to uncover mechanisms by which drugs relieve anxiety, tension, and related somatic symptomatology affecting muscular, cardiovascular, gastrointestinal, genitourinary, and autonomic systems. Since
stress affects all body systems and the minor tranquilizing agents act to
antagonize the physiological actions of stress, understanding the mechanism
by which this effect manifests itself is important to the development of
future minor tranquilizing agents.

V. SUMMARY

This brief review of the pharmacological properties of the minor tranquilizing agents was not intended to present all possible methods for the detection of anxiolytic activity. The methods are those which may be of use in

evaluating potentially active clinical entities and differentiating them from such other psychoactive agents as the major tranquilizers and sedative-hypnotics. The chapter illustrates the multiple activities of the minor tranquilizing agents and attempts to correlate some of these activities with anxiolytic effects in man.

REFERENCES

1. L. O. Randall, W. Schallek, G. A. Heise, E. F. Keith, and R. E. Bagdon, J. Pharmacol. Exp. Ther. 129, 163 (1960).

2. L. O. Randall, G. A. Heise, W. Schallek, R. E. Bagdon, R. F. Banziger, A. Boris, R. A. Moe, and W. B. Abrams, Curr. Ther. Res. 3, 405 (1961).

3. S. Irwin, in Psychopharmacology (E. H. Efron, ed.), Public Health Service Publ. No. 1836, 1968, pp. 185-204.

4. S. Norton and E. J. De Beer, Ann. N.Y. Acad. Sci. 65, 249 (1956).

5. R. N. Straw, in Hypnotics—Methods of Development and Evaluation (F. Kagan, T. Harwood, K. Rickels, A. D. Rudzik, and H. Sorer, eds.), Spectrum, New York, 1975, pp. 65-82.

6. D. G. Friend, Clin. Pharmacol. Ther. 5, 871 (1964).

7. J. B. Hester, A. D. Rudzik, and B. V. Kamdar, J. Med. Chem. 14, 1078 (1971).

8. E. A. Swinyard and A. W. Castellion, J. Pharmacol. Exp. Ther. 151, 369 (1966).

9. S. E. Svenson and L. E. Gordon, Curr. Ther. Res. 7, 367 (1965).

10. A. D. Rudzik, J. B. Hester, A. H. Tang, R. N. Straw, and W. Friis, in The Benzodiazepines (S. Garattini, E. Mussini, and L. O. Randall, eds.), Raven Press, New York, 1973, pp. 285-297.

11. L. O. Randall and B. Kappell, in The Benzodiazepines (S. Garattini, E. Mussini, and L. O. Randall, eds.), Raven Press, New York, 1973, pp. 27-51.

12. G. Zbinden and L. O. Randall, in Advances in Pharmacology (S. Garattini and P. A. Shore, eds.), Academic Press, New York, 1967, pp. 213-291.

13. R. D. Hudson and M. K. Wolpert, Neuropharmacology 9, 481 (1970).

14. L. O. Randall and W. Schallek, in Psychopharmacology (D. E. Efron, ed.), Public Health Service Publ. No. 1836, 1968, pp. 153-184.

15. A. D. Rudzik, W. Friis, and C. A. Solomon, Abstracts of the Fifth International Congress on Pharmacology, 1972, p. 197.

16. G. Chen and B. Bohner, Proc. Soc. Exp. Biol. Med. 106, 632 (1961).

17. R. F. Banziger, Arch. Int. Pharmacodyn. Ther. 154, 131 (1965).

18. R. N. Straw, Arch. Int. Pharmacodyn. Ther. 175, 464 (1968).

19. W. Schallek and A. Kuehn, Proc. Soc. Exp. Biol. Med. 105, 115 (1960).

20. S. Requin, J. Lanoir, R. Plas, and R. Naquet, Soc. Biol. (Paris) 157, 2015 (1963).

21. A. Morillo, Int. J. Neuropharmacol. 1, 353 (1962).

22. L. Valzelli, in The Benzodiazepines (S. Garattini, E. Mussini, and L. O. Randall, eds.), Raven Press, New York, 1973, pp. 405-417.

23. W. P. Heuschele, J. Am. Vet. Med. Assoc. 139, 996 (1961).

24. A. J. Christmas and D. R. Maxwell, Neuropharmacology 9, 17 (1970).

25. J. M. R. Delgado, in The Benzodiazepines (S. Garattini, E. Mussini, and L. O. Randall, eds.), Raven Press, New York, 1973, pp. 419-432.

26. I. Geller and J. Seifter, Psychopharmacologia I, 482 (1960).

27. I. Geller and J. Seifter, J. Pharmacol. Exp. Ther. 136, 284 (1962).

28. I. Geller, in Psychosomatic Medicine (J. H. Nodine and J. H. Moyer, eds.), Lea & Febiger, Philadelphia, 1962, pp. 267-274.

29. I. Geller, Arch. Int. Pharmacodyn. Ther. 149, 243 (1964).

30. L. Cook and A. B. Davidson, in The Benzodiazepines (S. Garattini, E. Mussini, and L. O. Randall, eds.), Raven Press, New York, 1973, pp. 327-345.

31. J. R. Vogel, B. Beer, and D. E. Clody, Psychopharmacologia 21, 1 (1971).

32. H. M. Hanson and C. A. Stone, in Animal and Clinical Pharmacologic Techniques in Drug Evaluation (J. H. Nodine and P. E. Siegler, eds.), Yearbook, Chicago, 1964, p. 317.

33. B. P. H. Poschel, Psychopharmacologia 19, 193 (1971).

34. K. M. Taylor and R. Laverty, Eur. J. Pharmacol. 8, 296 (1969).

35. K. M. Taylor and R. Laverty, in The Benzodiazepines (S. Garattini, E. Mussini, and L. O. Randall, eds.), Raven Press, New York, 1973, p. 191.

36. A. Pletscher, in International Symposium on Psychotropic Drugs in Internal Medicine (A. Pletscher and A. Marino, eds.), Excerpta Medical Foundation, Amsterdam, 1969, p. 1.

37. T. N. Chase, R. I. Katz, and I. J. Kopin, Neuropharmacology 9, 103 (1970).

38. J. W. Mason, J. V. Brady, and M. Sidman, Endocrinology 60, 741 (1957).

39. A. Pekkarinen, Acta Pharmacol. Toxicol. (Suppl.) 28, 71 (1970).

40. R. A. Lahti and C. Barsuhn, Psychopharmacologia 35, 215 (1974).

41. R. A. Lahti and C. Barsuhn, Res. Commun. Chem. Pathol. Pharmacol. 11, 595 (1975).

Chapter 8

ANTIDEPRESSANTS

Dewey H. Smith, Jr., and Vernon G. Vernier

Pharmaceuticals Division
E. I. du Pont de Nemours & Company, Inc.
Stine Laboratory
Newark, Delaware

I. INTRODUCTION

Depression is the most common psychiatric disorder and is a major public
health problem in many countries today. There are now nearly 100 million
depressed people in the world, and this number is expected to increase [1].
Medical treatment for depressed patients then must necessarily rely heavily
on chemical antidepressant therapy. The primary purpose of this chapter
is to provide a reference source of pharmacological and biochemical methodology for the detection and evaluation of new antidepressant drug therapies.
To do this effectively requires an acquaintance with the disease itself, the
technical jargon that surrounds it, and a brief survey of the present modes
of treatment.

II. THE DISEASE

Depression or melancholia is an affective or primary mood disorder [2]; it
is neither a single disease nor a discretely defined group of diseases. In
clinical psychiatry, depression can imply "a normal mood state, a pathological symptom, one or more clinical syndromes, or one or more disease
entities" [3]. The common symptoms include sadness, listlessness,
apathy, definite feelings of unworthiness, insomnia, anorexia, weight loss,
diminished libido, preoccupation with hypochrondriacal thoughts, and preoccupation with thoughts of suicide. Since the nomenclature in this field is
varied and not altogether consistent, the following scheme is offered as an
aid to reading and understanding the vast and varied literature.
    Depressions may be classified as endogenous (or vital) in which the
patient's condition is unaffected by environmental factors. Endogenous
depressions are characterized by a clear-cut onset; classical symptoms
include psychic retardation, loss of initiative, and preoccupation with suicidal thoughts. Endogenous depressions may be further classified as bipolar
(or manic-depressive) in which there is a known history of manic or hypo-
manic episodes, and unipolar depression in which there is no known history
of mania. Endogenous depressions are recurrent more often than nonre-
current. Endogenous depressions are sometimes classified as involutional
in which delusions of guilt or paranoia may be present. Involutional

depressions usually occur after age 45. Patients with endogenous depression generally respond well to antidepressant therapy, better than depressed patients of all other types.

Some depressions are reactive (neurotic, situational), i.e., they occur in response to some acute stress situation. Reactive depression (including pathological grief) usually remit spontaneously and therefore the clear-cut efficacy of antidepressant therapy is difficult to demonstrate unless patient group size is large.

Depressions also may be schizoaffective, i.e., a depressed condition that is a secondary feature of a schizoid type of illness. Schizoaffectives generally respond better to treatment with neuroleptics (major tranquilizers) than to treatment with antidepressants.

Neurasthenics, or patients with chronic characterological depressions, have chronic personality problems. These types respond briefly to almost all forms of therapy but are particularly suited to psychotherapy for long-term improvement.

Endogenous and reactive depressions together may be further classified as agitated or retarded. In agitated forms there is considerable anxiety present; these types respond better to therapies which include a sedative or tranquilizer component. The retarded forms respond better to treatments which avoid sedation.

And finally, depression may be merely a "normal" mood state. In such instances the somatic components of depression, anorexia, weight loss, dizziness, headache, fear, and trembling are usually absent [4].

III. THERAPIES

Although depression has been recognized for over 2000 years [5], probably the earliest recorded treatment (and of doubtful value) was the use of hellebore prescribed for "melancholia" in the early eighteenth century [6]. In 1927, with the discovery of the mood-elevating and euphoric effects of amphetamine, the age of chemical antidepressant therapy was born [7]. During the 1930s many modifications were made on the phenethylamine skeleton. These amphetamine-type stimulants found some use in the treatment of reactive depression but most were of little value in treating endogenous depression. Electroconvulsant therapy (ECT) came into use in the early 1930s and was tried in the treatment of all types of mental illness. The greatest success of ECT was found in the treatment of endogenous depression. After the discovery of the monoamine oxidase inhibitors and the tricyclic antidepressants in the late 1950s the popularity of ECT declined considerably. Later with the advent of good skeletal muscle relaxants interest in the use of ECT resumed. Because of its reputedly early onset of action and its high improvement rate (nearly 90%) ECT still remains the treatment of choice with some clinicians in potentially suicidal patients [8].

The early onset of therapeutic effect may be debated but the usual concomitant hospitalizing of the patient gives control and assurance against
early suicide.

Most effective antidepressants fall into two classes, the monoamine
oxidase inhibitors (MAOI) and the thymoleptics. The latter are a group
largely of tricyclic and tetracyclic compounds, most of which are somewhat
structurally related to the phenothiazine neuroleptics. Both types have been
reviewed extensively [9,10]. The discovery of antidepressant activity in
both the MAOI and the thymoleptics occurred rather serendipitously and
almost simultaneously. Kuhn [11] in 1957 noted that imipramine, an imino-
dibenzyl being tested as an antipsychotic, was inactive as such but was
effective in the treatment of depression. Kline et al. [12] in the same year
found that iproniazid, an MAOI originally synthesized for the treatment of
tuberculosis, was effective in depressed patients. The MAOI, although by
many reports as effective in man as the thymoleptics and ECT, are more
risky to use because they can cause hypertensive crises. Because of this
and because the thymoleptics have played a major role in antidepressant
therapy, particularly in the United States, the thymoleptics are treated here
in more detail than the MAOI and the other agents used in the treatment of
depression.

Other treatments which have met with varying degrees of success in
treating affective disorders include lithium and rubidium salts, cyclic AMP,
thyrotropin-releasing hormone (TRH), and certain narcotics and narcotic
antagonists. Lithium treatment was introduced into psychiatry in 1969 [13].
Its subsequent use has proved it valuable for the treatment of mania and it
appears to be useful prophylactically for the prevention of depression.
Rubidium in 1969 and later cesium were suggested for the treatment of
depression.

A. Depressants

Sedatives have been used for many years in the treatment of agitated depressions particularly. Phenothiazine neuroleptics, especially thioridazine,
have also been used in anxious depressed patients. The most successful
thymoleptics, amitriptyline and imipramine, have neuroleptic and sedative
activity in addition to their antidepressant effects. Some success has also
been reported in the therapy of agitated neurotic depression using simultaneous treatment of a thymoleptic (protriptyline) and an anxiolytic (meprobamate) [14]. Diazepam and phenobarbital also appear to be effective in
neurotic depressives [15].

A relatively new drug, clozapine (1), a neuroleptic with some anticholinergic activity, may also be an antidepressant. In an uncontrolled study
[16] of 54 women and 22 men clozapine reportedly gave complete remission
in 50% of the cases and partial improvement in an additional 21%. As might
be expected the drug was more effective in atypical, anxious, and agitated
forms of depression rather than in retarded endogenous depressions.

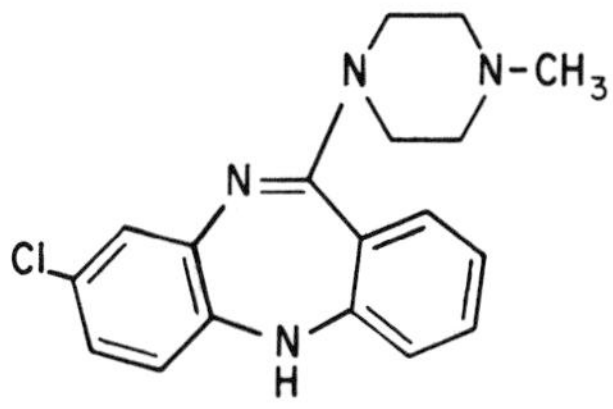

CLOZAPINE (1)

Trazodone (2) is the first representative of a new class of psycholeptic drugs which has clinically shown marked antidepressant activity [17]. In several controlled double blind studies, trazodone was as effective as imipramine and amitriptyline. Improvement in depressed patients has been reported as early as the second day of treatment but patients' conditions deteriorated upon withdrawal of the drug [18].

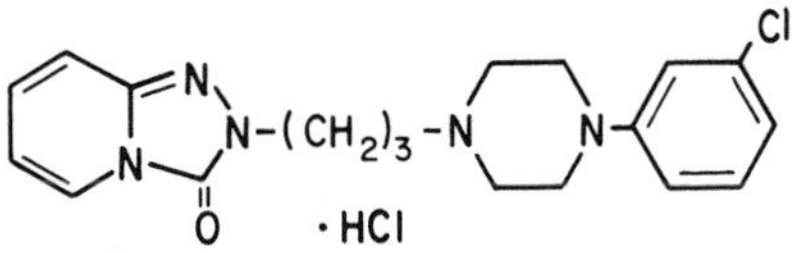

TRAZODONE (2)

In many parameters in animal studies, trazodone looks like a neuroleptic [19], but it does not reduce body temperature nor cause catalepsy. It decreases spontaneous motor activity and potentiates hexobarbital sleeping time. Trazodone is neither an MAOI nor does it potentiate catecholamines [20]. It was inactive in the mouse reserpine antagonism test and did not potentiate either 5-hydroxytryptamine (5HT) in mice nor amphetamine in rats; in fact, trazodone blocked amphetamine toxicity in grouped mice. Trazodone is not anticonvulsant and is very weak as a muscle relaxant.

Sulpiride (3) is a benzamide type of neuroleptic. When compared to amitriptyline in a single blind, 12-patient study, sulpiride appeared slightly more effective than the latter on depressive symptomatology [21], in particular as psychomotor retardation.

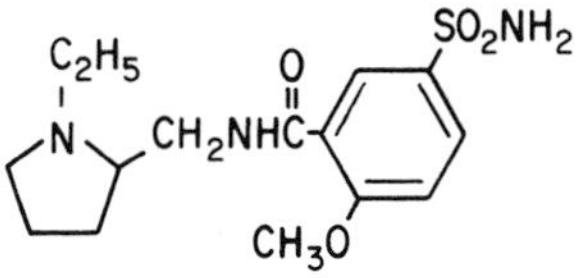

SULPIRIDE (3)

B. Stimulants

Many CNS stimulants including the amphetamines, methylphenidate, and pipradrol have been tried clinically in treatment of depression with limited success. These drugs produce alertness and some mood elevation but also cause anxiety and irritability. The stimulation and mood elevation are frequently followed by fatigue and exacerbation of the depressive symptomatology. The stimulants have the advantage of early onset of action but tolerance develops rapidly, and the drugs usually become ineffective after a few days. One psychomotor stimulant, cocaine, with a biochemical mode of action different from that of the amphetamines and similar to that of the thymoleptics, will probably never be tested as an antidepressant clinically because of abuse liability.

Pure stimulant amines may yet find a place in antidepressant therapy as well as for use in the treatment of minor reactive episodes. In an uncontrolled study of patients [22] with endogenous depression which previously did not respond to thymoleptic nor MAOI therapy, dl- or l-phenylalanine (precursor of phenethylamine, levodopa, dopamine, and norepinephrine) was given orally for 15 days. A complete euthymia was obtained in 17 of 23 subjects in 1 to 13 days. Further studies are needed.

Other studies of amino acid precursors of biogenic amines have not been as successful. In a double blind placebo-controlled study [23] of hospitalized depressed patients, relatively large doses of levodopa and l-tryptophan yielded only minor clinical improvement in a few patients; in no case was the improvement sufficient to warrant the patient's discharge.

C. Monoamine Oxidase Inhibitors

The MAOI are clearly effective as antidepressants, and in most studies have been equal in efficacy to the thymoleptics. These have been reviewed in detail [9,10]. Because the mechanism of action of the MAOI is not currently considered a desirable one, at least in the United States, discussion of this class of antidepressants is brief.

From the horde of MAOI that have been synthesized in the last 40 years, only five are now marketed in the United States. Three of these, phenelzine (4), isocarboxazide (5), and nialamide (6), are hydrazine derivatives, the other two, tranylcypromine (7) and pargyline (8), are not. Phenelzine

PHENELZINE (4)   ISOCARBOXAZIDE (5)

NIALAMIDE (6)

TRANYLCYPROMINE (7)   PARGYLINE (8)

and tranylcypromine are clinically effective as antidepressants but the efficacy of isocarboxazide and nialamide is less clear. Pargyline is primarily used as an antihypertensive, but appears to have some effect as an antidepressant [24].

Monoamine oxidase (MAO) in human brain is a complex of isoenzymes, each apparently having different abilities to metabolize various substrate amines [25]. The ability of MAOI to block oxidation of substrate varies with the identity of the substrate, e.g., tranylcypromine and isocarboxazide block oxidation of tyramine, tryptamine, and kynuramine more potently than they block oxidation of dopamine. Norepinephrine and serotonin unfortunately were not studied as substrates. The lack of desirable substrate and organ specificities of the MAOI limits their usefulness and has led to toxicological and regulatory problems.

D. Thymoleptics

This large group of antidepressants includes the classical tricyclics, some newer tetracyclics, and certain others, all of which do not inhibit MAO in their pharmacologically effective dose range and have virtually none of the CNS stimulant actions of direct and indirect acting amines. Most of these drugs do inhibit the presynaptic uptake of catecholamines.

The clinical efficacy of the thymoleptics is well established. In an extensive review [26] thymoleptics were considerably more effective than placebo in 61 of 93 studies, whereas in no study was placebo more effective than a thymoleptic. Six compounds of this class are now being sold in the United States. Of these, amitriptyline and imipramine are the most important; the others are desipramine, nortriptyline, protriptyline, and doxepin.

The tricyclic antidepressants have replaced the psychomotor stimulants for the treatment of various depressive states and in general they are considered at least as effective as and much safer to use than the MAOI [27].

Thymoleptics are particularly effective in endogenous depressions, and recently imipramine has been found useful in childhood enuresis, hyperactivity, and school phobia. Side effects from tricyclic therapy usually stem from cholinergic blockade; reversal of the toxic effects can be accomplished with physostigmine [28,29].

1. Tricyclics

    a. Imipramine and related drugs   Many analogs of imipramine (9) have been synthesized in the search for improvement in clinical efficacy of this original example of the iminodibenzyls, but none has been found superior. Since most of these have been well reviewed [9,10], only a few of the more significant ones are considered here.

    Imipramine is an active antidepressant per se but also is active through its primary metabolite, desmethylimipramine [desipramine (10)]. The pharmacology of imipramine is typical of most of the iminodibenzyls. It is

IMIPRAMINE (9)   DESIPRAMINE (10)

weakly neuroleptic and causes depression in cats, dogs, and monkeys, and at high doses in rats and mice also [30]. Motor deficit is seen in rodent inclined screen and rotorod tests but high doses are required. Imipramine blocks fighting in isolated mice (ED50 = 31 mg/kg) and muricidal rat behavior, but unlike neuroleptics, it does not affect exploration of rats in a Y-maze. Neither imipramine nor desipramine blocks active or passive avoidance in rats but the former blocks Sidman avoidance in squirrel monkeys (at 20 mg/kg). Various cat EEG studies also suggest mild phenothiazinelike activity for imipramine and desipramine. Paradoxical sleep periods are reduced by both agents and the usefulness of imipramine in childhood enuresis may be related to this property. Imipramine and desipramine weakly block apomorphine-induced emesis in dogs. Both partially inhibit EST convulsions in rats but are ineffective against pentylenetetrazol in mice. Both partially block chlorpromazine-induced catalepsy in mice but not the effects of bulbocapnine. Imipramine somewhat prolongs hexobarbital sleeping time in rodents, has local anesthetic activity, and is active in the antiphenylquinone writhing analgesic test.

Imipramine and most other tricyclics potentiate exogenous norepinephrine responses, including pressor response in dogs, contractions of the
nictitating membrane in cats, and contractions of isolated rat vas deferens.
Imipramine also potentiates endogenously released norepinephrine in a
variety of preparations. The phenothiazines behave similarly at some
doses but the effect is masked by adrenergic receptor blockade at others.
Imipramine and desipramine inhibit mouse heart catecholamine depletion
induced by a variety of depletors, inhibit the postganglionic blockade by
guanethidine on nictitating membrane, and block the effects of carotid
occlusion.

Imipramine and other iminodibenzyls inhibit uptake of norepinephrine
through cell membranes, as do cocaine, the phenothiazines, and other
potentiators of norepinephrine responses. The iminodibenzyls slightly
depress epinephrine pressor responses and markedly and most characteristically block pressor action of indirect acting amines by blocking their
uptake into the norepinephrine stores. The iminodibenzyls also potentiate
many of the effects of the amphetamines such as increased motor activity
in rodents and hyperthermia; in most cases this is due to inhibition of
p-hydroxylase which metabolizes amphetamines. Certain antihistaminics
and anticholinergics potentiate the amphetamines also.

Imipramine and desipramine also potentiate the stereotypic and hyper-
thermic effects of levodopa in mice pretreated with a threshold dose of an
MAOI; anticholinergics do this as well. Other interactions of MAOI and
tricyclic antidepressant abound; e.g., imipramine and etryptamine in inactive doses separately, together cause fighting and squeaking in mice; tranylcypromine induces EEG arousal in dogs pretreated with imipramine.

Imipramine and related drugs block many effects of the amine-depleting
agents, reserpine and tetrabenazine. In animals whose brains have been
depleted by α-methyl-m-tyrosine prior to reserpinization, however, the
tricyclics are ineffective. The tricyclics generally do not block amine
depletion by reserpine in brain as the MAOI do but desipramine does slow
norepinephrine depletion by reserpine.

Imipramine and desipramine potentiate serotonin (5HT)-induced contraction of cat nictitating membrane; chlorpromazine diminishes the response.
Other effects of 5HT such as rat paw edema and contraction of the isolated
guinea pig ileum are diminished by the action of tricyclics. 5HT uptake
into blood platelets is inhibited by imipramine, chlorpromazine, and cocaine.
5HT hyperthermia in rabbits is augmented by imipramine and desipramine
but blocked by thioridazine. Like the phenothiazines, imipramine and
desipramine block 5-hydroxytryptophan (5HTP) stereotypies and convulsions
in mice, but large doses are required [31].

Imipramine potentiates acetylcholine at low doses and inhibits it at
higher doses both centrally [32] and peripherally [33]. Most tricyclics have
some anticholinergic activity similar to the phenothiazines. They cause

mild mydriasis in mice, block pilocarpine-induced salivation, and in vivo antagonize the hypotensive actions of acetylcholine and vagal stimulation. The tricyclics block tremorine-induced tremors in rodents apparently by inhibiting tremorine metabolism. They block oxotremorine-induced tremors only at high doses but more potently antagonize oxotremorine hypothermia. The tricyclics, like chlorpromazine, attenuate EEG arousal evoked by physostigmine.

Chlorimipramine (11), in a study of 138 episodes of endogenous depression in 107 subjects, was antidepressant in 84% and anxiolytic in 80% of the cases [34]. Improvements seen with imipramine and imipramine

CHLORIMIPRAMINE (11)

plus ECT were about equal. In another study of 24 subjects with endogenous depression, chlorimipramine was about equal to imipramine in both antidepressant and anxiolytic efficacy [35].

Chlorimipramine was more potent than imipramine or desipramine in blocking attack behavior in cats induced by hypothalamic stimulation [36]. p-Chlorophenylalanine (PCPA), which selectively depletes 5HT, antagonized the effect of chlorimipramine and the blocking action was restored by giving 5HTP. 6-Hydroxydopamine, which lowered hypothalamic norepinephrine, did not antagonize chlorimipramine. Chlorimipramine blocked fenfluramine-induced depletion of rat brain 5HT but imipramine and desipramine did not [37]. Chlorimipramine also blocked fenfluramine anorexia. Similarly chlorimipramine but not desipramine blocked PCPA depletion of brain 5HT [38]. Chlorimipramine also inhibited reuptake of 5HT much more potently than reuptake of norepinephrine [39].

Dimethacrine (12), homomeric with imipramine, was less antidepressant and less sedative than imipramine in a double blind clinical study [40]. Previously reported early onset of action [41] was not confirmed. Dimethacrine was less anticholinergic than imipramine and altered liver function more. It is reportedly equipotent with imipramine in the antitetrabenazine test.

Iprindole (13) was equal to imipramine in efficacy in a study of 100 depressed and anxious depressed patients [42] but yielded less sedative and autonomic side effects. Iprindole was particularly effective in patients with little or no anxiety and was ineffective in the anxious group whereas

DIMETHACRINE (12)   IPRINDOLE (13)

imipramine was effective in the latter. Iprindole differs from imipramine
in pharmacological action since it does not block norepinephrine uptake.
It is not active in the antitetrabenazine test but does potentiate amphetamines.
This latter property apparently is due to inhibition of the p-hydroxylase
enzyme which metabolizes amphetamines.

b. Amitriptyline and related drugs   Amitriptyline (14) therapeutically
is undoubtedly the most useful thymoleptic marketed today. Most major
pharmacological actions of amitriptyline are similar to those of imipramine

AMITRIPTYLINE   (14)

but the sedative and neuroleptic potencies of amitriptyline are greater.
Clinically, the antidepressant potency of amitriptyline is about the same as
that of imipramine [43]. Orally, in mice amitriptyline was about half as
potent as imipramine for antagonism of tetrabenazine-induced ptosis and
locomotor deficit (Table 1), and was less potent than imipramine in a reserpine ptosis test [44].

All aspects of depression are not affected to the same degree by amitriptyline (and probably other tricyclics). In a study of 172 depressed
women given amitriptyline for 4 to 6 weeks rapid improvement was seen in
the first week in suicidal feelings, insomnia, and anorexia, but impaired
work and interest, retardation, and pessimism improved more slowly [45].
Neurotic depressives improved dramatically in the first week but psychotic
depressives did not show marked improvement until the third week.

Amitriptyline poisonings have been reported to cause arrhythmias and
coma. These are apparently due to anticholinergic actions and are counteracted by physostigmine [28]. Imipramine and chlorimipramine also have
anticholinergic and cardiovascular side effects in man.

TABLE 1   Primary Antidepressant Tests

Drug[a]	Antitetrabenazine test ED50 (mg/kg, p.o.)				ED50, p.o. for prevention of haloperidol catalepsy in mice[c]
	Mouse		Rat[b]		
	Explor.	Ptosis	Explor.	Ptosis	
Imipramine	2.7	1.0	13.7	0.6	16.3
Amitriptyline	4.7	1.7	50.0	3.8	5.6
Protriptyline	0.61	0.47			
Doxepin	>125.0	12.0			
Maprotiline	8.0	3.9			2.6
Pheniprazine*	2.2	2.2			
Phenelzine*	17.0	17.0			
Pargyline	34.0	30.0			
Cocaine	8.1	3.2			
d-Amphetamine*	0.63	0.43			
Meperidine	13.3	6.9			
Tripelennamine	3.0	1.6			
Molindone[d]	11.1	8.5			

[a]HCl salts, except those marked with an asterisk are sulfates.
[b]Data from Dr. M. Cohen, Endo Laboratories.
[c]Data from S. Ueki et al. [60].
[d]At 2 hr.

Protriptyline (15) is an effective antidepressant in man and is potent in animal model systems, but it is without sedative action in either man or animal. It is four times as potent as amitriptyline in the mouse antitetrabenazine test and 10 times as potent as the latter in the dog pressor response test. Because protriptyline lacks any sedative or tranquilizing ability it is not useful in agitated forms of depression.

Butriptyline (16) is in many respects pharmacologically similar to imipramine and amitriptyline [46]. However, in a double blind study of 28 neurotic depressives, butriptyline appeared significantly superior to imipramine in improving symptoms of depression and anxiety while causing fewer side effects.

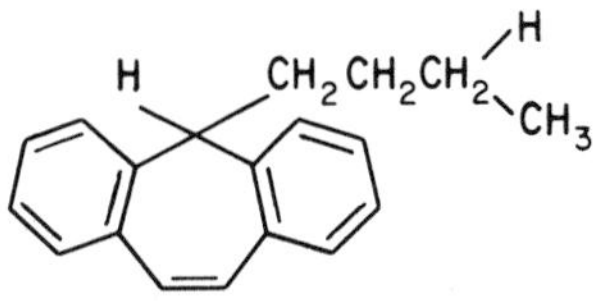

PROTRIPTYLINE (15) 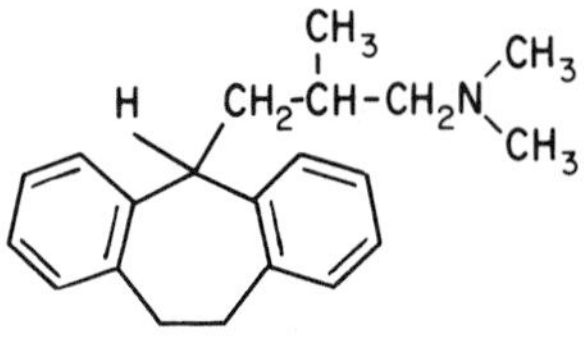   BUTRIPTYLINE (16)

Unlike most thymoleptics [48], butriptyline in cats did not potentiate the effects of norepinephrine or 5HT in causing contractions of the nictitating membrane. Butriptyline also did not antagonize guanethidine-induced blockade of electrically stimulated contraction of guinea pig vasa deferentia. In rabbits, however, butriptyline, like imipramine and amitriptyline, caused synchronization of the EEG and antagonized physostigmine-induced arousal.

Octitriptyline (17) was reported [49] to be extremely potent in blocking reserpine-induced hypothermia in mice. It was 500 times as potent as protriptyline orally but equipotent to the latter intraperitoneally.

Doxepin (18) differs structurally from amitriptyline only in the oxygen atom of the cycloheptadiene ring. Because it is more depressant in animal tests than amitriptyline and has neuroleptic activity, doxepin was expected

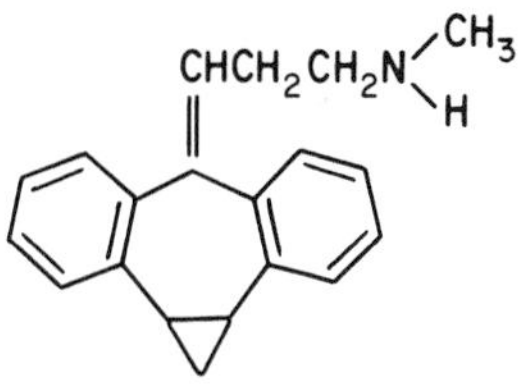

OCTITRIPTYLINE (17) 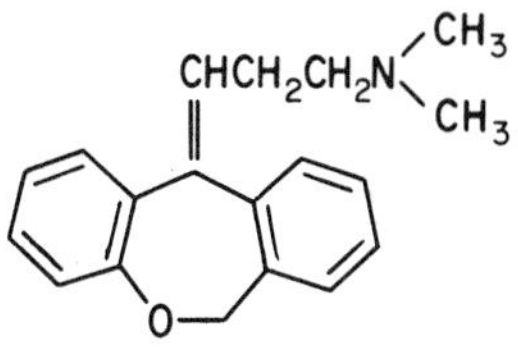   DOXEPIN (18)

to be particularly suitable for the treatment of patients with agitated forms of depression. The present clinical status has been reviewed [50]:

"Numerous clinical studies indicate that doxepin is not significantly different from other antianxiety and antidepressant drugs but their design was such that the null hypothesis was not likely to be rejected. Although doxepin can be used to treat both anxiety and depression it may present more hazards than the benzodiazepines and lack enough potency to treat severe depressions."

Both cis and trans isomers of doxepin were active in animal studies [51]. The cis isomer potentiated amphetamine and was strongly neuroleptic.

It also had antidepressant activity in man. In mice, doxepin was only moderately potent in blocking tetrabenazine-induced ptosis (Table 1) and failed to prevent the locomotor deficit. This mouse test appears to have predicted the degree of clinical antidepressant efficacy achieved.

Thiothixene (19) is basically a major tranquilizer but several studies have reported it to be useful as an antidepressant. In one 50-patient double blind study [52] of largely reactive depressions, thiothixene appeared at least as effective as protriptyline and perhaps was more so.

OI 77 (20) is a new type of tricyclic which antagonized reserpine-induced hypothermia in mice and blocked muricidal behavior in rats [53].

THIOTHIXENE   (19)   OI 77   (20)

It potentiated amphetamine-induced gnawing in rats and amphetamine-induced hyperactivity in mice, and antagonized perphenazine-induced cata-lepsy in mice. OI 77 also reduced aggression of isolated mice and prevented restraint ulcers in rats. It potentiated the nictitating membrane response in cats induced by electrical stimulation or 5HT injection. OI 77 is not an MAOI.

2. Tetracyclics

Maprotiline (21) is the prototype for one group of tetracyclic antidepressants with tranquilizing properties.

In a double blind clinical trial of 135 hospitalized patients, 104 with endogenous depressions and 31 with neurotic depressions, maprotiline appeared more effective against the neurotic depressions [54]. Overall activity and onset of action were equal to those of imipramine and amitriptyline. In a similar small study [55], maprotiline was at least as effective

MAPROTILINE   (21)

as amitriptyline; however, three of four bipolar depressives given maprotiline developed hypomania. Other studies [56-58] have reported an earlier onset of action for maprotiline than for the tricyclics. Maprotiline was well tolerated in repeated doses and apparently caused fewer side effects (heartburn, tachycardia, excitement, and sweating) than imipramine [59].

In mice, maprotiline antagonized reserpine-induced hypothermia [60] and ptosis but less potently than imipramine. Also in mice, it potentiated methamphetamine and levodopa and was six times as potent as imipramine against haloperidol-induced catalepsy (Table 1) and 2.5 times as potent as amitriptyline against rat muricidal behavior. Maprotiline lacks anticholinergic activity since it does not block physostigmine as do amitriptyline and imipramine. It inhibits reuptake of norepinephrine much more potently than reuptake of 5HT.

Mianserin (22), a tetracyclic with a fused piperazine moiety, was selected for clinical study based on its EEG effects in normal volunteers [61]. In a clinical trial [62] mianserin reportedly elevated mood, was effective

MIANSERIN   (22)

in agitated depressions, and had early onset, usually 2 to 3 days. Pharmacologically, mianserin differs from most tricyclics and somewhat resembles minor tranquilizers [63,64]. It is neither anticholinergic nor neuroleptic but causes α-adrenergic receptor blockade at high doses. Unlike tricyclics, mianserin potentiated α-methyl-p-tyrosine (AMPT)-induced catecholamine release in rats [65]. Mianserin itself did not affect catecholamine turnover acutely but upon dosing for 21 days, it did increase turnover. Both chronically and acutely, mianserin slowed 5HT turnover.

Mianserin partly blocked d-amphetamine-induced circling in rats with unilateral striatal lesions. It was inactive in many standard antidepressant screening tests, including reserpine antagonism and muricidal rat tests. Although a potent antiserotonin agent in several tests, mianserin did not inhibit 5HT uptake by human blood platelets as do amitriptyline and other tricyclics.

3. Others

Oxaflozane (23) blocked reserpine-induced ptosis (0.25 X imipramine) in mice and antagonized prochlorperazine catalepsy (1.0 X imipramine)

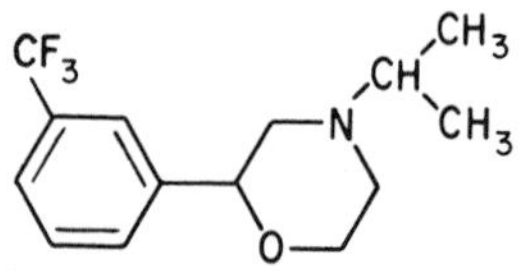

OXAFLOZANE (23)

in rats [66]. At high dose, oxaflozane per se was cataleptogenic. It very weakly potentiated amphetamine-induced stereotypies in rats and failed to block 5HT depletion in mice. Oxaflozane weakly decreased locomotor activity and potentiated barbiturate-induced sleep. It was 15 times as potent as imipramine and twice as potent as chlordiazepoxide in a rat anti-aggression test, suggesting possible anxiolytic activity. Oxaflozane lacks neuroleptic activity since it failed to antagonize amphetamine toxicity in grouped mice. It antagonized oxotremorine less potently than amitriptyline or imipramine.

Viloxazine (24) is hard to classify; it has some amphetaminelike properties at low doses in animals but generally its pharmacological profile

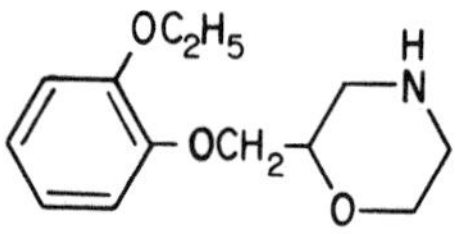

VILOXAZINE (24)

differs from those of CNS stimulants [67]; like the thymoleptics it is not an MAOI. At high doses in animals it is a central depressant. In man, viloxazine is less anticholinergic than imipramine [68], but more frequently causes nausea and vomiting [69]. Though it is an effective antidepressant it does not offer advantages over established thymoleptics.

Nomifensine (25) is a thymoleptic with some CNS stimulant activity. Like nortriptyline and protriptyline it inhibited norepinephrine uptake by

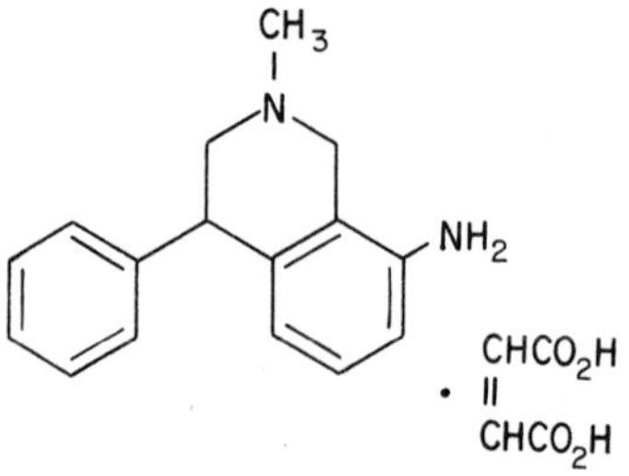

NOMIFENSINE (25)

synaptosomes [70] from rat hypothalamus and like amphetamine but unlike
known tricyclics it potently inhibited norepinephrine uptake by synaptosomes
from whole brain, and mildly inhibited 5HT uptake.

E. Univalent Cations

1. Lithium

The pharmacology of lithium has been reviewed in detail [71-74]. Lithium
salts are now recognized as effective treatment for mania and hypomania
of bipolar endogenous depressions [75-78] but the effectiveness of lithium
treatment for unipolar depressions is less certain. Early reports indicated
that lithium not only lacked efficacy but in some cases aggravated the depressed state. Recently [79], however, of over 300 depressed patients,
56% were improved by lithium treatment to some extent; some of these patients had failed to improve on ECT therapy. Most of the successes were
in bipolar endogenous depressions. With lithium, the onset of action was
1 to 2 weeks, similar to that of thymoleptics and MAOI. On the other hand,
lithium in eight double blind studies [26] was conclusively beneficial in none.
In one study [80] of 45 depressed patients combined therapy of lithium plus
a thymoleptic or an MAOI appeared more effective than thymoleptic or
MAOI alone.

The prophylactic value of lithium against both manic and depressed
phases of manic-depressive psychosis seems clear. In an extensive 6.5-
year study [81] of 88 manic-depressives, mean relapse time was stretched
from 8 months for controls to 72 months for lithium-treated patients. Although lithium treatment is effective therapeutically for mania and prophylactically for both mania and depression, its use is risky because the
effective dose is very close to the toxic dose. Thus lithium therapy requires
close monitoring of plasma lithium levels and the clinical effects produced.

Lithium appeared to increase neuronal uptake of amines but decrease
vesicular binding since chronic pretreatment of rats with LiCl increased
uptake and retention of (-)-erythrometaraminol but not (-)-m-octopamine
[82]. Lithium increased uptake of norepinephrine into synaptosomes [83]
and increased norepinephrine intracellular metabolism and turnover rate
in brain tissue [84,85], thus decreasing the availability of norepinephrine
at adrenergic receptor sites. These actions are in direct contrast to those
of typical thymoleptic and MAOI antidepressants and to those of rubidium.
Lithium also inhibited electrically evoked release of norepinephrine and
5HT in rat brain slices [86].

In mice [87] treated daily for 7 days, subcutaneous LiCl depressed
spontaneous motor activity in a dose-related manner whereas similar
treatments with RbCl and CsCl augmented motor activity; KCl treatment
had no effect.

In preliminary testing, lithium appeared to potentiate the antidepressant effect of desipramine and other thymoleptics [80].

2. Rubidium and cesium

In early studies in the 1880s many patients had reported a sense of well-being while being treated with RbCl. These reports were virtually unnoticed until the rebirth of medical interest in metal ions in the late 1960s.

The behavioral, EEG, and biochemical properties of rubidium salts are in direct contrast to those of lithium salts. Rubidium and cesium act like antidepressants in certain animal model systems but not in others. Rb_2CO_3 and CsCl both increased motor activity in mice when given subcutaneously for 7 days [87]. Rubidium also potentiated the locomotor stimulant action of morphine in mice [88]. In rats, RbCl given for 10 days increased metanephrine content of brain stem whereas similar LiCl treatment reduced it [83]. In other rat studies, rubidium increased norepinephrine turnover while cesium was ineffective; cesium, however, increased 5HT turnover 40% [89, 90].

RbCl elevated adrenal enzymes involved in catecholamine biosynthesis [91] and this may in part contribute to increased norepinephrine turnover. Rubidium potentiated shock-induced aggression in rats but cesium did not.

Clinical data are scanty. In one small clinical study, five depressed patients improved on rubidium [92]. Since the biological half-life of rubidium is 50 to 60 days, weekly or bimonthly dosing might be feasible, but if adverse effects were encountered the long half-life could be a serious problem. The status of rubidium as an antidepressant has been reviewed [91] with special emphasis on safety.

F. Cyclic AMP

Adenosine 3':5'-cyclic monophosphate (cyclic AMP), which has been suggested as a neurotransmitter [93], is abundantly present in brain. Cyclic AMP is formed from ATP by the enzyme adenylcyclase and is degraded by cyclic AMP phosphodiesterase; both also are abundant in brain. The phosphodiesterase is inhibited by tricyclic antidepressants and by chlorpromazine, leading to an increase in the cyclic AMP supply. Lithium, which is antimanic, inhibits the production of cyclic AMP. Cyclic AMP is reported to prevent or reverse reserpine-induced ptosis in mice [94]. Urinary cyclic AMP is decreased in both endogenous and neurotic depressions [95].

In a controlled 2-week clinical study of 26 depressed (or manic) female patients and 18 healthy adult females, 13 depressed subjects who had improved symptomatology also had more than doubled excretion of urinary cyclic AMP. The manic patients who had improved or became depressed had decreased excretions of cyclic AMP, and the healthy control subjects showed no change in urinary cyclic AMP. In another clinical study [96] of manic-depressives urinary excretion of cyclic AMP on the day of "switch" from depression to mania was significantly greater than the "preswitch" level. Treatment of four depressed patients with levodopa greatly increased cyclic AMP excretion and the two with the highest cyclic AMP excretion showed the greatest clinical improvement. Finally, in 13 patients [97], ECT increased urinary cyclic AMP 310% over preshock levels while four patients prepared for treatment but not shocked had slightly reduced cyclic AMP excretions.

G. Thyrotropin-Releasing Hormone

As yet there has been no convincing evidence of thyroid dysfunction in depressions [2], however, thyrotropin-releasing hormone (TRH) may have antidepressant action of its own.

TRH, produced in the hypothalamus, potently stimulates thyrotropin (TSH) and prolactin formation in the pituitary in man [98,99]. Prange et al. [100] in treating 10 euthyroid women with unipolar depressions reported that TRH gave prompt but brief improvement without significant side effects. Some investigators [101,102] have provided confirmatory evidence for the efficacy of TRH but many others found TRH only mildly effective in a few cases [103] or totally ineffective [104] as an antidepressant in man. TRH was reported active, however, in the pargyline-primed levodopa potentiation test [105] which is used in many antidepressant screening programs. The effect probably was not due to TSH release since TRH was also active in hypophysectomized mice. TRH did not potentiate yohimbine in conscious dogs [106], a test reportedly positive for thymoleptics and negative for CNS stimulants.

H. Narcotic Analgesics and Narcotic Antagonists

Cyclazocine has been reported clinically to have antidepressant activity [107] and to antagonize reserpine- and tetrabenazine-induced depressions in mice [108]. Morphine and naloxone also have been reported to have anti-reserpine activity. Meperidine in combination with d-amphetamine appeared effective in an uncontrolled study of 22 depressed patients [109]. Meperidine has antitetrabenazine activity (Table 1).

I. Electroconvulsive Shock Therapy

Electroconvulsive shock therapy (ECT) today is still one of the most effective treatments for endogenous depressions [110,111], in which 88% of the patients show improvement. ECT is effective in both manic and depressed

phases of bipolar depression [112]. Improvement after ECT has been noted
as early as Day 3 and most responders show improvement by Day 7. Because
of this relatively early onset of effect, ECT is currently the method of
choice for cases in which suicide is likely. However, the many CNS disrup-
tive effects of ECT (memory and subtle cognitive functions) are now becoming
better recognized. These effects plus the general aversiveness of the treatments to the patients and other hazards such as fractures (although fairly
well controlled by a muscle relaxant, e.g., succinylcholine) bring to question the desirability of using ECT.

Electroshock lowers rabbit brain norepinephrine [113] and raises
brain serotonin [114]. Overall ECT appears to promote release of norepinephrine in brain [115,116]. For example, when [^{3}H]norepinephrine was
given intracisternally and followed by ECT, the [^{3}H]norepinephrine content
of brain decreased and the [^{3}H]normetanephrine content increased.

The use of ECT in combination with antidepressant drugs has been reviewed [117]. Although the available information is scanty the combination
of methods appears to lower the relapse rate [118] and reduce the number
of ECT treatments necessary [119]. There is a great need for well-designed
studies of ECT and antidepressant drug combinations employing double blind
techniques.

J. Combination Treatments

A recent review [120] points out that despite all the individual therapies
available, 10 to 28% of depressed patients remain refractory. Because of
the high suicide risk more severe therapeutic techniques may be justified.
A first approach is to increase dosages, and this has met with some success.

Although it is generally considered dangerous to combine antidepressant drug therapies, especially when one component is an MAOI, solid evidence that combinations are unsafe appears lacking [121,122]. Several
investigators found no serious side effects from combined administration of
thymoleptics and MAOI. In one study [121] of 84 patients in which combination therapies included carefully controlled doses of thymoleptics and MAOI
plus ECT, 82 patients showed some degree of improvement; none were
worsened. The patients were warned not to eat the tyramine-containing
foods and not to take other medications without the physician's approval,
and they suffered no ill effects.

Similarly, combinations of thymoleptics with d-amphetamine or methylphenidate [123] have been tried with some success. Others have reported
that Li$_2$CO$_3$ plus an MAOI [124] or a thymoleptic [125] was effective in alleviating depressions. Pretreatment or simultaneous treatment with reserpine can make depressed patients more sensitive to treatment with thymoleptics [126]. Onset of action with imipramine was decreased to 1 to 2 days
by means of concomitant artifically induced pyrexia [127].

Combination therapies of a thymoleptic plus triiodothyronine (T3) have been the subject of many trials; the results of most have suggested earlier onset of antidepressant action. In a recent study of 44 depressed patients, all of whom were refractory to thymoleptics alone or thymoleptics plus tranquilizer treatments, 35 improved on a thymoleptic plus T3. TSH could replace T3 but the long duration of action of TSH makes dose control difficult. TRH has been reported to work also [128].

Combinations of antidepressants and vitamins have been suggested because various vitamins have been found deficient in depressed patients. These include folic acid, pyridoxine, and tryptophan. Some investigators have reported success with combinations of tranylcypromine plus large doses of tryptophan, with clinical improvement appearing in 2 to 3 days [129,130].

Combinations of steroids plus antidepressant therapy have some reported success. Dexamethasone plus imipramine, amitriptyline, or nialamide was better than antidepressant alone; clinical responses in some cases appeared as early as 3 days [131]. Estrogen therapy has been successful in treating menopausal depression [132]; data on estrogen-antidepressant combinations are not yet available.

Certain other drugs may be useful in antidepressant combination therapies. The anti-parkinsonian drug, amantadine, showed significant antidepressant activity [133]. The neuroleptic, molindone, also may be an antidepressant [134]. Molindone antagonized tetrabenazine in mice (Table 1). S-Adenosylmethionine was reported to have a rapid and intense antidepressant effect in over 80% of 49 depressed patients [135].

Patients with endogenous depression appear to benefit from sleep deprivation [136]. Combined treatments of sleep deprivation plus antidepressant therapy apparently have not yet been tried.

IV. MECHANISMS OF ANTI-
     DEPRESSANT ACTION

Depressed patients have been shown to have greatly reduced biogenic amine metabolite concentrations in their tissues. In susceptible persons with a prior history of depression, reserpine has been known to precipitate the depressed state. Since reserpine can also totally deplete the biological stores of catecholamines and indolamines, it has been logical to associate the existence of affective disorders with an insufficiency of one or more biogenic amines. More selective depletions of norepinephrine and dopamine by α-methyl-p-tyrosine (AMPT), which inhibits tyrosine hydroxylase, or of 5-hydroxytryptamine (5HT) by p-chlorophenylalanine (PCPA) have not been associated with human depression. In animals AMPT does cause sedation and decreased motor activity and suppresses conditioned avoidance responses, but PCPA in animals causes hyperaggressive behavior reminiscent of mania rather than depression [137].

It seems clear that in depressed patients there are decreased turn-over rates for central catecholamines and indolamines. In a study of 38 depressed and 12 control patients treated with probenecid, which blocks transport of acid metabolites from the CNS to the bloodstream, the accumu-lations in the cerebrospinal fluid (CSF) of homovanillic acid (HVA) from dopamine and 5-hydroxyindoleacetic acid (5-HIAA) from 5HT were less in the depressed group than in the controls [139]. The 14 patients with de-creased HVA all exhibited motor retardation, suggesting the involvement of dopamine in this feature of depression. In probenecid-treated patients given oral tryptophan, the content of this amino acid in the CSF of depressed patients tripled but was hardly changed in the controls, and 5-HIAA content in the CSF of the depressed group was less than that of the controls. Thera-peutic response to nortriptyline, which more potently blocks catecholamine reuptake than indolamine reuptake, is less in patients with low 5-HIAA in the CSF [138]. In 10 depressed patients, 5 with low CSF levels of HVA and 5 with normal HVA, treatment with levodopa and a peripheral carboxylase inhibitor nearly abolished motor retardation in the low HVA group but not in the others; no effect was seen on mood.

Coppen hypothesized that affective disorders result from abnormal tryptophan metabolism [139]. As positive support for this, certain types of depressed patients have decreased tryptamine excretion and decreased 5HT levels in the CSF [140,141].

It has been suggested that reduced phenethylamine (PE) levels may be directly involved in some cases of depression [142]. Brain PE is lowered by reserpinelike drugs and is raised by MAOI and thymoleptics. Its pre-cursor, phenylalanine, raises cerebral PE and antagonizes reserpine tremor and rigidity in the rat but neither causes hyperkinesis nor antagonizes reserpine hypokinesis [142]. Of 11 depressed patients (mostly endogenous) with low urinary PE output who were treated 15 days orally with d-phenyl-alanine, all showed some improvement paralleling increased urinary PE levels. Complete euthymia was achieved within 10 days in five cases.

In spite of the diversity of agents which have been more or less suc-cessful in the treatment of depression, the actions of most of these can be related to biogenic adrenergic amine metabolism. The catecholamine hypothesis, which has been excellently reviewed [143], evolved 10 years ago as the etiological basis for affective disorders. It remains neither proved or disproved but is as useful today as it was then. Norepinephrine appears to be the major neurotransmitter involved in depression, but dopa-mine and 5HT also may play a role, at least in some cases [138,140,141, 144]. Norepinephrine and possibly 5HT levels contribute to mood while dopamine deficit may be responsible for motor retardation. Reserpine-induced depression in animals appears to be the result of norepinephrine depletion. In reserpinized rabbits pargyline could not reverse the depres-sion in the presence of resynthesized dopamine and 5HT, but only did so when norepinephrine had risen to about 50% of the prereserpine level.

Additionally, levodopa, the precursor of the dopamine and norepinephrine, counteracted reserpine-induced depression, but 5HTP, the precursor of 5HT, did not [145-147].

An enormous amount of research has been done to relate the actions of antidepressants to the function of one or more of these amines.

Amphetamine and other drugs with a β-phenethylamine skeleton are presumed to be "antidepressant" mainly by stimulating the release of norepinephrine from its presynaptic bound state. However, catecholamine-depleting agents such as reserpine, tetrabenazine, and α-methyl-m-tyrosine do not block the stimulation of amphetamine. To account for this it has been necessary to postulate two presynaptic catecholamine "pools," one a smaller functional pool affected by amphetamines and other indirect acting amines, and a larger storage pool which is drained by the major depletors and not affected, except at very high doses, by the amphetamines. Some β-phenethylamines also may be "antidepressant" by direct stimulation of central adrenergic receptors. Amphetamine also can block uptake of norepinephrine and this may in part contribute to its action [148].

The action of MAOI appears mainly due to prevention of norepinephrine destruction by MAO. The slow onset of action of these drugs may reflect the time needed to build the neurotransmitter supply up to threshold level. MAOI also may act through prevention of destruction of other monoamines which in turn either release the natural neurotransmitter or per se activate the receptors.

The mechanism of action of the thymoleptics is not known. From data on the cat nictitating membrane response, Sigg [149] first proposed that the tricyclics act by sensitizing central adrenergic receptor sites. Later it was shown that tricyclics blocked neuronal uptake of norepinephrine peripherally and centrally [150-152]. From these findings it was hypothesized that tricyclics were antidepressant because they blocked the presynaptic reuptake of catecholamines. Most thymoleptics block indolamine uptake also.

It has also been suggested that 5HT may be involved in the antidepressant action of imipramine and other thymoleptics [153]. Depression returned to patients on imipramine when given small doses of PCPA, a specific 5HT depletor, for a few days, but similar patients given AMPT, which depletes mostly norepinephrine and dopamine, in large doses for several weeks showed no signs of returning depression. In a repeated dose test in rats, imipramine was more effective in blocking 5HT depletion of PCPA than it was in blocking norepinephrine and dopamine depletion by AMPT. Imipramine, per se, slowed 5HT turnover; other tricyclics are reported to do this also [154]. Chlorimipramine, in contrast to imipramine and desipramine, blocked rat brain 5HT depletion by fenfluramine [37].

Most thymoleptics also have both central and peripheral anticholinergic effects. It has been proposed that the central anticholinergic activity may be responsible for the antianxiety and antiagitation effects of these drugs [155].

Less is known of the mechanism by which other antidepressant medication and therapies act. ECT appears to promote release of norepinephrine [115,116]. Cyclic AMP may be a neurotransmitter [93] and is reported to antagonize reserpine in mice [94]. The enzymatic destruction of cyclic AMP is inhibited by thymoleptics, and lithium inhibits its production. Lithium appears to increase catecholamine uptake and increase intracellular turnover whereas rubidium appears to act oppositely [84,85].

V. ANIMAL MODELS AND TEST SYSTEMS

The ideal animal model test system for antidepressants is not yet available because a true animal model of human mental depression does not exist. Most available methods for the detection and evaluation of antidepressants rely on drug interaction studies, and most of those are based on the catecholamine hypothesis for mood [143,156]. Although some of these tests have been fruitful in providing new antidepressants they are likely to produce only those drugs which alter catecholamine metabolism and will not likely detect any which may operate by some other mechanism.

This section is meant to contain all the currently used antidepressant screening and evaluation methods of merit plus a few which need further development and validation.

A. Antagonism of Reserpine or Tetrabenazine

Reserpine can precipitate mental depression in man [157-159]. Reserpine and related drugs cause profound (blepharo) ptosis, depression of locomotor or exploratory activity, and hypothermia in mice and rats and thus have provided a well-known "model of depression" in laboratory animals. The locomotor depression and ptosis are central effects but the hypothermia may be peripheral [160]. Prevention or reversal of these effects has been used widely as the foundation of methods for detection of new antidepressant species [161]. All thymoleptics and MAOI of proven antidepressant efficacy in man and psychomotor stimulants and some narcotic agonists, antagonists [107,162], and antihistamines prevent the induction of ptosis. In mice the depression of locomotor activity is prevented by most tricyclic antidepressants such as imipramine and amitriptyline. Pretreatment of mice with an MAOI followed by tetrabenazine results in frank psychomotor stimulation such as is seen with an amphetaminelike drug per se. In rats excitement of manic proportions is produced when repeated doses of desipramine are followed by a large intravenous dose (32 mg/kg) of tetrabenazine.

All antidepressants and psychomotor stimulants both prevent and reverse the hypothermia of reserpine and tetrabenazine [163]. In mice but not in rats, reserpine hypothermia also is blocked by chlorpromazine [164] and by such diverse drugs as aspirin, diethyldithiocarbamate, pentylene-tetrazol, morphine, and LSD 25.

1. Ptosis and locomotor depression

Both of these parameters are easily measured in a modification of a test described by Vernier et al. [161]. Tetrabenazine rather than reserpine is used because of its rapid onset of action and decreased peripheral autonomic actions.

Mice or rats deprived of food for 2 hr are dosed orally with test drug followed at an appropriate time, usually 0.5 hr, by tetrabenazine methane-sulfonate (free base weight 32 mg/kg for mice, 20 mg/kg for rats). In mice 30 min later the test animal is placed in the center of a 12 × 8 × 1-in. screened animal box lid on the bench top and locomotor and exploratory activity are observed for 10 sec. Relief of locomotor depression is scored when a mouse either moves to the edge of the screen or moves its head at least 30° to each side (minimum 60° of arc) of center. To determine ptosis in mice the animal is grasped by the tail and nape of the neck and held facing the observer. Two seconds later relief of ptosis is scored when both eyelids are >50% open. To determine ptosis in rats the animals are held by the tail on the bench top facing the observer but otherwise are scored the same as are mice. The data for blockade of both exploratory loss and ptosis are treated quantally and the ED50 (median effective dose) values and confidence limits are calculated according to the method of Thompson and Litchfield [175] respectively.

2. Hypothermia in mice

In spite of its nonspecificity, reversal of reserpine-induced hypothermia is useful as a crude screening method for antidepressant activity. From a method of Askew [166] mice are given reserpine (5 mg/kg, i.p.) followed 2 to 18 hr later by oral test drug. Rectal temperatures are taken at 0.5, 1, 2, and 4 hr after test drug and these are compared to the predrug values or to values of concurrent vehicle-treated controls. To get meaningful results ambient temperature must be controlled and mice must be equilibrated, preferably at 20 ± 1°C. The criterion of antidepressant activity is a statistically significant reversal of the hypothermia and so quantitative sensitivity becomes a direct function of the number of animals tested. By use of a large number of control animals (30 or more) and suitable transforms ED50 values can be calculated.

It has been reported recently [167] that thymoleptics also prevent apomorphine-induced hypothermia in mice. The hypothermic mechanism involved is probably dopaminergic or serotonergic but certainly not cholinergic since atropine is not effective. Additional studies are needed to

determine if there is the nucleus of an antidepressant evaluation method
here since pimozide and spiroperidol are reportedly active also.

B. Antagonism of Adrenergic
    Blocking Agents

In recent years two new tests for antidepressants have been reported which
are based on the prevention or reversal of the action of adrenergic blocking
agents. Haloperidol or a phenothiazine such as prochlorperazine has been
used in test procedures similar to the antitetrabenazine test. The parameters measured are ptosis, exploratory activity, hypothermia, and especially catalepsy. In the second test pimozide, a dopamine-blocking agent,
produces similar symptomatology.

1. Haloperidol-induced catalepsy

Haloperidol, a potent α-adrenergic blocking agent, causes profound depression of locomotor activity, loss of muscle tone, catalepsy, and marked
hypothermia. Reversal of catalepsy makes a convenient endpoint to use as
an indicator of antidepressant activity. Test drugs are given orally to mice
followed by an ED98 intraperitoneal dose of haloperidol. Thirty min or so
later the mice are tested for catalepsy. Maprotiline [60] and amitriptyline
are reportedly more potent than imipramine in this test (Table 1).

2. Antipimozide test in mice

Pimozide is a dopamine receptor blocking agent which at 12.5 mg/kg, i.p.,
in mice gives marked behavioral depression and decreases locomotor activity, muscle tone, and body temperature [108]. Tests with a limited number of drugs suggest that a pimozide depression assay may separate thymoleptics from central stimulants, MAOI, and certain narcotic analgesics
and narcotic antagonists, all of which are active in the antitetrabenazine or
antireserpine mouse tests. More data are needed to assess the true value
of a pimozide depression assay in sorting out antidepressant drugs.

C. Potentiation of CNS Stimulants

The excitement, locomotor stimulation, anorexia, and other properties of
amphetaminelike drugs are thought to be due to catecholamine relase.
Levodopa, the biological precursor of dopamine and norepinephrine, is
thought to act pharmacologically through these amines. Both thymoleptics
and MAOI actively potentiate amphetamines and levodopa; the thymoleptics
probably act by blockade of catecholamine reuptake but they may also

potentiate methamphetamine by blocking its metabolism [168]. Promethazine, which is an antihistaminic, potentiates methamphetamine by this mechanism [169]. Activity in the methamphetamine potentiation test should be confirmed by some other antidepressant test.

1. Dopa potentiation in mice

MAOI markedly potentiate the excitatory effects of levodopa, and a standard in vivo test (see Section V.I.2.b) for MAOI activity is based on this property. By threshold priming with a low dose of an MAOI the levodopa potentiation test has been adapted [170] for the additional detection of thymoleptic drugs which per se will not potentiate levodopa.

In a modified protocol groups of four mice housed in wire-topped cages (8 × 5 × 4 in.) are intubated with 40 mg/kg pargyline hydrochloride 18 hr prior to test. Test drugs are given orally, symptoms from them are recorded, and 1 to 4 hr later 100 mg/kg levodopa is given intraperitoneally. The mice are scored 0.25, 0.5, and 1.0 hr after levodopa for increased irritability, reactivity, jumping, squeaking, and fighting behavior. Data for some thymoleptics and phenelzine are shown in Table 2 in which the MAOI primer was nialamide [171].

2. Methamphetamine potentiation in rats

Thymoleptics enhance behavioral effects of the amphetamines whereas neuroleptics antagonize them [172-174]. Amphetamine potentiation has been useful in characterizing iprindole which is antidepressant clinically but is inactive against tetrabenazine. Certain anticholinergics and antihistamines also potentiate amphetamine but these can be sorted out in other tests. The following modified test procedure is suited for detection of thymoleptic activity.

Rats, four per group, are intubated with test drug and are challenged intraperitoneally at 1.5 hr with 3 mg/kg methamphetamine or d-amphetamine. At 2, 4, and 6 hr after test drug the rats are observed and scored for increased motor activity, stereotyped head movements, continuous licking, biting, and gnawing. The number of rats showing at least one stereotypy is counted, the data are analyzed quantally, and the ED50 values are calculated [165,175] for each time period of observations. Alternatively, the various behavioral signs may be graded and quantitative data analysis may be used.

A variation of the methamphetamine potentiation test involves self-stimulation testing in rats [176]. In these tests, rats with electrodes implanted in the median forebrain bundle or the lateral hypothalamus are taught to press a lever to receive a "reward" of electrical stimulation. Antidepressants per se are ineffective but they increase markedly the self-stimulation rate of the threshold dose of 0.25 mg/kg, i.p., methamphetamine.

TABLE 2   Antidepressant and Stimulant Tests

Drug[a]	Picrotoxin potentiation[b] s.c.		Dopa potentiation[c] p.o.
	ED50 (mg/kg)	Time (hr)	ED50 (mg/kg)
Imipramine	15.2[d]	2	35.0
Desipramine	14.2	2	9.0
Amitriptyline	—	—	10.0
Doxepin	—	—	35.0
Viloxazine	18.9	1	—
Phenelzine	—	—	8.0
Tranylcypromine[*]	13.4	2	2.2
Nialamide	5.6	1	—
Pargyline	—	—	50.0
Morphine[*]	25.2	0.5	—
Diphenylhydantoin[†]	4.6	4	—

[a]HCl salts except (*) = sulfates and (†) = sodium.
[b]Data from Cowan and Harry [179].
[c]Data from Gouret and Reynaud [171]; the MAOI primer was nialamide.

Complex in design, this test version is less practical than others for use in a broad antidepressant screening program.

Another variation of the methamphetamine potentiation test involves enhancement of anorexia [177]. Rats are weighed before and 6 hr after various doses of oral drug and 0.75 mg/kg, i.p., methamphetamine. In a 400 g rat methamphetamine alone causes a 5 g weight loss which can be boosted to 13 g by imipramine. The test is sensitive but lacks specificity since in addition to antidepressants, central stimulants, many depressants, and purely anorectic drugs also can cause or enhance anorexia.

D.   Potentiation of Convulsants

Two convulsant tests have come into use for the detection of antidepressant activity. These have the advantage of a clear-cut endpoint. More data are needed to assess their usefulness in an antidepressant program.

1. Yohimbine-induced convulsions in mice

Imipramine appears to potentiate the autonomic and psychic effects of yohimbine in man and to increase yohimbine lethality in mice [178]. Yohimbine causes intermittent clonic convulsions in mice which last several hours.
The effects of yohimbine differ from those of amphetamine as evidenced by
the lack of continuous hyperactivity and lack of increased mortality in
grouped animals.

Many drugs have been found to cause increased yohimbine toxicity,
including thymoleptics, some phenothiazine tranquilizers, especially chlorpromazine, certain MAOI, and most adrenergic stimulants. Cholinergic
blocking agents and α-adrenergic blocking agents are weakly active, but
β-adrenergic blockers are inactive.

Although it is easily performed and the endpoint is clear, this test appears to be of limited usefulness because of the apparent lack of specificity.

2. Picrotoxin-induced convulsions in mice

Picrotoxin produces convulsions in mice and rats and these convulsions are
potentiated by imipramine [162,179]. Diphenylhydantoin potentiates the
convulsive effect of picrotoxin but trimethadione does not. Diphenylhydantoin also is active in the mouse reserpine-reversal test [180].

Male albino 20 to 24 g mice, 10 per group, are dosed orally or subcutaneously with test drug at 0.5 to 4 hr prior to a challenge with 3.5 mg/kg,
i.p., picrotoxin. The number of mice convulsing within 45 min is scored
and ED50 values are calculated quantally [165,175]. The ED50 values for
several antidepressants are shown in Table 2. Morphine was active but
other narcotic analgesics and narcotic antagonists were not. Representative
major tranquilizers, anxiolytics, psychomotor stimulants, and antihistamines also appeared to be inactive. Pending additional evaluation this test
could be a useful adjunct to an antidepressant screening program.

E. Behavioral Tests

Ideally, tests for antidepressant effects should be based on behavioral models free of interactions with other drugs. Since endogenously depressed
rats or mice are not available we must turn to tests which measure effects
on normal or conditioned behavior in normal animals. Of the several tests
listed here the most successful has been the use of muricidal behavior inherent in some rats.

1. Unconditioned behavior in rats

Two tests have been described which measure the effects of drugs on exploratory activity, general locomotor activity, and emotional reactivity [181].

These are the Novelty Preference Test and the Open Field Test. By these two tests imipramine is clearly differentiated from amphetamine. Both drugs inhibit exploratory behavior but amphetamine stimulates locomotor behavior whereas imipramine depresses it. Imipramine blocks defecation but amphetamine does not.

a. <u>Novelty preference test</u>   A Y-maze with arms 150 mm high × 300 mm × 400 mm is used. Two arms are neutrally colored and the third arm, separable by a removable partition, is striped black and white. The maze is lighted (40 W) at 3 ft above the arms' intersection.

Initially the third arm is blocked off and the rat is placed in one of the other arms for 40 min, during which time it is injected with drug or placebo. At 40 min, the partition is removed and the number of arms entered (locomotor activity) and the total time spent in the striped arm (exploratory activity) are recorded for a 10-min observation period.

b. <u>Open field test</u>   In a white circular arena, 83 cm in diameter with walls 33 cm high, the floor is divided into 19 equal sections. A 70 dBA background white noise at floor level and a background light (5 × 200 W) 4 ft above the floor are used throughout the test. At a suitable time after dosing with drug or placebo the rat is placed in the center of the open field and is observed for 5 min. The numbers of crossing made and fecal boluses dropped are scored.

2.   Muricidal rat test

A small percentage of rats will spontaneously and instinctively kill a mouse within minutes of presentation [182]. Antidepressants and certain antihistamines (e.g., tripelennamine) and anxiolytics selectively block this behavior at doses which do not cause motor deficit. Muricidal behavior appears to involve a discrete brain sector, the amygdala, since bilateral lesions in this sector abolish muricidal behavior. Because amygdaloid afterdischarge is depressed by antidepressants [183], the amygdala may be involved in depression and in antidepressant function. One advantage of the test is that it does not involve drug interactions. One disadvantage of the test is its lack of specificity; another is that the preparation and maintenance of a supply of mouse-killing rats requires considerable preselection effort.

In one version of the test [169], male rats are isolated in individual cages, fasted 24 hr, and then each rat is challenged by placing a mouse in his cage. Those rats which kill the mouse within 30 min are selected for further intensification of their mouse-killing behavior. Eventually these preselected rats will kill mice within 30 sec of presentation without prior fasting and will continue to kill mice if presentations are spaced a few minutes apart. Muricidal rats rarely eat the mice.

In a typical protocol, five rats per intraperitoneal dose of test drug are presented at 30-min intervals with mice. Mouse-killing behavior is considered blocked when the mouse is not attacked within 30 sec of presentation. Quantal ED50 values for prevention of muricidal behavior are calculated based on the 30-sec cutoff [175]. An advantage of this procedure is that both dose- and time-response data are available in a single test.

3. Others

a. Rat swim-stress-fatigue test   A test has been proposed [184] in which rats are made to swim in a 7 × 8 × 24-in. container filled with water at 30°C. Predosing orally with imipramine or amitriptyline at 3 mg/kg increased swim time from a baseline of 100 min to about 200 min. Desipramine (10 mg/kg), ipronazid (10 mg/kg), and metrazol (30 mg/kg) also were active orally, and morphine (0.3 mg/kg) was active subcutaneously. Tranylcypromine, pheniprazine, anxiolytics, neuroleptics, and cholinolytics apparently were inactive. A detailed follow-up evaluation of this test has not been reported, but such a method might merit further examination.

b. Motor activity and aggressiveness in 3-day-old chicks   In 3-day-old chicks which have an inefficient blood-brain barrier [185], imipramine, desipramine, and amitriptyline all increase motor activity whereas imipramine and desipramine but not amitriptyline cause aggressiveness as evidenced by "attack pecking." Only transient sedation was elicited by the three drugs in 4-week-old chicks.

c. Mouse rotorod test [186]   A 1-in.-diameter dowel divided into 10 equal 3.5-in. spaces by 8-in.-diameter plastic disks is operated by a kymograph motor rotated at 11 to 12 rpm. Average performance time for a mouse at 11.44 rpm is 30.2 ± 2.2 min. Pheniprazine intraperitoneally at 2 hr after dose was effective (ED50 = 0.8 mg/kg) in prolonging performance time on the rotorod as was intraperitoneal amphetamine (ED50 = 5.1 mg/kg); caffeine was inactive up to 20 mg/kg. A further look at this test and the effects of other types of antidepressants seems warranted.

F. Autonomic Tests

1. Amine pressor responses in vivo

Effects on the pressor responses to norepinephrine and to indirect acting amines such as phenethylamine and tyramine in dogs and cats have been used to characterize antidepressants [187,188]. In these tests the tricyclic antidepressants mimic the effects of the stimulant cocaine. At doses at which they per se have no effect on blood pressure, the tricyclics potentiate

the pressor effect of norepinephrine and antagonize the pressor effects of
the indirect acting amines. Certain antihistaminics, e.g., tripelennamine,
which potently block amine uptake in adrenergic neurons are also active in
the test. The frankly stimulant direct and indirect acting amines potentiate
pressor responses of both norepinephrine and phenethylamine and also have
considerable pressor response of their own. The MAOI act differently than
the thymoleptics in these tests. For example, phenelzine intravenously in
the "ganglion blocked" dog has little effect on the response to norepinephrine
but augments the pressor effects of phenethylamine. Chlorpromazine at
low doses blocks both norepinephrine and phenethylamine but at high doses
the blockade of the norepinephrine effect disappears. Many thymoleptics
also have α-adrenergic blocking activity which to some extent obscures the
potentiation of the norepinephrine response. In the ganglion-blocked dog,
amitriptyline at 1 mg/kg, i.v., potentiates norepinephrine pressor response
25% but at 3 mg/kg the response to norepinephrine appears unpotentiated.
The test dose range must be carefully chosen so that thymoleptic-type activity will not be missed. One advantage of this test is that it distinguishes
among thymoleptics, MAOI, and stimulant amines. A disadvantage is that
it will detect and characterize only those antidepressants which affect catecholamine disposition.

   In a typical protocol four dogs are used per test drug and the data are
compared to those of at least as many control animals. The dogs are anesthetized with pentobarbital and the carotid or femoral artery is cannulated.
Blood pressure is measured directly by means of a Statham transducer and
is recorded on a Grass polygraph. The femoral vein is cannulated for administration of drugs. Ganglionic blockade is effected by 2 mg/kg, i.v.,
mecamylamine 15 min before injection of the other drugs. Then 1 μg/kg
norepinephrine is given followed at a suitable later time by 150 μg/kg
phenethylamine. After these "priming" doses a schedule of norepinephrine,
phenethylamine, and test drug is followed with increasing cumulative doses
of test drug. Potentiation and antagonism are expressed as the percentage
of mean control pressor response and the ED50% values are estimated
graphically.[1] Typical data are shown in Table 3.

2.   Antagonism of adrenergic neuronal blockade in vivo

The adrenergic neuronal blocking effect of guanethidine on the cat nictitating
membrane has been used to help define the action of thymoleptics, and the
method has been described in detail [189]. This method also is based on the
ability of these drugs to block the presynaptic uptake of biogenic amines and

---

[1] ED50% refers to the amount of drug needed to give a response 50% different from the mean response of control animals.

TABLE 3   Autonomic Tests

| Drug | ED50 for pressor effects in dogs[a] (mg/kg, i.v.) | | | | ED50 for potentiation of cat nictitating membrane response |
| | Norepinephrine potentiation[b] | Phenethylamine | | | |
		Antagonism[b]	Potentiation[b]	Drug only	
Imipramine	3.0	1.5		—	>2.0
Amitriptyline	1.0[c]	1.1		—	>2.0
Protriptyline	0.04	0.03		—	0.23
Pheniprazine	←		0.9		
Phenelzine[d]	No effect		2.0[e]	0.15	
Cocaine[f]	0.3	0.9		—	
Amphetamine[d]	No effect	0.3		0.014	
Chlorpromazine	→	0.4		↑	
Tripelennamine	←	1.0			

[a] In ganglion-blocked dogs.
[b] Stone [188] except as noted.
[c] This is an ED25% since an ED50% was not reached (see text).
[d] Data of J. M. Stump, Stine Laboratory, E. I. du Pont de Nemours & Company, Inc.
[e] Data for tyramine response instead of phenethylamine.
[f] Data of V. G. Vernier, Stine Laboratory, E. I. du Pont de Nemours & Company, Inc.

has advantages and disadvantages similar to the amine pressor response
tests in the ganglion-blocked dog.

3. Potentiation of yohimbine in conscious dogs

It has been reported [190] that thymoleptics and MAOI antidepressants potentiate pressor and behavioral responses of conscious dogs to intravenous yohimbine. Amphetamine and cocaine were essentially inactive in the test.
Data on other standard drugs are needed to determine the usefulness of this
test as part of an antidepressant drug program.

4. In vitro tests

Satisfactory in vitro tests for the potentiation of norepinephrine or the
blockade of phenethylamine and tyramine have not been worked out. In the
isolated rat vas deferens with mainly α-adrenergic receptors the doses at
which imipramine and amitriptyline inhibit norepinephrine uptake are not
separated sufficiently from the doses which block α-adrenergic receptors
[191]. Desipramine, chlorimipramine, and cocaine significantly potentiate
the norepinephrine-induced contractile response, however [192], and norimipramine blocks it. Imipramine, amitriptyline, and desipramine do
antagonize tyramine in this preparation but apparently by means of α-adrener-
gic blockade, rather than blockade of norepinephrine release [193]. Cocaine
is inactive in the tyramine test.
      Amitriptyline and chlorimipramine potently block 5HT-induced contrac-
tions of rat uterus; protriptyline and orphenadrine block less potently; and
imipramine, norimipramine, and tofenacine moderately inhibit this system.
      In the isolated guinea pig atrial strip test with mainly β-adrenergic re-
ceptors, amitriptyline blocked tyramine response [194]. Amitriptyline also
was reported to potentiate the effects of nerve stimulation in the isolated
guinea pig hypogastric nerve-vas deferens preparation at 0.01 times the
concentration that antagonizes nerve stimulation. More work is needed to
define the limits of usefulness of such in vitro tissue assays.

G. Inhibition of Catecholamine Uptake or Release

1. Inhibition of [7-^{3}H]norepinephrine uptake

      a. Mouse cerebral cortex slices   Test drugs are usually given in
vivo but an in vitro version of the test may be used [195]. In a modified in
vivo version mice are dosed orally or intraperitoneally with test drug or
vehicle and 1 hr later are killed. The brains are removed quickly and 100-
mg slices are prepared. These are incubated 5 min in 2 ml Krebs-Hense-
leit buffer containing 0.1 nmole/ml dl-[7-^{3}H]norepinephrine using a Dubnoff

metabolic incubator in an atmosphere of 93.5% O_2 and 6.5% CO_2. The slices then are blotted, weighed, and homogenized in 2 ml absolute ethanol. Then 0.1 ml of incubation medium is also mixed with 2 ml ethanol. All extracts are centrifuged and the tritium content is assayed by liquid scintillation counting.

The ratio of [7-^{3}H]norepinephrine in the slices to that in the medium is taken as a measure of norepinephrine uptake. Percent inhibition (P_I) due to test drug is calculated:

$$P_I = \frac{(R_c - R_i) \cdot 100}{R_c - 1}$$

where R_c is the control ratio of uptake and R_i is the ratio with inhibitor present. An ED50 is determined graphically. The ED50 values for intraperitoneal imipramine and desipramine are 6 and 2 mg/kg, respectively [195]. These values are somewhat larger than the corresponding oral ED50 values for prevention of ptosis in the mouse antitetrabenazine test.

b. Mouse heart   Good procedures also are available for determining drug effects on [7-^{3}H]norepinephrine uptake in mouse heart [196]. However, with the brain cortex slice methods available, uptake studies in peripheral organs assume lesser importance.

2. Antagonism of 6-hydroxydopamine or guanethidine

6-Hydroxydopamine and guanethidine peripherally deplete norepinephrine and the depletion is counteracted by thymoleptics [189]. In a modified protocol, test drugs are given orally or intraperitoneally to mice 1 hr prior to 7 mg/kg, i.p., 6-hydroxydopamine. Sixteen hours later the mice are killed, the hearts are removed and pooled in groups of five, and are homogenized in 6 ml wet butanol/g tissue. The homogenates are centrifuged and the clear supernatants are extracted with 0.1 N HCl (6 ml/10 ml butanol). The norepinephrine content is determined photofluorimetrically [197]. The amount of antagonist to inhibit depletion by 50% (ED50%) is estimated by linear regression analysis of percent inhibition versus log dose. All major thymoleptics are active; protriptyline is especially potent (ED50% = 0.09 mg/kg, i.p.).

H.   Encephalographic Activity

Imipramine and amitriptyline produce characteristic alterations of the EEG pattern in man [61]; these include "increased slow waves and superimposed fast activity." The effects on EEG patterns in human volunteers were helpful in predicting antidepressant activity for mianserin and OI 77 as well as cyclazocine (a narcotic agonist-antagonist). The use of encephalography in man or animals should provide a useful addition to the armamentarium currently available to the standard antidepressant screening programs. Drugs such as mianserin are inactive in most animal antidepressant tests.

I. Unwanted Side Effects

The current trend is to select antidepressants which are free of or have very little central stimulant activity and which are not long-acting MAOI. The following tests sort out these types of drug action.

1. Psychomotor stimulation

CNS stimulant effects are detected conveniently by measuring locomotor activity. A satisfactory procedure is described in Section V. J. 2; typical data for stimulants, thymoleptics, neuroleptics, and anxiolytics are given in Table 4.

2. Monoamine oxidase inhibitors

Most of the procedures already mentioned detect MAOI. In these tests, e.g., the antitetrabenazine test, the MAOI generally can be identified by their time of peak effects. In mice, thymoleptics and CNS stimulants usually peak at 30 to 90 min after oral dosing and are ineffective after 4 to 5 hr, whereas the irreversible MAOI usually peak at 4 to 8 hr and may still be at peak effect up to 48 hr. Confirmation of MAOI activity can be had by any of the following fairly specific tests.

   a. 5HTP and tryptamine potentiation tests   5-Hydroxytryptophan (5HTP), the biological precursor of 5HT, elicits a head twitch and convulsion in mice which correspond to increased free 5HT in the brain. The effect is strongly aggravated by pretreatment with an MAOI [31] and appears to be attenuated by thymoleptics and stimulants and by certain narcotic analgesics and antagonists [198]. The protocol involves 10 nonfasted 18 to 20 g mice per dose of test drug which is given subcutaneously 30 min before 200 mg/kg, i.p., 5HTP. Two-minute counts of head twitches are made at 9, 14, 19, 24, 29, and 34 min after 5HTP and the total number of twitches are summed. The data are treated quantitatively and an ED50% is calculated.
   An alternative test [199] employs 60 mg/kg tryptamine hydrochloride given intravenously 55 min after oral test drug. At 5 min after tryptamine injection the mice are observed for 30 sec for stereotyped head turning, twitching, and convulsings with "piano player" type movements of the front feet and for flaccid paralysis of the hindlimbs. Tryptamine alone, 60 mg/kg, causes this syndrome but it lasts for less than a minute, and usually only a

TABLE 4 Stimulant, Depressant, Neuroleptic, and Anxiolytic Tests

| Drug | Mouse ED50 values (mg/kg, p.o.) | | | | | Rat MED, p.o. Conflict[d] |
| | Locomotor activity of mice in pairs[a] | Catalepsy | Antagonism of | | | |
			Tryptamine[b]	5HTP[c]	PTZ	
Imipramine		245.0		59.0	Inactive	Inactive
Amitryptyline	35.0 ↓	70.0		1.4	90.0	—
Protriptyline	16.0 ↓	Inactive			Inactive	—
Doxepin	26.0 ↓	209.0			Inactive	—
Maprotiline		450.0			Inactive	—
d–Amphetamine	0.8 ↑	Inactive		5.6	—	—
Meprobamate		—			50.0	63.0
Chlordiazepoxide		—		36.0	7.5	2.2
Diazepam	2.0 ↓	108.0			1.2	0.63
Chlorpromazine	6.6 ↓	52.0	9.0	0.86	Inactive	Inactive
Haloperidol	0.5 ↓	3.2			Inactive	Inactive
Trifluoperazine		—	14.0		Inactive	0.17

[a]Free base basis.
[b]From Tedeschi et al. [199].
[c]From Corne et al. [31], ED50 for subcutaneous route.
[d]From Cook and Davidson [209].

few seconds. The data are analyzed quantally and ED50 values and confidence limits may be calculated [165,175]. Data for several drugs are shown in Table 5. All MAOI are active in this test whereas thymoleptics and psychomotor stimulants are inactive. The ED50 values of irreversible MAOI parallel those found in the antitetrabenazine test but the reversible MAOI, e.g., harmine, are several-fold weaker as tryptamine potentiators of head twitch than they are as tetrabenazine antagonists. However, ED50 values of the reversible MAOI for prevention of tetrabenazine-induced ptosis and for potentiation of tryptamine-induced hindlimb paralysis correlate closely.

b. Dopa potentiation   Potentiation of dopa-induced excitation and autonomic effects has been used as an in vivo assay of MAOI activity and for detection of thymoleptics [170]. The simplified versions described herein detect only the MAOI; the modification which detects thymoleptics also is discussed in Section V.C.1.

Mice, four per wire-topped (8 × 5 × 4 in.) cage, are dosed orally with test drug, and 4 or 24 hr later are challenged intraperitoneally with 100 mg/kg levodopa. The mice are scored at 0.25, 0.5, and 1.0 hr for increased irritability, reactivity, jumping, squeaking, lacrimation, salivation, and fighting behavior. Scores (0 to 3+ basis) for each treated group are compared to those of known saline vehicle controls (score = 0) and to a standard 100 mg/kg, p.o., dose of pargyline hydrochloride (score = 3+). Data are treated quantitatively and ED50% values are calculated by linear regression analysis. In a modified version of the test, levodopa is given intravenously 55 min after oral test drug and the mice are observed for 10 sec at 5 min after levodopa. Responses are scored quantally. Using salivation as the endpoint, quantal ED50 values for several MAOI and thymoleptics are shown in Table 5.

c. In vivo/vitro MAOI tests   In vivo/vitro methods involve giving the drug orally or intraperitoneally to the test animal, then isolating a tissue from which a crude homogenate enzyme system is prepared. The enzyme activity is measured in vitro against a suitable substrate. Since there are at least four MAO isoenzymes with possible different substrate and inhibitor specificities, it is best to use crude tissue homogenates and an appropriate substrate such as phenethylamine or tyramine when searching for undesirable MAOI activity. Brain MAO preparations are usually used, but the liver enzyme system probably is more germane. A manometric method using tyramine has been described [200].

In a modified protocol, two to four rats per test drug dose are intubated or injected intraperitoneally. One hour later the rats are killed and the brains or livers are excised quickly and homogenized in 10 ml of ice-cold distilled water per gram of tissue. The particulate fraction is separated by centrifugation and resuspended in ice-cold 0.67 M phosphate (pH 7.2) at 2.5 ml buffer/g tissue. The Warburg flask side arm is loaded with 0.2 ml of 0.032 M KCN and 0.2 ml of 0.15 M tyramine hydrochloride, then 1.0 ml

TABLE 5   MAOI Activity of Various Antidepressants

Drug	Mouse ED50 values					Mouse MAOI in vitro vs. 5HT KI50% (M/L)
	Tetrabenazine antagonism		Tryptamine potentiation		Dopa potentiation for MAOI[a]	
	Explor.	Ptosis	Stereotyp.	Paralysis		
Non-MAOI						
Imipramine	2.7	1.0	>120.0	>120.0	>135.0	2.8×10^{-3}
Amitriptyline	4.7	1.7	>120.0	>120.0	>135.0	4.0×10^{-3}
Protriptyline	0.61	0.47	>80.0	>80.0	>81.0	2.3×10^{-3}
Maprotiline	8.0	3.9	>135.0	>135.0	>135.0	2.3×10^{-3}
MAOI						
Tranylcypromine	3.0	2.2	2.6	1.9	1.6	2.8×10^{-6}
Pheniprazine	2.2	2.2	3.0	1.7		3.5×10^{-6}
Phenelzine	17.0	17.0	26.0	16.0	13.0	1.8×10^{-6}
Pargyline	34.0	30.0	61.0	19.0	30.0	2.0×10^{-5}
Nialamide	6.5	6.5	10.6	5.0	3.3	3.7×10^{-5}
Harmine	4.2	3.7	20.0	2.3		$<1.0 \times 10^{-7}$
Stimulants						
d–Amphetamine	0.63	0.43	>27.0	>27.0		1.0×10^{-4}

[a]Salivation endpoint.

homogenate and 1.6 ml pH 7.2 phosphate are put in the main compartment. The center well contains 0.2 ml 1 N KOH plus filter paper and the system is gassed with 100% O_2 and equilibrated to 38°C. The side arm contents are tipped into the main compartment and readings are taken at 0, 10, 20, and 30 min. Results are expressed in microliters O_2 consumed per gram of wet tissue per hour and the percent inhibitory activity is calculated relative to O_2 consumption of controls.

    d. In vitro MAOI tests   If an antidepressant fails to inhibit MAO in vitro, it probably is safe to assume it will not inhibit in vivo or in an in vivo/vitro test, but the in vitro methods for measuring MAO inhibition are not recommended as a final means of identifying possibly undesirable MAOI activity. This is because occasionally there are discrepancies noted between the effects in vitro and those observed in vivo and in the in vivo/vitro tests [200, 201]. In addition, appropriate substrates, such as tyramine and phenethylamine, are not useful in the sensitive fluorimetric methods employed in the usual in vitro methods.

    In vitro MAO studies might be useful, however, as a means of detecting types of MAOI with favorable specific activities by the choice of appropriate substrates. That is, antidepressant drugs which strongly inhibit destruction of norepinephrine or 5HT in vitro but fail to inhibit tyramine destruction may be desirable and perfectly safe to use.

    In a modified protocol [202] for brain MAO studies, 10 20 g mice or 3 100 g rats are killed. The brains are excised quickly and dropped into ice-cold 0.1 M phosphate pH 7.4, 10 ml/g wet tissue, and are homogenized for 5 min with ice chilling. The homogenate is stored at ice temperature until used. Test beakers (20 ml) are prepared with 1 ml homogenate and 0.5 ml test drug or water and are preincubated 10 min at 37°C with shaking in air using a Dubnoff metabolic incubator; 0.5 ml of the substrate 5HT, 2×10^{-4} M, is added and the samples, three per dose and three with substrate but no enzyme, are incubated for 60 min. The reaction is stopped by addition of 2 ml 0.5 M borate, pH 10.5. NaCl (2 g) is then added and the samples are extracted with 7 ml borate-washed n-butanol and centrifuged. Three milliliters of each n-butanol extract plus 5 ml of HCl-washed n-heptane are back-extracted with 1.5 ml 0.1 N HCl and centrifuged. The organic layer is aspirated off and 1 ml of each 0.1 N HCl extract is mixed with 1 ml 6 N HCl. Fluorescence is measured at 540 nm with excitation at 290 nm and mean values are determined. Percent inhibition P_I is calculated by

$$P_I = \frac{F_I - F_0}{F_S} \cdot 100$$

where F_I is the fluorescence of the test drug sample, F_0 the fluorescence of the uninhibited sample, and F_S the fluorescence of the substrate-only sample. Percent inhibition versus inhibitor concentration is plotted and the

KI50% (concentration for 50% inhibition) is estimated either graphically or by linear regression analysis. Data for typical MAOI, thymoleptics, and other drugs are listed in Table 5.

J. CNS Depressant Effects

The most successful antidepressants or antidepressant drug combinations also have some sort of sedative or "tranquilizing" action. Protriptyline, which is totally devoid of sedative or tranquilizing properties, has not been useful in agitated or anxious depressives. Amitriptyline, the most widely used antidepressant to date, has considerable sedative and neuroleptic activity, and admixture with the neuroleptic perphenazine appears even more effective in some agitated depressed patients. Similarly, combination therapies with an anxiolytic, meprobamate, also have been reported to be effective [114]. Since the "ideal" antidepressant may be visualized (Section VI) to have some additional "calming" property, the following tests are included here.

1. Potentiation of hexobarbital sleep

Prolongation of sleep time from a fixed dose of a barbiturate can indicate the degree of potency of a drug as a CNS depressant or it can mean that the drug blocks metabolism of the barbiturate [53]. Compounds which prolong the sleep time therefore should be tested also for the ability to reduce threshold barbiturate dose as well since threshold is independent of drug half-life.

In a typical protocol male rats in randomized groups of 10 are injected intravenously with 25 mg/kg hexobarbital sodium 30 min after oral or intraperitoneal test drug or vehicle. Sleep duration is measured from time of loss to time of return of the righting reflex. An ED50%, the dose which increases sleep time to 150% of controls, may be calculated.

To check for interference with barbiturate metabolism, a side-by-side dose-response of intravenous hexobarbital is done in untreated rats given the ED50% dose of oral or intraperitoneal drug. A significantly lowered ED90 for hexobarbital sleep threshold (3 sec to righting) for the drug-treated group eliminates metabolism blockade as a mode of action.

2. Locomotor activity in mice

General depressant effects on locomotor activity can be measured in mice or rats in a number of ways involving some sort of activity cage or chamber and a mechanical, photoelectric, or electromagnetic recording of movement. The mechanical and photoelectric systems are preferable to the electromagnetic ones because the latter are sensitive to all types of movement, including tremors, sniffing, and respiration.

A typical protocol uses 24 mice per dose, fasted 16 to 22 hr, intubated in pairs at suitable doses such as 0, 1, 3, 9, 27, and 81 mg/kg in 10 ml/kg of aqueous 1% Methocel. Twenty minutes after intubation the pairs of mice are put in opaque, covered Woodard photoelectric activity chambers and 10 min later a 5-min count is taken. Counting-chamber characteristics are balanced out by counting two paris of mice at each dose in each of six different chambers. The activity counts do not distribute normally, but their square roots nearly do [203]; thus, statistical significance of the data at any dose may be determined either nonparametrically [204] or the data must be "pseudonormalized" prior to parametric treatment. ED50% values for decrease or increase from controls are calculated. Values for several antidepressants are given in Table 4.

3. Mouse tryptamine and 5HTP antagonism test[2]

Tryptamine convulsions [199] in mice are blocked by neuroleptics and anxiolytics and 5HTP head twitch is attenuated by thymoleptics, 5HT antagonists, stimulants, certain antihistaminics, narcotic analgesics, and narcotic antagonists [31]. The following two tests can aid in characterizing antidepressant drugs with some depressant character in their pharmacological action.

   a.   Tryptamine blockade   An intravenous ED98 for head stereotypies and convulsions is determined [199]. Mice are dosed orally or intraperitoneally with graded doses of test drug or vehicle. After 59 min, an intravenous ED98 dose of tryptamine hydrochloride is given and the mice are observed for 1 min for the appearance of the stereotypies. Failure of stereotypies to appear during this time constitutes blockade of tryptamine. ED50 values and confidence limits may be calculated [165,175]. Selected data are shown in Table 4.

   b.   5HTP blockade in mice   The protocol is the same as that described in Section V.I.2.a; a few data are given in Table 4.

4. Catalepsy in mice and rats

All major tranquilizers cause pronounced catalepsy in mice and rats. Other depressant drugs, including anxiolytics and some thymoleptics, cause varying lesser degrees of catatonia. This property is readily and easily measured (see also Section V.B.1). Selected data are listed in Table 4.

---

[2]See also Section V.I.2.a.

5. Conditioned avoidance
    response in rats

A simplified rat conditioned avoidance response (CAR) procedure has been
described [205] which detects major and minor tranquilizers and distinguishes
them from sedative-hypnotics. The animals are trained and tested on the
same day and then are discarded. At the time of peak drug effect the ratios
of escape failure ED50 to avoidance failure ED50 are >4 for major and minor
tranquilizers, ≤ 2 for most sedative-hypnotics, and about 1 for other types
of drugs.
    The method merits further evaluation. Of particular advantage is the
small (2%) rejection rate of animals which do not learn to avoid shock and
the small number of animals (<1%) which fail to avoid on subsequent testing.

6. Amphetamine toxicity in
    grouped mice [206]

This test has been called a "model of agitation." The LD50 of amphetamine-
treated mice can be reduced up to sixfold by confining the animals in a
small space. The "grouped effect" is counteracted by chlorpromazine and
reserpine at low doses, by phenobarbital at high doses, and not at all by
pentobarbital.
    In a typical protocol doses of test drug or vehicle are given orally or
subcutaneously to groups of 18-hr fasted mice, 0.5 or 1.0 hr prior to intraperitoneal dl-amphetamine sulfate (AMP) at 10, 30, and 90 mg/kg. Four
hours after AMP, the dead mice are counted, and the LD50 values and
confidence limits are calculated [165,175].

7. Antagonism of amphetamine-
    induced hypermotility

Neuroleptics such as chlorpromazine block amphetamine-induced hypermotility in grouped mice much more potently than they decrease endogenous
locomotor activity [207]. Anxiolytics such as chlordiazepoxide have little
effect on grouped amphetamine hypermotility but do decrease endogenous
locomotor activity of single mice.
    In a modified procedure [63], 20 g male mice in groups of 4 to 10 are
dosed orally or intraperitoneally with drug or vehicle followed at a suitable
time, usually 0.5 or 1.0 hr, by oral or subcutaneous amphetamine sulfate
at 3 or 6 mg/kg. The animals in groups are put in locomotor activity
measuring devices and are "counted" for 60 min. The data are treated in
the same fashion as other locomotor activity data. A good dose-response
requires at least five groups of mice per dose.

8. Aggression of isolated mice [63]

Aggressiveness in isolated male mice is potently antagonized by centrally active anticholinergic agents such as atropine and cyproheptadine and less potently by anxiolytics such as chlordiazepoxide which have no anticholinergic activity.

    To prepare animals for drug evaluation, male mice are individually caged for 3 weeks, then placed together for a 30-min test. Three days later the active "fighters" are used for drug evaluation, 10 pairs for each dose and 20 pairs for placebo controls. After use the animals are returned to their home cages for 7 days prior to selection for a new test. During the 3-min test the frequency and duration of attacks are recorded and the mean "fighting time" per dose is calculated from which ED50% values may be derived.

9. Punished behavior in mice

Minor tranquilizers are best detected and studied in tests which use punished behavior. A test in which normal exploratory activity is suppressed by electric shock punishment has been described [208]. Antianxiety drugs apparently suppress the "fear" of being shocked. The test needs further development.

10. Rat conflict test

This is a more specialized form of punished behavior test which involves both positive (food) and negative (electric shock) reinforcements to develop a "conflict" situation. This test is especially suited for characterizing drugs with an anxiolytic component to their action spectrum. The following protocol is a modification of the original Geller lever press test [209].

    Male rats are reduced to and maintained at 80% of free-feeding weight (about 250 g). The test chamber ($25.5 \times 25.5 \times 23$ cm), containing a response lever, food-delivery mechanism, an electrifiable grid floor, and a stimulus light, is enclosed in a sound-resistant, ventilated box. Positive reinforcement is food pellets available by pressing the response lever. Initially rats are trained to 10 lever presses (FR 10) for each food pellet reward in the presence of flashing light. When performance becomes stable, 5-min periods with pellet reinforcement at variable intervals in the presence of steady light are alternated with 2-min periods of FR 10. The mean variable interval is 30 sec (VI 30). When performance on the combined schedules stabilizes, electric shock punishment is added to the FR 10. Daily test sessions consist of six FR 10 periods and seven VI 30 periods.

    Drugs are given orally to three rats per dose; each rat is dosed only once each week. Each rat serves as its own control, averaging responses of the 3 days prior to treatment and comparing to the responses following treatment on the fourth day. Data are analyzed by analysis of variance and MED values are calculated as the lowest dose at which a significant ($P < 0.05$)

attenuation of shocks is seen. The MED values for several drugs are shown
in Table 4.

11. Antagonism of pentylenetetrazol
     in mice

Pentylenetetrazol (PTZ) causes tonic and clonic convulsions in mice. The
convulsions can be prevented by many depressant drugs but not by diphenylhydantoin [210], a typical anticonvulsant drug, potent against electroshock
convulsions, and in use for treatment of grand mal epilepsy. The potencies
of many anxiolytic drugs for PTZ antagonism parallel their potency for
antagonism of conflict in rats and their efficacy in man in the treatment of
anxiety. The following protocol provides a simple convenient quantal assay
of antipentylenetetrazol activity.

Female white mice fasted for 18 hr are dosed orally with test drug
and 30 min later are injected intravenously with 40 mg/kg PTZ. Immediately after PTZ each mouse is put on a 4 × 4-in. platform 16 in. above the
bench top. Unprotected mice fall off the platform within 20 sec. Quantal
ED50 values are calculated (Table 4).

K. Anticholinergic Tests

It has been suggested that the sedative or tranquilizing properties of amitriptyline may be due to its central anticholinergic activity. Most of the
side effects and toxicities of the thymoleptics are due to peripheral anticholinergic activity for which physostigmine has been a successful antidote.
The "ideal" antidepressant may possess a moderate amount of central anticholinergic activity but should be devoid of peripheral anticholinergic activity.
The latter may be estimated by measurement of pupillary diameter in mice
or rats under a low-power microscope fitted with a 0.1 mm × 30 scale in
the eyepiece. As a quantal endpoint 1.5 mm pupillary diameter is considered mydriasis. Typical data are given in Table 6. Peripheral anticholinergic activity may also be estimated in the mouse pilocarpine test whereas
the central anticholinergic effect is estimated by oxotremorine antagonism.

1. Pilocarpine antagonism in mice

Pilocarpine, a potent cholinomimetic, induces copious salivation in mice.
In a typical protocol [63] male mice are anesthetized with 0.4 ml of 9% urethane and 5 min later are injected subcutaneously with drug or vehicle.
Fifteen minutes later 0.02% pilocarpine hydrochloride is given subcutaneously after which the mouse is placed head down on a sloping board covered
with filter paper. Twenty minutes after pilocarpine the wetted area of the
paper is measured. Mean wetted areas are calculated and drug effect is
expressed as ED50%. Alternatively, test drugs are given orally to conscious
mice and 50 min later the mice are injected subcutaneously with 15 mg/kg
pilocarpine hydrochloride. Ten minutes after pilocarpine the mice are

248   D. H. SMITH AND V. G. VERNIER

TABLE 6   Anticholinergic Tests in mice

Drug	Mydriasis,[a] p.o.	ED50 (mg/kg, p.o.) Antag. pilocarpine	Antag. oxotremorine[b]
Imipramine	159.0	81.0	18.0
Amitriptyline	23.0	11.0	6.0
Protriptyline	20.0	15.0	
Doxepin	60.0	160.0	
Iprindole		320.0	
Maprotiline	260.0		
Butriptyline	36.0	144.0	
Tranylcypromine	324.0		—
Atropine	3.0	0.8	3.4

[a]Pupil size ≥ 1.5 mm at peak time (usually 30 min).
[b]Calculated from data of Levy and Michel-Ber [215]; route was intraperitoneal.

checked for salivation quantally by their ability to produce a 0.25-in.-diameter wet spot on Whatman #1 filter paper. Some typical data are shown in Table 6.

2. Oxotremorine antagonism

Oxotremorine-induced tremor is a direct CNS effect since ablation of the midbrain tegmentum (rats) prevents the tremors [211], and spinal cord transection limits tremor to the region above the cut. Mice probably are a better choice for oxotremorine studies than rats since in the latter at least one thymoleptic (desipramine) inhibits oxotremorine by blocking its metabolism [212].

Mice are dosed orally with test drug at doses such as 0, 1, 3, 9, 27, and 81 mg/kg, in 10 ml 1% Methocel/kg, and 45 min later are injected intraperitoneally with an ED95 dose of oxotremorine (0.4 mg/kg). Mice are observed 15 min later for tremors and salivation. Atropine is used as a comparative standard. ED50% values are calculated for both parameters. Data for some antidepressants and for atropine are given in Table 6.

L. New Models of Depression

The first of these is an attempt at providing an animal model with a "conditioned" depression. The second is an in vitro model which allows study of antidepressants on various aminergic systems.

1. Depression conditioning

The production of an animal model of depression using rats with a buzzer as conditioned stimulus (CS) and a tetrabenazine injection as an unconditioned stimulus (US) has been reported [213]. When conditioned, which required many trials, the rats became and remained motionless at the sound of the buzzer. The "motionlessness" was antagonized by imipramine treatment. At present this is not a practical test for an antidepressant screening program but is a step in the right direction. A more rapid-acting US might greatly enhance conditioning speed.

2. In vitro models

Synaptosomes are "pinched off" nerve endings which biochemically and histologically look like in vivo nerve endings. Synaptosomes can be used to study overall amine uptake, i.e., membrane transport plus vesicular storage [214]. Thymoleptics are extremely potent inhibitors of 5HT uptake into synaptosomal preparations with KI50% values of about 1×10^{-6} M whereas the MAOI per se are virtually inactive. Neuroleptics also are active in the test but are less potent, having KI50% values generally $>1 \times 10^{-5}$ M.

VI. THE IDEAL ANTIDEPRESSANT

Could there be an ideal antidepressant drug useful in all patients? Probably not, and the most cogent reason lies in the nature of the disease itself. Depression is not a discrete disease of a singular biochemical or physiological etiology, but rather a continuum of diseases with perhaps several biochemical origins. Nevertheless there are many characteristics to look for in a search for new drugs which can make an antidepressant more desirable, or less so.

First, the new drug candidate should have a novel chemical structure. So much effort already has been spent on the innumerable "variations on a theme" as in the tricyclics, the phenethylamines, and the hydrazine MAOI; the improvements from such efforts lie mainly in potency variations and provide little new in therapeutic approach.

New antidepressant candidates should be "antidepressant" in one and preferably more animal models of depression and in more than one species.

An ideal antidepressant must have a good therapeutic ratio in all species in which it is tested. If possible, it should be "antidepressant" in at least one test not involving drug interactions and should be active in one nonrodent species.

It should be virtually free of purely stimulant capability, or mechanistically, should not be a direct or indirect acting amine. Such compounds generally have not been successful in providing more than temporary improvement in the endogenously depressed. Some psychostimulant activity (e.g., potentiation of amphetamine) may be desirable and could help provide a desirable early onset of action. It also should not be a long-acting MAOI because of the ever present danger of hypertensive crisis if the patient ingests tyramine-containing foods during or following treatment.

An ideal antidepressant should have some sedative, neuroleptic, or anxiolytic activity. A large proportion of depressed patients also are agitated or anxious. These respond best to the more "depressant" antidepressants such as amitriptyline and respond less favorably, sometimes unfavorably, to drugs such as protriptyline which are free of depressant capabilities.

The ideal antidepressant should have some purely central anticholinergic activity as this is thought by some to provide the sedation needed in agitated depressives even though centrally active anticholinergics are somewhat disruptant in man and in animal tests. It should not have peripheral anticholinergic activity as this is the basis of the undesirable side effects and toxicities from which the currently used thymoleptics suffer.

The ideal antidepressant should have an early onset of action, preferably within minutes or hours of the time of medication. The onset time for all currently accepted therapies is from several days to 2 to 4 weeks. At present, however, there is no meaningful way to study onset time of antidepressant action in animal test systems.

All of these are requirements of a good antidepressant, suitable for treatment of all forms of depression. When better, more biochemically specific diagnoses of the various depressions become readily available, it may be possible to tailor antidepressants more precisely to fit the disease. One may then consider specific blockers of norepinephrine, dopamine, or 5HT reuptake, or substrate- or organ-specific reversible MAOI suited to the patient's diagnosis. It may be feasible then to choose combination therapies to suit an individual patient's needs. Until such time the searcher for a new and better antidepressant must try to juggle the properties, good and bad, of known treatments with the hope of arriving at some sort of optimum.

ACKNOWLEDGMENTS

The authors thank Mrs. Susan Zehnder for valuable assistance in unearthing the information on which this chapter is based, Mrs. Betty Fitzgerald who patiently persisted through retypings of the manuscript, and Dr. J. M. Stump, Dr. E. N. Goldschmidt, and Dr. W. F. Herblin for their suggestions on the text.

REFERENCES

1. F. J. Ayd, Dis. Nerv. Syst. 35, 475 (1974).

2. A. T. Beck, in Depression: Clinical, Experimental and Theoretical Aspects, Hoeber Med. Div., Harper & Row, New York, 1967, p. 141.

3. J. J. Schildkraut, J. M. Davis, and G. L. Klerman, in Psychopharmacology, a Review of Progress, 1957-1967 (D. H. Efron, ed.), Public Health Service Publ. No. 1836, 1968, pp. 625-648.

4. M. M. Weissman, B. Prusoff, and C. Pincus, J. Nerv. Ment. Dis. 160, 15 (1975).

5. A. T. Beck, in Depression: Clinical, Experimental and Theoretical Aspects, Hoeber Med. Div., Harper & Row, New York, 1967, pp. 3-4.

6. B. G. Adams, in Psychopharmacology, Dimensions and Perspectives (C. R. B. Joyce, ed.), Tavistock Publ., Lippincott, Philadelphia, 1968, p. 158.

7. G. A. Alles, J. Pharmacol. Exp. Ther. 32, 121 (1927).

8. B. G. Adams, in Psychopharmacology, Dimensions and Perspectives (C. R. B. Joyce, ed.), Chap. 5, Tavistock Publ., Lippincott, Philadelphia, 1968.

9. C. Kaiser and C. L. Zirkle, in Medicinal Chemistry (A. Burger, ed.), 3rd ed., Vol. 2, Wiley, New York, 1970, pp. 1470-1497.

10. C. Kaiser and C. L. Zirkle, Annu. Rep. Med. Chem. 8, 11 (1973).

11. R. Kuhn, Schweiz. Med. Wochenschr. 87, 1135 (1957).

12. H. P. Loomer, J. C. Saunders, and N. S. Kline, Am. Psychiatr. Assoc. Psychiat. Rep. 8, 129 (1957).

13. J. F. J. Cade, Med. J. Aust. 2, 349 (1949).

14. K. Rickels, E. Raab, R. DeSilverio, and B. Etemad, JAMA 201, 675 (1967).

15. K. Rickels, H. R. Chung, H. S. Feldman, P. E. Gordon, E. A. Kelly, and C. C. Weise, J. Nerv. Ment. Dis. 157, 442 (1973).

16. K. Nahunek, A. Rodova, J. Svestka, V. Kamenicka, and J. Misurec, Act. Nerv. Super. (Praha) 15, 111 (1973).

17. R. U. Udabe, Curr. Ther. Res. 15, Oct, Suppl., 755 (1973).

18. T. A. Ban, H. E. Lehmann, M. Amin, L. A. Bronheim, A. Klingner, N. P. V. Nair, L. Galvan, L. Vergara, and C. Zoch, Int. J. Clin. Pharmacol. 9, 23 (1974).

19. T. A. Ban, H. E. Lehmann, M. Amin, L. Galvan, N. P. V. Nair,
    L. Vergara, and C. Zoch, Curr. Ther. Res. 15, 540 (1973).

20. B. Silvestrini and R. Lisciani, Curr. Ther. Res. 15, Oct. Suppl., 749
    (1973).

21. P. Niskanen, T. Tamminen, and M. Viukari, Curr. Ther. Res. 17,
    281 (1975).

22. E. Fischer, B. Heller, M. Nachon, and H. Spatz, Arzneim. Forsch.
    25, 132 (1975).

23. J. Mendels, J. L. Stinnett, D. Burns, and A. Frazer, Arch. Gen.
    Psychiatry 32, 22 (1975).

24. J. M. Davis, G. L. Klerman, and J. J. Schildkraut, in Psychophar-
    macology, A Review of Progress, 1957-1967 (D. H. Efron, ed.), Public
    Health Service Pul. No. 1836, 1968, pp. 719-747.

25. M. B. H. Youdim, G. G. S. Collins, M. J. Sandler, A. B. B. Jones,
    C. M. B. Pare, and W. J. Nicholson, Nature 236, 225 (1972).

26. J. B. Morris and A. T. Beck, Arch. Gen. Psychiatry 30, 667 (1974).

27. AMA Drug Evaluations, 2nd ed., Publishing Sciences Group, Inc.,
    Mass., 1973, pp. 359-367.

28. B. D. Snyder, L. Blonde, and W. R. McWhirter, JAMA 230, 1433
    (1974).

29. J. S. Burke, J. E. Walker, B. M. Rumack, and J. E. Ott, JAMA 230,
    1405 (1974).

30. E. B. Sigg, in Psychopharmacology, A Review of Progress, 1957-1967
    (D. H. Efron, ed.), Public Health Service Publ. No. 1836, 1968,
    pp. 655-669.

31. S. J. Corne, R. W. Pickering, and B. T. A. Warner, Br. J. Phar-
    macol. 20, 106 (1963).

32. P. Bevan, C. M. Bradshaw, M. H. T. Roberts, and E. Szabadi,
    Br. J. Pharmacol. 49, 173P (1973).

33. M. Osborne and E. B. Sigg, Arch. Int. Pharmacodyn. Ther. 129, 273
    (1960).

34. B. Bergamasco, M. Chiusano, and G. Asteggiano, Acta Neurol.
    (Napoli) 29, 93 (1974).

35. D. J. McClure, G. L. Low, and M. Gent, Can. Psychiatr. Assoc. J.
    18, 403 (1973).

36. B. Dubinsky, J. K. Karpowicz, and M. E. Goldberg, J. Pharmacol.
    Exp. Ther. 187, 550 (1973).

37. D. Ghezzi, R. Samanin, S. Bernasconi, G. Tognoni, M. Gerna, and S. Garrattini, Eur. J. Pharmacol. 24, 205 (1973).

38. J. L. Meek, K. Fuxe, and A. Carlsson, Biochem. Pharmacol. 20, 707 (1971).

39. H. M. van Praag, Pharmakopsychiatrie 7, 281 (1974).

40. F. S. Abuzzahab, Sr., Int. J. Clin. Pharmacol. 8, 244 (1973).

41. E. Guth and G. Hoffmann, Wien. Klin. Wochenschr. 78, 14 (1966).

42. K. Rickels, H. R. Chung, I. Csanalosi, L. Sablosky, and J. H. Simon, Br. J. Psychiatry 123, 329 (1973).

43. G. L. Klerman and J. O. Cole, Pharmacol. Rev. 17, 101 (1965).

44. W. Theobald, O. Büch, H. A. Kunz, and C. Morpurgo, Med. Pharmacol. Exp. 15, 187 (1966).

45. D. S. Haskell, A. DiMascio, and B. Prusoff, J. Nerv. Ment. Dis. 160, 24 (1975).

46. S. Hernandez and J. H. Gonzales, Prensa Med. Mex. 38, 215 (1973).

47. B. Levinson, S. Afr. Med. J. 48, 873 (1974).

48. J. Jaramillo and R. Greenberg, Can. J. Physiol. Pharmacol. 53, 104 (1975).

49. W. E. Coyne and J. W. Cusic, J. Med. Chem. 17, 72 (1974).

50. L. E. Hollister, Ann. Intern. Med. 81, 360 (1974).

51. J. R. Tretter, J. F. Muren, B. M. Bloom, and B. A. Weissman, Am. Chem. Soc. Med. Symp., Bloomington, Indiana, 1966.

52. A. Kiev, Dis. Nerv. Syst. 33, 811 (1972).

53. H. van Riezen, W. J. vanderBurg, H. Berendsen, and M.-L. Jaspar, Arzneim. Forsch. 23, 1295 (1973).

54. A. Balestrieri, P. Benassi, G. B. Cassano, P. Castriogiovanni, A. Catalano, A. Colombi, C. Conforto, G. De Soldato, F. Gilberti, P. E. Luchelli, A. Muratorio, M. Nistri, and P. Sarteschi, Int. Pharmacopsychiatry 6, 236 (1971).

55. M. Amin, E. Brahm, L. A. Bronheim, A. Klingner, T. A. Ban, and H. E. Lehmann, Curr. Ther. Res. 15, 691 (1973).

56. O. Benesova and V. Benes, Act. Nerv. Super. (Praha) 16, 190 (1974).

57. N. G. Dionisio and H. Perez Rincon, Prensa Med. Mex. 38, 429 (1973).

58. G. F. T. Marais, S. Afr. Med. J. 48, 1530 (1974).

59. P. Castriogiovanni, G. Placidi, C. Maggini, B. Ghetti, and G. Cassano, Pharmacokopsychiatr. Neuropsychopharmakol. 4, 170 (1971).

60. S. Ueki, M. Fujiwara, and K. Inoue, Jap. J. Pharmacol. 24, Suppl. 66 (1974).

61. T. M. Itil, Dis. Nerv. Syst. 33, 557 (1972).

62. J. Fleischauer, B. Al-Schaltchi, and A. Brändli, Arzneim. Forsch. 23, 1808 (1973).

63. H. Van Riezen, Arch. Int. Pharmacodyn. Ther. 198, 256 (1972).

64. B. B. Vargaftig, J. L. Coignet, C. J. de Vos, H. Grisjen, and I. L. Bonta, Eur. J. Pharmacol. 16, 336 (1971).

65. B. E. Leonard, Psychopharmacologia 36, 221 (1974).

66. J. Hache, P. Duchene-Marullaz, and G. Streichenberger, Therapie 29, 81 (1974).

67. K. B. Mallion, A. H. Todd, R. W. Turner, J. G. Bainbridge, D. T. Greenwood, J. Madinaveitia, A. R. Somerville, and B. A. Whittle, Nature 238, 157 (1972).

68. P. F. C. Bayless and S. M. Duncan, Br. J. Clin. Pharmacol. 1, 431 (1974).

69. Drug Ther. Bull. 13, 39 (1975).

70. U. Schacht and W. Heptner, Biochem. Pharmacol. 23, 3413 (1974).

71. M. Schou, in Psychopharmacology, A Review of Progress, 1957-1967 (D. H. Efron, ed.), Public Health Service Publ. No. 1836, 1968, pp. 701-718.

72. J. Mendels, in Lithium, Its Role in Psychiatric Research and Treatment (S. Gershon and B. Shopsin, eds.), Plenum Press, New York, 1973, pp. 253-267.

73. J. M. Davis and W. E. Fann, Annu. Rev. Pharmacol. 11, 285 (1970).

74. S. Watanabe, H. Ishino, and S. Otsuki, Folia Psychiatr. Neurol. Jap. 28, 267 (1974).

75. C. H. Noack and E. M. Trautner, Med. J. Aust. 2, 219 (1951).

76. M. Schou, Psychopharmacologia 1, 65 (1959).

77. S. Gershon, Clin. Pharmacol. Ther. 11, 168 (1970).

78. R. F. Prien, E. M. Caffey, Jr., and C. J. Klett, Arch. Gen. Psychiatry 26, 146 (1972).

79. R. Noyes and G. M. Dempsey, Dis. Nerv. Syst. 35, 573 (1974).

80. O. Lingjaerde, A. H. Edlund, C. A. Gormsen, C. G. Gottfries,
    A. Haugstad, I. L. Hermann, P. Hollnagel, A. Makimattila, K. E.
    Rasmussen, J. Remvig, and O. H. Robak, Acta Psychiatr. Scand. 50,
    233 (1974).

81. P. C. Baastrup and M. Schou, Arch. Gen. Psychiatry 16, 162 (1967).

82. H. Komiskey and C. K. Buckner, Neuropharmacology 13, 159 (1974).

83. S. R. Platman, Dis. Nerv. Syst. 32, 604 (1971).

84. K. Greenspan, M. S. Aranoff, and D. F. Bogdanski, Pharmacology 3,
    129 (1970).

85. D. N. Stern, R. R. Fieve, N. H. Neff, and E. Costa, Psychopharma-
    cology 14, 315 (1969).

86. R. I. Katz, T. N. Chase, and I. J. Kopin, Science 162, 466 (1968).

87. Y. Yamauchi, M. Nakamura, and K. Koketsu, Kurume Med. J. 19, 175
    (1972); also CA 78, 314r (1973).

88. B. J. Carroll and P. T. Sharp, Science 172, 1355 (1971).

89. E. Eichelman, N. B. Thoa, and J. Perez-Cruet, Fed. Proc. 31, 289
    Abstr. (1972).

90. J. M. Stolk, W. J. Nowack, and J. D. Barchas, Science 168, 501
    (1970).

91. From Rubidium: Safety and Potential as an Antidepressant—Abridged
    Proceedings of a Workshop, Psychopharmacol. Bull. 10(1), 26-50
    (January 1974).

92. R. R. Fieve, H. Meltzer, D. L. Dunner, M. Levitt, J. Mendlewicz,
    and A. Thomas, Am. J. Psychiatry 130, 55 (1973).

93. E. W. Sutherland, G. A. Robison, and R. W. Butcher, Circulation 37,
    279 (1968)

94. Y. H. Abdulla and K. Hamadah, Lancet I, 378 (1970).

95. K. Sinanan, A. M. B. Keatinge, P. G. S. Beckett, and W. C. Love,
    Br. J. Psychiatry 126, 49 (1975).

96. M. I. Paul, H. Cramer, and F. K. Goodwin, Arch. Gen. Psychiatry
    24, 327 (1971).

97. K. Hamadah, H. Holmes, G. B. Barker, G. C. Hartman, and D. V. W.
    Parke, Br. Med. J. 3, 439 (1972).

98. M. S. Anderson, C. Y. Bowers, A. J. Kastin, D. S. Schlach, A. V.
    Schally, P. J. Snyder, R. D. Utiger, J. F. Wilber, and A. J. Wise,
    N. Engl. J. Med. 285, 1279 (1971).

99. L. S. Jacobs, P. J. Snyder, J. F. Wilber, R. D. Utiger, and W. H. Daughaday, J. Clin. Endocrinol. Metab. 33, 996 (1971).

100. A. J. Prange, Jr., P. P. Lara, I. C. Wilson, L. B. Alltop, and G. R. Breese, Lancet II, 999 (1972).

101. A. J. Kastin, R. H. Ehrensing, D. S. Schlach, and M. S. Anderson, Lancet II, 740 (1972).

102. M. J. E. Van der Vis Melsen and J. D. Weiner, Lancet II, 1415 (1972).

103. S. Takahashi, H. Kondo, M. Yoshimura, and Y. Ochi, Folia Psychiatr. Neurol. Jap. 27, 305 (1973).

104. C. Q. Mountjoy, M. Weller, R. Hall, J. S. Price, P. R. Hunter, and J. H. Dewar, Lancet I, 958 (1974).

105. N. P. Plotnikoff, A. J. Prange, Jr., G. R. Breese, M. S. Anderson, and I. C. Wilson, Science 178, 417 (1972).

106. B. Hine, I. Sanghvi, and S. Gershon, Life Sci. 13, 1789 (1973).

107. M. Fink, J. Simeon, T. M. Itil, and A. M. Freedman, Clin. Pharmacol. Ther. 11, 41 (1970).

108. N. S. Doggett, H. Reno, and P. S. J. Spencer, Neuropharmacology 14, 85 (1975).

109. H. E. Lehmann, J. V. Ananth, K. C. Geagea, and T. A. Ban, Curr. Ther. Res. 13, 42 (1971).

110. M. Greenblatt, G. H. Grosser, and H. Wechsler, Am. J. Psychiatry 120, 935 (1964).

111. I. S. Turek, Compr. Psychiatry 14, 495 (1973).

112. A. T. Beck, in Depression, Clinical, Experimental and Theoretical Aspects, Hoeber Med. Div., Harper & Row, New York, 1967, pp. 305-310.

113. A. A. Shatalova and E. K. Antonov, Psychopharmacol. Abstr. 1, 341 (1961).

114. C. Breitner, A. Picchioni, L. Chin, and L. E. Burton, Dis. Nerv. Syst. 22 (Suppl.), 93 (1961).

115. J. J. Schildkraut, S. M. Schanberg, G. R. Breese, and I. J. Kopin, Am. J. Psychiatry 124, 600 (1967).

116. S. S. Kety, F. Javoy, A.-M. Thierry, L. Julou, and J. Glowinski, Proc. Natl. Acad. Sci. U.S.A. 58, 1249 (1967).

117. J. Ravin, Br. J. Psychiatry 112, 501 (1966).

118. C. P. Seager and R. L. Bird, J. Ment. Sci. 108, 704 (1962).

119. L. Grinspoon and M. Greenblatt, Compr. Psychiatry 4, 256 (1963).

120. J. Ananth and R. Ruskin, Int. Pharmacopsychiatry 9, 218 (1974).

121. I. Ray, Can. Psychiatr. Assoc. J. 18, 399 (1973).

122. F. Winston, Br. J. Psychiatry 118, 301 (1971).

123. R. N. Wharton, J. M. Perel, P. G. Dayton, and S. Malitz, Am. J. Psychiatry 127, 1619 (1971).

124. J. M. Himmelhoch, T. P. Detre, D. J. Kupfer, M. Schwartzburg, and R. Byck, J. Nerv. Ment. Dis. 155, 216 (1972).

125. O. Lingjaerde, Lancet II, 1260 (1973).

126. L. Haskovec and K. Rysanek, Psychopharmacologia 11, 18 (1967).

127. H. E. Lehmann, Am. J. Psychiatry 117, 356 (1960).

128. C. M. Tiwary, J. L. Frias, and A. L. Rosenbloom, Lancet II, 1086 (1972).

129. H. C. Stancer, B. Quarrington, B. A. Cookson, G. M. Brown, A. Bonkalo, and W. A. L. Lyall, Arch. Gen. Psychiatry 20, 290 (1969).

130. A. Coppen, P. C. Whybrow, R. Noguera, R. Maggs, and A. J. Prange, Jr., Arch. Gen. Psychiatry 26, 234 (1972).

131. S. Kumar and R. B. Davis, Indian J. Psychiatry 12, 260 (1970).

132. E. L. Klaiber, D. M. Broverman, W. Vogel, Y. Kobayashi, and D. Moriarty, Am. J. Psychiatry, 128 1492 (1972).

133. S. Vale, M. A. Espejel, and J. C. Dominguez, Lancet II, 437 (1971).

134. A. A. Rubin, H. C. Yen, and M. Pfeffer, Nature 216, 578 (1967).

135. C. Fazio, V. Andreali, A. Agnoli, M. Cassachia, and R. Cerbo, Minerva Med. 64, 1515 (1973).

136. G. W. Vogel, F. C. Thompson, Jr., A. Thurmond, and B. Rivers, Psychosomatics 14, 104 (1973).

137. J. Mendels and A. Frazer, Arch. Gen. Psychiatry 30, 447 (1974).

138. M. Äsberg, L. Bertilsson, D. Tuck, B. Cronholm, and F. Sjoqvist, Clin. Pharmacol. Ther. 14, 277 (1973).

139. A. Coppen, Br. J. Psychiatry 113, 1237 (1967).

140. A. Coppen, D. M. Shaw, A. Malleson, D. Eccleston, and G. Grundy, Br. J. Psychiatry 111, 993 (1965).

141. G. W. Ashcroft and D. F. Sharman, Nature 186, 1050 (1960).

142. H. Spatz, B. Heller, M. Nachon, and E. Fischer, Biol. Psychiatry 10, 235 (1975).

143. J. J. Schildkraut and S. S. Kety, Science 156, 21 (1967).

144. D. J. McClure, Can. Psychiatr. Assoc. J. 18, 309 (1973).

145. A. Carlsson, M. Lindqvist, and T. Magnusson, Nature 180, 1200 (1957).

146. P. L. McGeer, E. G. McGeer, and J. A. Wada, Arch. Neurol. 9, 81 (1963).

147. J. A. Wada, J. Wrinch, D. Hill, P. L. McGeer, and E. G. McGeer, Arch. Neurol. 9, 69 (1963).

148. B. Bhagat, J. Pharmacol. Exp. Ther. 149, 206 (1965).

149. E. B. Sigg, Can. Psychiatr. Assoc. J. 4 (Suppl.), 75 (1959).

150. G. Hertting, J. Axelrod, and L. G. Whitby, J. Pharmacol. Exp. Ther. 134, 146 (1961).

151. J. Glowinski and J. Axelrod, Nature 204, 1318 (1964).

152. J. Glowinski and J. Axelrod, J. Pharmacol. Exp. Ther. 149, 43 (1965).

153. E. Friedman, B. Shopsin, M. Goldstein, and S. Gershon, J. Pharm. Pharmacol. 26, 995 (1974).

154. K. Modigh, J. Pharm. Pharmacol. 25, 926 (1973).

155. O. Benesova, in Proceedings of the First International Symposium on Antidepressant Drugs (S. Garrattini and M. N. J. Dukes, eds.), Excerpta Medica Foundation, Amsterdam, 1967, pp. 247-254.

156. H. E. Himwich and H. S. Alpers, Annu. Rev. Pharmacol. 10, 313 (1970).

157. R. W. P. Achor, N. O. Hanson, and R. W. Gifford, JAMA 159, 841 (1955).

158. T. H. Harris, Am. J. Psychiatry 113, 950 (1957).

159. J. C. Muller, W. W. Pryor, J. E. Gibbons, and E. S. Orgain, JAMA 159, 836 (1955).

160. A. Cowan and B. A. Whittle, Br. J. Pharmacol. 44, 353P (1972).

161. V. G. Vernier, H. M. Hanson, and C. A. Stone, in Psychosomatic Medicine (J. H. Nodine and J. H. Moyer, eds.), Lea & Febiger, Philadelphia, 1962, pp. 638-690.

162. N. S. Doggett, H. Reno, and P. S. J. Spencer, Br. J. Pharmacol. 50, 440P (1974).

163. P. S. J. Spencer, in Proceedings of the First International Symposium on Antidepressant Drugs (S. Garrattini and M. N. J. Dukes, eds.), Excerpta Medica Foundation, Amsterdam, 1968, pp. 194-204.

164. B. A. Whittle, Nature 216, 579 (1967).

165. W. R. Thompson, Bact. Rev. 11, 115 (1947).

166. B. M. Askew, Life Sci 2, 725 (1963).

167. J. Maj, P. Pawlowski, and G. Wiszniowska, Pol. J. Pharmacol. Pharm. 26, 329 (1974).

168. F. Sulser, M. H. Bickel, and B. B. Brodie, J. Pharmacol. Exp. Ther. 144, 321 (1966).

169. A. Barnett and R. I. Taber, in Screening Methods in Pharmacology II (R. A. Turner and P. Hebborn, eds.), Academic Press, New York, 1971, pp. 209-226.

170. G. M. Everett, in Proceedings of the First International Symposium on Antidepressant Drugs (S. Garrattini and M. N. G. Dukes, eds.), Excerpta Medica Foundation, Amsterdam, 1966, pp. 164-167.

171. C. Gouret and G. Reynaud, Therapie 30, 225 (1975).

172. C. Morpurgo and W. Theobald, Med. Pharmacol. Exp. 12, 226 (1965).

173. P. L. Carlton, Psychopharmacologia 2, 364 (1961).

174. A. Weissman, B. K. Koe, and S. S. Tenen, J. Pharmacol. Exp. Ther. 151, 339 (1966).

175. J. T. Litchfield, Jr., and F. Wilcoxon, J. Pharmacol. Exp. Ther. 96, 99 (1949).

176. L. Stein, in Recent Advances in Biological Psychiatry (J. Wortis, ed.), Vol. 4, Plenum Press, New York, 1962, pp. 288-309.

177. L. Stein, in Antidepressant Drugs of Non-MAO Inhibitor Type, Proc. 1966 Workshop (D. H. Efron and S. S. Kety, eds.), Workshop Series of Pharmacology Unit, NIMH, NIH, Bethesda, Maryland, pp. 111-114.

178. R. M. Quinton, Br. J. Pharmacol. 21, 51 (1963).

179. A. Cowan and E. J. R. Harry, Br. J. Pharmacol. 52, 432P (1974).

180. V. J. Lotti, M. L. Torchiana, and C. C. Porter, Arch. Int. Pharmacodyn. Ther. 203, 107 (1973).

181. T. Cox and N. Tye, Psychopharmacologia 40, 297 (1975).

182. Z. P. Horovitz, J. J. Piala, J. P. High, J. C. Burke, and R. C. Leaf, Int. J. Neuropharmacol. 5, 405 (1966).

183. J. H. Penaloza-Rojas, G. G. Bach-y-Rita, H. F. Rubio-Chevannier, and R. Hernandez-Peon, Exp. Neurol. 4, 205 (1961).

184. S. Irwin, D. Buxbaum, and G. Feinberg, Pharmacologist 7, 173 (1965).

185. R. J. Coppola, J. Am. Osteopath. Assoc. 73, 411 (1974).

186. N. Plotnikoff, D. Reinke, and J. Fitzloff, J. Pharm. Sci. 51, 1007 (1962).

187. M. Osborne and E. B. Sigg, Arch. Int. Pharmacodyn. Ther. 129, 273 (1960).

188. C. A. Stone, in Proceedings of the First International Symposium on Antidepressant Drugs (S. Garrattini and M. N. G. Dukes, eds.), Excerpta Medica Foundation, Amsterdam, 1967, pp. 158-163.

189. C. A. Stone, C. C. Porter, J. M. Stavorski, C. T. Ludden, and J. A. Totaro, J. Pharmacol. Exp. Ther. 144, 196 (1964).

190. I. Sanghvi and S. Gershon, Life Sci. 8, 449 (1969).

191. A. Barnett, S. Symchowicz, and R. I. Taber, Br. J. Pharmacol. 34, 484 (1968).

192. W. Van Dorsser and A. Dresse, Arch. Int. Pharmacodyn. Ther. 208, 373 (1974).

193. A. Barnett, M. Staub, and S. Symchowicz, Br. J. Pharmacol. 36, 79 (1968).

194. K. D. Cairncross, Arch. Int. Pharmacodyn. Ther. 154, 438 (1965).

195. S. B. Ross and A. L. Renyi, Eur. J. Pharmacol. 2, 181 (1967).

196. A. Carlsson and B. Waldeck, Acta Pharmacol. Toxicol. (Kobenhavn) 20, 47 (1963).

197. G. Brownlee and T. L. B. Spriggs, J. Pharm. Pharmacol. 17, 429 (1965).

198. N. S. Doggett, H. Reno, and P. S. J. Spencer, Neuropharmacology 14, 81 (1975).

199. D. H. Tedeschi, R. E. Tedeschi, and E. J. Fellows, J. Pharmacol. Exp. Ther. 126, 223 (1959).

200. L. O. Randall and L. E. Bagdon, Ann. N.Y. Acad. Sci. 80, 626 (1959).

201. J. A. Roth and C. N. Gillis, Mol. Pharmacol. 11, 28 (1975).

202. S. Udenfriend, H. Weissbach, and B. B. Brodie, in Methods of Bio-
     chemical Analysis (D. Glick, ed.), Vol. 6, Wiley-Interscience, New
     York, 1958, pp. 122-124.

203. S. Irwin, Rev. Can. Biol. 20, 239 (1961).

204. S. Siegel, in Non-Parametric Statistics, McGraw-Hill, New York,
     1956, pp. 184-194.

205. R. Clark, Psychon. Sci. 6, 11 (1966).

206. L. Lasagna and W. P. McCann, Science 125, 1241 (1957).

207. T. Ott and H. Matthies, Acta Biol. Med. Ger. 22, 815 (1969).

208. J. R. Boissier, P. Simon, and C. Aron, Eur. J. Pharmacol. 4, 145
     (1968).

209. L. Cook and A. B. Davidson, in The Benzodiazepines (S. Garrattini,
     E. Mussini, and L. O. Randall, eds.), Raven Press, New York, 1973,
     pp. 327-345.

210. E. A. Swinyard and A. W. Castellion, J. Pharmacol. Exp. Ther.
     151, 369 (1966).

211. R. George, W. L. Haslett, and D. J. Jenden, Life Sci. 8, 361 (1962).

212. F. Sjöqvist, W. Hammer, H. Schumacher, and J. R. Gillette, Bio-
     chem. Pharmacol. 17, 915 (1968).

213. R. Takahashi, H. Nagayama, A. Kido, and T. Morita, Biol. Psychi-
     atry 9, 191 (1974).

214. M. H. Kannengiesser, P. Hunt, and J.-P. Raynaud, Biochem. Phar-
     macol. 22, 73 (1973).

215. J. Levy and E. Michel-Ber, C. R. Soc. Biol. 159, 640 (1965).

Chapter 9

ANALGESICS

Jeffrey K. Saelens and Francis R. Granat

Pharmaceuticals Division
CIBA-GEIGY Corporation
Summit, New Jersey

I. INTRODUCTION

The field of analgesics represents an unusual one for the industrial pharmacologist. It differs from almost all other fields involving central nervous
system function in one very important way: The industrial pharmacologist
knows exactly what he is looking for. He wants an agent for the treatment
of moderate to severe pain which has no physical dependence liability and a
minimum of side effects. The agent simply has not been made or identified.
The test systems available to him are numerous and have good clinical predictive value. It is not the purpose of this chapter to review the pros and
cons of all these tests. This has been done many times. The reader is
referred to the review of Taber [1] for such comparisons. Presented here
is what we think are a coherent series of test systems which answer some
of the basic questions which arise in the search for new analgesics. These

tests enable the industrial pharmacologist to estimate first the potency, then the efficacy, and finally the physical dependence liability of new experimental compounds.

II. ANALGESIC ACTIVITY AND
     CLINICAL POTENCY ESTIMATE

To detect analgesic activity a modification of the phenylquinone writhing test in mice was chosen many years ago after careful scrutiny and/or experience with other test systems. The test, as we use it, is sensitive to all known analgesics including the narcotic antagonist analgesics. The simplicity of the procedure makes the phenylquinone writhing test an excellent primary screening test. However, it is not specific to analgesic agents in that drugs such as chlorpromazine and most other phenothiazines, imipramine, fenfluramine, chlorphentermine, and haloperidol are also active. There are other examples of false positives in the literature [2-4] but many of these would be excluded by our quantal approach. Additional specificity is ascertained by the use of other test systems.

Male mice, 14 to 25 g, are used. Our short version of the phenylquinone writhing test was adapted from the method of Taber et al. [5] with the phenylquinone solution prepared as reported by Blumberg et al. [6]. At various time intervals after administration of the test compound the animals receive intraperitoneally 0.1 ml/10 g body weight of an 0.25 mg/ml solution of phenyl-p-quinone (Eastman) in 5% aqueous ethanol (2.5 mg/kg). Five minutes later they are placed in observation cages and the number of animals which do not perform a characteristic writhe during the next 10 min are recorded. Under these conditions, we have found that phenylquinone induces one or more writhes in 95% of the injected mice. Test compounds are administered subcutaneously or by oral intubation in a volume of 0.1 ml/10 g body weight in an appropriate vehicle. Mice receive food and water ad libitum up until the time of testing. Ten mice are used for each dose of each agent at each time. Statistical analysis of the quantal data [(number of mice not writhing)/(total number of mice tested)] is performed by the logit method of Berkson [7] which generates an ED50, slope, and 95% confidence limits.

There have been various attempts to predict the parenteral clinical unit dose from phenylquinone data in mice. Pearl and Harris [8] noted that narcotic antagonist analgesics had shallow logit-log dose slopes, whereas analgesics without narcotic antagonist properties had steep slopes. In correlation with this, the observation was made that the phenylquinone test usually underestimates the relative analgesic potency of narcotic antagonist analgesics. For instance, in a paper by Pearl et al. [9] the phenylquinone ED50 for morphine was 1.1 mg/kg whereas the phenylquinone ED50 for nalorphine

was 10.0 mg/kg. However, morphine and nalorphine are approximately
equipotent in man [10,11]. The data of Pearl et al. [9] offer a convenient
opportunity to attempt a correction of the ED50 using the logit-log dose
slopes for a number of standard analgesic agents for which there are also
clinical unit dose values available. Review of the data suggests that the
parenteral clinical unit dose is approximately one to two times the subcutaneous ED_{50} (obtained at 30 min) multiplied by the logit-log dose slopes.
Using this equation, the values for a number of standard agents are shown
in Table 1. These data from our laboratories are consistent with observations in the literature [9].

Evaluation of phenylquinone data after oral administration of known
analgesics indicates no correlation between the logit-log dose slopes and
the presence of narcotic antagonist properties. All the agents tested have
similar and relatively steep logit-log dose slopes. Table 2 summarizes
the results obtained with a number of standard agents reputed to have oral
analgesic activity. Interestingly, the oral ED50 derived from the phenylquinone test follows closely the oral clinical unit dose of the agents tested.
That is, an oral ED50 of 50 mg/kg, for example, would be equivalent to an
oral clinical unit dose of 50 mg.

TABLE 1   Estimate of the Parenteral Clinical Unit Dose

Agent	Mouse analgesic (PQW) ED50 (mg/kg, s.c.)	Slope	Estimated clinical unit dose (mg)	Recommended clinical unit dose (mg)
Levorphanol	0.24	5.5	1.3-2.6	2.5
Meperidine	1.7	4.0	6.9-13.8	50.0
Methadone	0.9	5.1	4.6-9.2	2.5-10.0
Morphine	1.0	4.2	4.2-8.4	8.0-12.0
Nalorphine	10.0	0.9	9.0-18.0	10.0-15.0
Pentazocine	3.3	4.6	15.2-30.4	30.0
Phenazocine	0.25	5.3	1.3-2.7	2.0-4.0
Profadol	2.8	4.3	12.0-24.1	30.0-50.0

TABLE 2　Estimate of the Oral Clinical Unit Dose

Agent	Mouse analgesic (PQW) ED50 (mg/kg, p.o.)	Estimated clinical unit dose (mg)	Recommended clinical unit dose (mg)
Aspirin	396.0	400.0	300.0-450.0
Codeine	42.0	42.0	30.0-60.0
Levorphanol	2.6	2.6	2.5
Meperidine	42.0	42.0	50.0-100.0
Methadone	14.5	14.5	2.5-10.0
Phenazocine	10.0	10.0	10.0
Pentazocine	100.0	100.0	50.0-100.0
Profadol	8.4	9.0	50.0
d-Propoxyphene	40.0	40.0	65.0
Tilidine	43.0	43.0	50.0-100.0

III. ANALGESIC EFFICACY AND DEPTH OF EFFECT

The data summarized in Table 2 suggest that meperidine and d-propoxy-phene are roughly equipotent in the phenylquinone test and the recommended clinical unit dose ranges are also similar. But it is generally accepted that meperidine is a "deeper" analgesic than d-propoxyphene and is usually pre-scribed for more severe pain. Further, agents such as fenfluramine (an anorexic) and chlorpromazine (an antipsychotic) are more potent than either meperidine or d-propoxyphene in the phenylquinone writhing test and have not found their way into the pain-relieving armamentarium of the physician. To what extent then can we expect to identify a centrally acting analgesic and characterize its effective depth of analgesia?

There is one test system which appears to be specific for centrally acting analgesics, the tail flick test as originally described by D'Amour and Smith [12]. The test is operationally selective for the opiates and opiate-type analgesics. It does not detect those milder analgesics such as aspirin, indomethacin, chlorphentermine, and imipramine which are all active in the phenylquinone test. The tail-flick reflex requires CNS involve-ment, albeit predominantly by a spinal mechanism.

Grumbach [13] and Gray et al. [14] investigated the relationship between intensity of pain and analgesic activity in rats. Grumbach was the first to report that the potency of an analgesic agent (meperidine) decreased with increased stimulus intensity in the rat tail-flick procedure. Gray et al. showed essentially the same thing for pentazocine, modifying the prevailing consensus that pentazocine was inactive in the tail-flick procedure [15,16]. Granat and Saelens [17] have extended the observations of Grumbach and Gray and developed a model specifically designed for industrial screening which, in effect, determines the maximum intensity of pain an agent is capable of suppressing without inducing undesirable neurological effects.

Male mice, 18 to 22 g, are used. The animals are allowed food and water up until the time of testing. In a typical experimental run, five groups of 10 mice receive orally either the test agent dissolved in an appropriate vehicle or the vehicle alone in a volume of 0.1 ml/10 g body weight. A short predetermined interval separates the dosing of each group of 10 mice. After dosing, each mouse is placed in a separate restraining cylinder and the tails are blackened with India ink. Each test agent is evaluated as close to its time of peak effect as possible using a modification of the "tail flick" technique described for rats by D'Amour and Smith [12].

As in the original technique, the basic parameter measured is the reaction time (RT) which is defined as the interval from the onset of the heat stimulus to the "flick" of the tail from the focal point of a converging light beam. An arbitrary cutoff time of 10 sec is used. In our modification of the original technique, each group of 10 mice is tested over a range of heat intensities. This is accomplished by varying the voltage on the power supply of the Schaer algesiometer used, usually in the range of 50 to 80 V, in steps of 5 V. Experience has shown that it is more convenient and the results are more reproducible if all five groups of 10 mice are studied at one voltage step before going on to the next voltage step. Also, the studies are started at the lowest and finished at the highest voltage step to minimize the chance of damaging the animals' tails early in the experiment.

The ED50 is determined as follows using an endpoint of 50% of the maximum change in the control animals' reaction time:

$$\left[\frac{10 - C\overline{x}}{2} \right] + C\overline{x} = endpoint$$

where $C\overline{x}$ is the average reaction time of control animals at any given voltage setting. Quantal data are then obtained by the following formula:

$$\frac{\text{Number of mice with RT at or above endpoint}}{\text{Number of mice treated}}$$

The quantal dose-response data are plotted on logarithmic probability paper and an ED50 estimated by eye fit of the data. An ED_{50} can also be obtained by the method of Berkson [7] as used in the phenylquinone test, already described. Each study should be replicated until at least three doses are used within the dose-response range.

In order to determine the maximum oral dose free of unacceptable neurological effects, test agents are examined separately for their ability to induce a neurological deficit in mice. The method is essentially the same as that of Irwin [18] with the exception that the data are scored in an all-or-none fashion. The criteria for the scoring roughly correspond to a change of two units in Irwin's system. Ataxia, sluggish righting reflex, changes in muscle tone, and catalepsy are considered detrimental signs. For these parameters, the quantal dose-response data are plotted on logarithmic probability paper and the ED50 estimated by eye fit of the data. The Berkson technique may also be used. For other more extreme signs of neurotoxicity such as tremors, convulsions, and death, the maximum noneffective dose is determined. This value (ED8.3) is determined in a similar quantal plot of the data, and, since six animals are usually used at each dose of each agent tested, the ED8.3 is theoretically the dose at which one-half of one animal is affected ($1/12 = 0.083$ or 8.3%). The dosing volume and route of administration are the same as in the tail-flick portion of the studies. The observations are made at 0.5, 1, and 2 hr.

As noted by others [1,13,14], the reaction time of control animals ($\overline{Cx}$) varies with the voltage setting on the algesiometer. When the voltage is low, the heat intensity is less and the reaction time is longer. This inverse relationship is apparently linear in the voltage range normally employed. Thus in the analysis of the data from drug-treated animals, it is convenient and considered reasonable to use $1/\overline{Cx}$ as an index of heat intensity rather than the voltage setting. Then each experimental run has its own internal control which theoretically reduces between-experiment variation. It also eliminates any changes in heat intensity at the same voltage setting due to aging of the movie projector bulb used in the algesiometer.

When the intensity of the heat source is increased, the amount of test agent necessary to reach an oral analgesic ED50 also increases. This phenomenon is illustrated in Figure 1 for codeine. The relationship appears to be curvilinear in nature, particularly for those agents with a wide spread of ED50 values within the intensity range studied. Further, the exponential characteristics of the relationship suggest that the analgesic ED50 is asymptotic at some index of heat intensity value. Double reciprocal plots of the data are shown in Figure 2 for codeine and a number of other standard analgesic agents reputed to have oral activity in man. There is the expected linear relationship between the reciprocals of the index of heat intensity and the oral analgesic ED50 values for all agents tested. Further, asymptotic values (intercept on X axis) are obtained for four of the six agents: codeine, meperidine, pentazocine, and d-propoxyphene.

The asymptotic values may represent the maximum heat intensity that an infinite dose of test agent is capable of protecting against. In medical

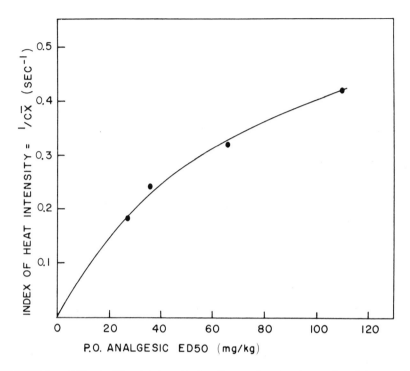

FIGURE 1. Effect of heat intensity on the analgesic ED50 of codeine in the mouse tail-flick procedure.

use, however, none of these agents is used at an infinite dose. Practically speaking, the agents can only be used at, or below, a dose which causes acceptable side effects. Therefore, a more realistic endpoint is the intercept of the linear regression for each agent with the respective maximum dose that is free of intolerable neurological effects. This index of heat intensity at a maximum tolerable dose is called the maximum intensity score (MIS).

The MIS for a number of standard analgesic agents and other nonanalgesic psychotropic agents is shown in Table 3. Operationally, the MIS is $1/C\overline{x}$ at the maximum tolerated dose and its units are in reciprocal seconds. For example, an MIS of 0.2 means that the voltage setting on the algesiometer would be set for a control reaction time of 5.0 sec (1/0.2) in order for the compound to reach its ED50 at the maximum tolerable dose. It is clear from Table 3 that the "true" centrally acting analgesics have MIS scores ≥ 0.19 whereas other psychotropic agents have lower scores. Further, once beyond 0.19, the analgesics are distributed in approximately the

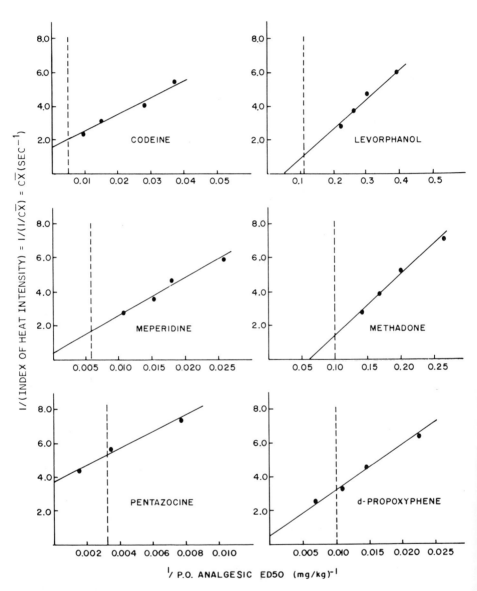

FIGURE 2.   Double reciprocal plots of heat intensity versus analgesic ED50 values. Data from the mouse tail-flick procedure.

TABLE 3   Maximum Intensity Score (MIS) for Various Analgesic Agents

Analgesic agent	MIS (sec^{-1})
Aspirin	0.00
Chlorpromazine	0.07
Clozapine	0.09
Codeine	0.46
Diviminol	0.25
Fenfluramine	0.16
Fentanyl	0.59
Imipramine	0.00
Indoramine	0.00
Levorphanol	0.91
Meperidine	0.56
Methadone	0.71
Methotrimeprazine	0.13
Methoxamine	0.00
Pentazocine	0.19
Propiram	0.23
d-Propoxyphene	0.30
Tilidine	0.47

same rank order as that for clinical efficacy; methadone and levorphanol at the top, meperidine, tilidine, and codeine in the middle; and pentazocine, propiram, and diviminol at the bottom, the latter group being the least capable of producing effective analgesia.

IV.   PHYSICAL DEPENDENCE

Clearly the most serious drawback in the treatment of pain with currently available deep analgesics is the risk of physical dependence development. Both governmental and medical concern for this issue dictates that new deep analgesics be virtually free of physical dependence liability. The need for

deep analgesics which do not cause physical dependence is as old as the use
of the agents which cause it, not something that arose with the current wave
of drug abuse.

In their pursuit of separating analgesic efficacy and physical dependence,
medicinal chemists and pharmacologists have pointed to the reduced physical
dependence capacity of codeine as compared to morphine. More recently,
they have concentrated on the fact that the N-allyl derivative of morphine,
nalorphine, does not cause any appreciable physical dependence and·yet has
deep analgesic properties. Although limited therapeutically by serious side
effects, nalorphine, a narcotic antagonist, has become the pharmacological
prototype for renewed efforts in the analgesic field.

The most prominent antagonist analgesic developed thus far is the ben-
zomorphan, pentazocine. The parenteral efficacy of pentazocine is reflected
in its widespread use as a morphine substitute. Its lack of appreciable
physical dependence capacity has resulted in its exclusion from government
control. Nevertheless, pentazocine's relatively limited oral efficacy and
its disturbing side effects make it a suitable target for analgesic research
programs.

The preceding two sections were concerned with finding and then determining the potency and efficacy of a potential analgesic agent. With regard to physical dependence evaluation, the National Institutes of Health have
established a program to test experimental compounds free of charge in
(a) a single-dose suppression test in morphine-dependent rhesus monkeys,
and if appropriate (b) a primary physical dependence test also in rhesus
monkeys. Similar studies are conducted for a modest fee in private research centers such as the International Center of Environmental Safety in
New Mexico. The advantages of contracting with private centers are the
shorter turn-around time for testing (2 to 4 weeks versus 6 to 8 months) and
control over protocol design. These alternatives are still not of sufficient
capacity to the industrial pharmacologist who may be responsible for evaluating 10 or more experimental agents a month from an active chemical
series. He needs a rapid, purely objective animal model for screening a
large number of compounds in his own laboratory at a minimum of cost.

It was observed in the early 1960s by Huidobro and Maggiolo [19-22]
and more recently by Way and his coworkers [23,24] that mice physically
dependent on morphine manifest antagonist-precipitated withdrawal by a
characteristic jumping episode. These mice literally leap into the air or
off a platform. In our laboratories, we have recorded jumps as high as 2.5
ft straight up from a crouched position on a bench top. Siegel et al. [25]
suggest that the jumping phenomenon is a behavioral manifestation of an
escape attempt from an aversive situation.

In all the early work a pellet containing approximately 75 mg of morphine base was implanted under the skin in the cervical region of the neck.
Within a few days the mice would maximally respond to a parenteral injection
of nalorphine or naloxone by jumping. It was also noted that if the pellet was

removed the jumping phenomenon would spontaneously appear 6 to 8 hr later. The correlation between mice and man as to the abstinence syndrome precipitated by a narcotic antagonist and withdrawal due to lack of remedication was excellent.

The studies of Saelens et al. [26] modified and expanded this earlier work. It was the specific purpose of these studies to determine if mice chronically treated with other agents known to cause physical dependence would also exhibit the jumping phenomenon when challenged with a morphine antagonist. The results so clearly indicated the strong relationship between known narcotic analgesics and physical dependence capacity in man that the procedure is now used to estimate the physical dependence capacity of unknown compounds which have activity in the standard analgesic screening tests.

Male CF_1 mice are used but other strains of mice have also been used successfully. The MAG and SPF strains in Europe may be even more sensitive than the CF_1 mice. The use of a pellet is not recommended, considering the problems of incorporating various materials with different toxicities, absorption rates, and compacting properties. An intraperitoneal injection schedule is the most efficient and allows the administration of both solutions and suspensions.

The mice are dosed for either 2 or 4 days. In the 2-day test, mice receive seven intraperitoneal injections. Five are given on the first day at 9:00 a.m., 10:00 a.m., 11:00 a.m., 1:00 p.m., and 3:00 p.m., and two on the second day at 9:00 a.m. and 11:00 a.m. In the 4-day test, mice receive 15 intraperitoneal injections. The injection schedule for the first day is identical to that of the first day of the 2-day test. Four injections are given on the second and third day at 9:00 a.m., 11:00 a.m., 1:00 p.m., and 3:00 p.m. On the fourth day, two injections are given at 9:00 a.m. and 11:00 a.m. Experimental agents are given in increasing increments usually starting in the analgesic range until a maximally tolerated dose is reached. The maximally tolerated dose is approached by injecting a small number of animals, usually five, with the next dose increment and waiting 15 min. If two or more mice die, the remaining mice are maintained on the previous dose for the rest of the dosing schedule.

The rationale for using this type of dosing schedule is that the potential human abuser would, by choice, progressively increase the dose of narcotic in order to obtain the desired effect. In the animal model, the mice are not offered a choice and their tolerance, rather than their desire, is used to determine dosage. This seemingly trivial point is really quite important. In man, the degree of physical dependence depends on the amount of drug taken and the frequency of its administration. An agent with inherent physical dependence properties may nevertheless be nonabusable because of noxious side effects that preclude its consumption at high doses or regular intervals. Such an agent may be highly active in animal tests for physical dependence and yet escape detection in man.

Two hours after the last dose of test agent (in both the 2- and 4-day tests) mice receive either nalorphine or naloxone intraperitoneally and are placed in separate Plexiglas cylinders, 16 in. high and 10 in. in diameter. The number of jumps (all four paws off the bottom surface) made by each mouse is recorded during the 10-min period following the administration of the narcotic antagonist. Experience has shown that jumping will occur, if it is to occur, within 1 to 2 min after administration of the narcotic antagonist and will not persist much longer than 10 min. After this time period, the mice usually become semicomatose, and diarrhea, ptosis, and tremors are prominent.

Results of the 2-day test with a number of centrally acting agents including several narcotic analgesics are shown in Table 4. The nalorphine challenging dose was 50 mg/kg and the naloxone challenging dose 100 mg/kg, i.p. Among the known analgesics, pronounced jumping was precipitated with nalorphine after chronic dosing only with compounds of high physical dependence capacity. Morphine, phenazocine, and myfadol are prime examples. Some jumping was precipitated with nalorphine after chronic administration of methadone, profadol, and methazocine but nalorphine seemed to have no effect on mice treated with codeine, cyclazocine, diviminol, fentanyl, meperidine, pentazocine, propiram, or USV-E142.

Naloxone is a more potent and generally considered a "purer" narcotic antagonist than nalorphine. That is, unlike nalorphine, naloxone does not have any analgesic properties of its own. Naloxone proved to be considerably more effective in precipitating the jumping phenomenon. It easily detected morphine, phenazocine, and myfadol but now also codeine, fentanyl, meperidine, methadone, pentazocine, profadol, propiram, tilidine, and USV-E142. Lesser and questionable jumping responses were elicited from animals treated with carbiphene, methazocine, and d-propoxyphene. Nalorphine was not antagonized by naloxone in this 2-day test.

Other known CNS stimulants and depressants with no history of morphinelike physical dependence capacity were also tested. Most were completely inactive. Some elicited jumping after several injections prior to administration of the nalorphine, thus invalidating the test. Others such as d-amphetamine, fenfluramine, and hexobarbital were associated with minimal naloxone-induced jumping. The latter may have occurred by chance since occasionally saline-treated animals have been observed to jump once or twice. We have therefore considered a response to be positive only if the average jumping rate is ≥ 4.0 jumps per mouse with $\geq 3/10$ mice jumping. One observation that cannot be ignored or explained at this time is the high jumping rate observed after administration of naloxone to mice which have been chronically treated with dl-dopa. This interaction is quite dramatic and reproducible provided the naloxone is given within 30 min after the last dose of dl-dopa. The role of catecholamines in analgesia and physical dependence is the subject of many articles, too numerous to mention here. The dl-dopa-naloxone interaction may represent still another aspect of this hypothesis.

TABLE 4 Two-Day Test Results with Various Compounds Known to Affect the CNS

Agent	Total dose (mg/kg, i.p.)	Nalorphine challenge incidence		Naloxone challenge incidence	
		Average jumps per mouse	No. mice jumped per no. tested	Average jumps per mouse	No. mice jumped per no. tested
d-Amphetamine	22	—	—	3.3	2/10
Aspirin	1800	—	—	0.0	0/10
Caffeine	450	—	—	0.1	1/10
Carbiphene	150	—	—	2.1	3/10
Chlordiazepoxide	450	0.0	0/10	0.0	0/10
Chlorphentermine[a]	300	16.5	6/10	0.2	1/10
Chlorpromazine	450	0.0	0/10	0.0	0/10
Clozapine	250	0.0	0/8	0.1	1/15
Cocaine	225	0.0	0/10	0.0	0/10
Codeine	400	0.0	0/10	26.1	9/10
Cyclazocine	225	0.0	0/10	0.1	1/10
Diethyldithiocarbamate	450	0.0	0/10	0.0	0/10
dl-Dopa (see text)	1600	—	—	7.5	6/10
Diviminol[a]	150	0.0	0/6	3.0	3/10
Fenfluramine[a]	140	0.0	0/10	1.2	2/10
Fentanyl	2	0.0	0/10	17.4	8/10

TABLE 4 (Cont.)

Agent	Total dose (mg/kg, i.p.)	Nalorphine challenge incidence Average jumps per mouse	Nalorphine challenge incidence No. mice jumped per no. tested	Naloxone challenge incidence Average jumps per mouse	Naloxone challenge incidence No. mice jumped per no. tested
Haloperidol	125	0.0	0/10	0.0	0/10
Harmaline	200	—	—	0.0	0/8
Harmalol[a]	225	—	—	0.0	0/10
Harmane	150	—	—	0.0	0/10
Hexobarbital[a]	450	—	—	2.1	2/10
l-5HTP	94	—	—	0.0	0/10
Imipramine	450	0.0	0/10	0.0	0/10
Laudanosine	200	0.0	0/10	0.0	0/10
Laudanosoline	350	0.0	0/10	0.0	0/10
Meperidine	300	0.0	0/10	25.2	9/10
Meprobamate	350	0.0	0/10	0.0	0/10
Mescaline	225	0.0	0/10	0.0	0/10
Methadone	63	1.0	2/10	20.3	8/10

Methazocine	300	1.6	1/10	2.2	4/10
Methotrimeprazine	163	0.0	0/10	0.0	0/10
Morphine	450	48.9	10/10	55.7	10/10
Myfadol	450	11.2	6/10	33.8	9/10
Nalorphine	2 225	—	—	0.0	0/10
Pentazocine	175	0.0	0/10	7.0	4/10
Phenazocine	56	10.2	8/10	81.4	9/10
Physostigmine	2	0.0	0/10	0.0	0/10
Profadol	300	1.3	3/10	12.8	6/10
Propiram	450	0.0	0/10	8.9	4/10
d–Propoxyphene	150	0.0	0/10	2.4	2/10
Salsolidine	450	0.0	0/10	0.0	0/8
Theophylline	575	—	—	0.0	0/10
Tilidine	225	—	—	4.8	4/10
USV–E142	100	0.0	0/10	8.5	4/10

[a] Some jumping seen without antagonist challenge.

TABLE 5   Four–Day Test Results with Known Analgesic Compounds

Compound	Total dose (mg/kg, i.p.)	Nalorphine (mg/kg, i.p.)	Nalorphine challenge incidence		Naloxone (mg/kg, i.p.)	Naloxone challenge incidence	
			Average jumps per mouse	No. mice jumped per no. tested		Average jumps per mouse	No. mice jumped per no. tested
Codeine	1119	3	0.0	0/6			
		10	3.3	1/6			
		30	8.5	3/6			
		100	22.2	6/6			
Meperidine	969	3	0.0	0/7	3	6.0	3/10
		10	3.6	1/7	10	12.4	5/10
		30	3.0	1/7	30	10.3	4/10
		100	4.7	1/7	100	16.4	6/10
Morphine	1470	3	24.2	8/10	3	Seizures	
		10	30.4	9/10	10		
		30	27.7	10/10	30		
		100	35.0	10/10	100		

Drug		Dose			Seizures	
Nalorphine	625	3	1.1	2/10	1.9	3/10
		10	2.8	2/10	4.0	3/10
		30	0.0	0/10	9.6	5/10
		100	1.8	2/10	12.1	8/10
Pentazocine	425	3	0.0	0/10		
		10	0.0	0/10		
		30	0.0	0/10		
		100	0.0	0/10		
Phenazocine	350	3	4.5	2/5		
		10	51.4	5/5		
		30	43.4	5/5		
		100	96.4	5/5		
d-Propoxyphene	300	3	9.0	2/11		
		10	2.6	2/11		
		30	5.1	5/11		
		100	1.5	5/11		

Mice treated with narcotic analgesics for 4 days are more sensitive to nalorphine-induced jumping than those on the 2-day schedule. Results of these experiments are summarized in Table 5. In a dose range of 3 to 100 mg/kg, nalorphine not only induced jumping after morphine and phenazocine but also after codeine, meperidine, and d-propoxyphene. The important exception is pentazocine which is still nalorphine resistant even after 4 days of chronic administration.

There is little qualitative difference between the results obtained after 2 or 4 days when naloxone is used as the narcotic antagonist. Quantitatively, however, naloxone produces such a severe withdrawal reaction in those mice receiving morphine and phenazocine that seizures, convulsions, and death preempt coordinated jumping. One notable qualitative difference between the 2- and 4-day results is that naloxone does precipitate some jumping in mice which were chronically treated with nalorphine for 4 days but not for 2 days. Physical dependence has been demonstrated for nalorphine in man [27]. Because of side effects, however, nalorphine has no history of abuse in man.

The data in Tables 4 and 5 suggest that the various mouse jumping test designs have the following order of sensitivity: 4-day naloxone challenge > 2-day naloxone challenge > 4- day nalorphine challenge > 2-day nalorphine challenge. The use of all four jumping test designs permits a ranking of unknown compounds among the various agents whose physical dependence capacity has been studied in man. For instance, among the morphinans, morphans, and benzomorphans, the target comparison may be pentazocine. Mice which do not exhibit jumping when dosed for 4 days with compounds from these series and then challenged with nalorphine would be predicted to have the same or lower physical dependence capacity than pentazocine. If no jumping is observed in the 2-day naloxone test, then test compounds would be predicted to have less physical dependence capacity than pentazocine.

In testing compounds with chemical structures somewhat different from that of morphine (e.g., meperidine, methadone, and d-propoxyphene analogs) naloxone is the preferred challenging agent. Considering the marked physical dependence liability of meperidine and methadone in man and the fact that these compounds cause no reproducible jumping in the 2- or 4- day nalorphine tests, analogs would have to be evaluated in the naloxone test in order to safely predict physical dependence liability in man.

Information accumulated thus far with the mouse jumping test may complement and supplement data obtained in the rhesus monkey. Mice appear to be particularly sensitive to benzomorphans such as pentazocine whereas rhesus monkeys are surprisingly insensitive to such compounds [28]. The reverse situation appears to be true with meperidine. The rank order of physical dependence liability for meperidine in the mouse jumping test is much lower than it is in man. On the other hand, rhesus monkeys are quite sensitive to meperidine [29]. Perhaps borderline compounds should be tested in both species. Because of time and expense consideration, however, the mouse jumping test should be used first.

V. SUMMARY

A specific series of test systems is described which enable the industrial pharmacologist to estimate the potency, efficacy, and physical dependence liability of potential analgesic agents. All the test systems place emphasis on efficiency, cost, and reliability. Taken together they represent a reasonable industrial screening approach to the search for new analgesic drugs.

REFERENCES

1. R. I. Taber, in Advances in Biochemical Psychopharmacology: Narcotic Antagonists (E. Costa and P. Greengard, eds.), Vol. 8, Raven Press, New York, 1973, p. 191.

2. L. O. Randall, in Physiological Pharmacology, Vol. 1, Central Nervous System Drugs (W. S. Root and F. G. Hofmann, eds.), Academic Press, New York, 1963, p. 313.

3. L. C. Hendershot and J. Forsaith, J. Pharmacol. Exp. Ther. 125, 237 (1959).

4. H. I. Chernov, D. E. Wilson, F. Fowler, and A. J. Plummer, Arch. Int. Pharmacodyn. 167, 171 (1967).

5. R. I. Taber, D. D. Greenhouse, and S. Irwin, Nature 204, 189 (1964).

6. H. Blumberg, P. S. Wolf, and H. B. Dayton, Proc. Soc. Exp. Biol. Med. 118, 763 (1965).

7. J. Berkson, J. Am. Statist. Assoc. 48, 565 (1953).

8. J. Pearl and L. S. Harris, J. Pharmacol. Exp. Ther. 154, 319 (1966).

9. J. Pearl, H. Stander, and D. B. McKean, J. Pharmacol. Exp. Ther. 167, 9 (1969).

10. L. Lasagna and H. R. Beecher, J. Pharmacol. Exp. Ther. 112, 356 (1954).

11. A. S. Keats and J. Telford, J. Pharmacol. Exp. Ther. 117, 190 (1956).

12. F. E. D'Amour and D. L. Smith, J. Pharmacol. Exp. Ther. 72, 74 (1941).

13. L. Grumbach, personal communication, as reported in Drug Addiction and Narcotics, Appendix 26, 3987 (1964).

14. W. D. Gray, A. C. Osterberg, and T. J. Scuto, J. Pharmacol. Exp. Ther. 172, 154 (1969).

15. S. Archer, N. F. Albertson, L. S. Harris, A. K. Pierson, J. G. Bird, A. S. Keats, J. Telford, and C. N. Papadopoulos, Science 137, 541 (1962).

16. L. S. Harris and A. K. Pierson, J. Pharmacol. Exp. Ther. 143, 141 (1964).

17. F. R. Granat and J. K. Saelens, Arch. Int. Pharmacodyn. 205, 52 (1973).

18. S. Irwin, Science 136, 123 (1962).

19. F. Huidobro, J. P. Huidobro, and G. Larrain, Acta Physiol. Lat. Am. 18, 59 (1968).

20. F. Huidobro and C. Maggiolo, Acta Physiol. Lat. Am. 11, 201 (1961).

21. F. Huidobro and C. Maggiolo, Arch. Int. Pharmacodyn. 158, 97 (1965).

22. C. Maggiolo and F. Huidobro, Acta Physiol. Lat. Am. 11, 70 (1961).

23. E. L. Way, H. H. Loh, and F. H. Shen, Science 162, 1290 (1968).

24. E. L. Way, H. H. Loh, and F. H. Shen, J. Pharmacol. Exp. Ther. 167, 1 (1969).

25. R. K. Siegel, B. E. Gusewelle, and M. E. Jarvik, J. Pharmacol. 5 (Suppl. 2), 92 (1974).

26. J. K. Saelens, F. R. Granat, and W. K. Sawyer, Arch. Int. Pharmacodyn 190, 213 (1971).

27. W. R. Martin and C. W. Gorodetzky, J. Pharmacol. Exp. Ther. 150, 437 (1965).

28. N. B. Eddy and E. L. May, Synthetic Analgesics, Part IIB, 6, 7-Benzomorphans (J. Rolfe, ed.), 1st ed., Pergamon Press, London, 1965, p. 192.

29. L. B. Mellett and L. A. Woods, Progress in Drug Research, Birkhauder Press, Basel, 1963, p. 155.

AUTHOR INDEX

Numbers in brackets are reference numbers and indicate
that an author's work is referred to although his name is
not cited in the text. Underlined numbers give the page
on which the complete reference is listed.

290

Friis, W., 191-193[10,15], <u>199</u>, <u>200</u>
Frohlich, E. D., 83[104], <u>92</u>
Fry, G. A., 109[67], <u>121</u>
Fujii, J., 62[26], <u>88</u>
Fujita, T., 163[58], 166, <u>183</u>, <u>184</u>
Fujiwara, M., 214[60], 217[60], 228[60], <u>254</u>
Fukui, H., 64[79], <u>91</u>
Fuller, W. M., 109[67], <u>121</u>
Fulton, J. F., 156, <u>180</u>
Funderburk, W. H., 157[15], 164[67], 170[67], 171[15,96], 173[15], <u>181</u>, <u>183</u>, <u>184</u>
Furman, S., 127, 142[134], 143[134], <u>147</u>, <u>153</u>
Fuxe, K., 169[85,86], <u>184</u>, 212[38], <u>253</u>

G

Gabbiana, G., 42[53], 43[53], <u>56</u>
Gaffney, R., 142[132], <u>153</u>
Gaffney, T. E., 86[112], <u>93</u>
Gagen, D., 65[97], <u>92</u>
Gallant, D. M., 158[25], <u>181</u>
Galvan, L., 207[18,19], <u>251</u>, <u>252</u>
Ganellin, C. R., 30[5], <u>54</u>
Ganz, W., 101, <u>120</u>
Garcia Ramos, J., 131, <u>148</u>
Gardocki, J. F., 159[36], <u>182</u>
Garrattini, S., 212[37], 225[37], <u>253</u>
Gautier, J., 158[26], <u>181</u>
Geagea, K. C., 221[109], <u>256</u>
Geivers, H. A., 174[103], <u>185</u>
Gelbart, A., 141[123,124], <u>152</u>
Gell, P. G. H., 31[7], <u>54</u>
Geller, I., 195[26,27], 196[28,29], <u>200</u>
Geller, R., 62[36], <u>89</u>
Gelok, R., 143[139], <u>153</u>
Gent, M., 212[35], <u>252</u>

George, A., 130[40], 131[40], <u>148</u>
George, R., 248[211], <u>261</u>
Germain, G. S., 62[9], 65[96], <u>88</u>, <u>92</u>
Gerna, M., 212[37], 225[37], <u>253</u>
Gershon, S., 219[77], 221[106], 225[153], 236[190], <u>254</u>, <u>256</u>, <u>258</u>, <u>260</u>
Ghetti, B., 217[59], <u>254</u>
Ghezzi, D., 212[37], 225[37], <u>253</u>
Gibbons, J. E., 226[159], <u>258</u>
Gifford, R. W., 226[157], <u>258</u>
Gilbert, J. L., 136[89], <u>151</u>
Gilberti, F., 216[54], <u>253</u>
Gildiz, M., 133[56], <u>149</u>
Giles, R. E., 37[30], 51[30], <u>55</u>
Gillam, P. M. S., 118[100], <u>123</u>
Gillette, J. R., 248[212], <u>261</u>
Gillis, C. N., 242[201], <u>260</u>
Gillis, R. A., 99[21,23], <u>119</u>
Gimenez, J. L., 112[79], <u>122</u>
Ginocchio, S., 159[35], <u>181</u>
Giudicelli, J. F., 138[106], <u>151</u>
Giudicelli, R., 86[109], <u>92</u>
Glava, E., 64[66,67], <u>90</u>
Glaviano, V. V., 164[54], <u>182</u>
Glavas, E., 64[67,68], <u>90</u>, <u>91</u>
Gliklich, J. I., 142[132], <u>153</u>
Glowinski, J., 222[116], 225[151, 152], 226[116], <u>256</u>, <u>258</u>
Gluckman, M. I., 86[111], <u>93</u>
Glynn, I. M., 140[117], <u>152</u>
Gobel, F. L., 96[5], 108[5], <u>118</u>
Goetzl, E. J., 42[50], <u>56</u>
Gold, W. M., 40[32], <u>55</u>
Goldberg, M. E., 213[36], <u>252</u>
Goldblatt, H., 61[7], <u>87</u>
Goldreyer, B. N., 129[23,24], <u>148</u>
Goldschlager, N., 100[30], <u>120</u>
Goldstein, B. J., 157[20], <u>181</u>
Goldstein, L., 159[36], <u>182</u>
Goldstein, M., 225[153], <u>258</u>
Goldstein, P. E., 118[101], <u>123</u>
Goldstein, R. E., 96, 102[35], 104[42], 106[42], 108[9], <u>118</u>, <u>119</u>, <u>120</u>

Koetschet, P., 158[27], 163[27],
   167[27], 181
Kojima, S., 49[70], 57
Koketsu, K., 219[87], 220[87], 255
Kokubo, T., 157[23], 181
Kolsky, M., 158[27], 163[27],
   167[27], 181
Komiskey, H., 219[82], 255
Koretsky, S., 107[54], 121
Kopin, I. J., 197[37], 201,
   219[86], 222[115], 226[115],
   255, 256
Kondo, H., 221[103], 256
Kramer, M., 157[21], 181
Kramer, P., 62[30], 88
Kraupp, O., 111[75], 122
Kreiskott, H., 166[77], 184
Krell, R. D., 37[31], 55
Krisiak, M., 175, 185
Kuehl, F. A., Jr., 4[1], 26
Kuehn, A., 193, 200
Kuhn, R., 206, 251
Kuhn, W. J., 110[68], 121
Kulczycki, A., 42[48], 56
Kumar, S., 223[131], 257
Kunz, H. A., 213[44], 253
Kupfer, D. J., 222[124], 257
Kurihara, H., 62[26], 88
Kus, T., 129[31,32], 148
Kusner, E. J., 42[52], 46[56],
   48[56], 49[56,66], 56, 57

L

L'Abbate, A., 110[69], 121
Laborit, H., 157, 180
Laddu, A. R., 133, 138[108], 149,
   151
Lagerquist, B., 134[69], 150
Lagunoff, D., 48[65], 57
Lahti, R. A., 198[40,41], 201
Laidlaw, P. P., 30, 54
Lakdensus, A., 40[36], 56
Lal, H., 159[34,35], 181

Lambelin, G., 92
Lang, T., 99[22], 119
Lange, G. G., 136[89], 151
Langston, M. F., Jr., 117[99], 123
Lanoir, J., 193[20], 200
Lantsber, L., 62[12], 88
Lanzoni, V., 140[116], 152
Lara, P. P., 221[100], 256
Laragh, J. H., 87[122], 93
Lare, S. H., 132[50], 149
Larrain, G., 272[19], 282
Larsson, K., 169[85], 184
Lasagna, L., 143[147], 153, 159,
   181, 245[206], 261, 265[10],
   281
Lau, S. H., 132[49], 138[100], 149,
   151
Laverty, R., 197[34,35], 200
Lawson, J. W., 134[74], 150
Lazzara, R., 129[30], 148
Leach, B. E., 62[9], 65[96], 88,
   92
Leach, G. D. H., 64[62], 90
Leaf, R. C., 232[182], 260
Lee, J. B., 62[11], 88
Lee, R. J., 114, 115, 122
Leenen, F. H., 61[3], 87
Lefebvre, Y., 142[128], 153
Lehmann, H. E., 207[18,19],
   216[55], 221[109], 222[127],
   251, 252, 253, 256, 257
Lehr, D., 144[155], 154
Lehrer, S. B., 41, 56
Lehtosuo, E. J., 117[93], 123
Leinbach, R. C., 142[136], 153
Leitl, G., 64[81], 91
Leonard, B. E., 217[65], 254
Leonard, C. A., 163[58], 183
Lessin, A. W., 167, 168[83], 184
Leth, A., 65[91], 92
Leveque, P. E., 134[77,78], 150
Levine, B. B., 42[44], 56
Levinson, B., 253
Levitt, B., 137[90], 151
Levitt, M., 220[92], 255

Rakkolainen, V. , 178[119], <u>186</u>
Randall, L. O. , 187[1,2], 191–
193[11,12,14], 195[12,14],
196[1,12], <u>199</u>, 240[200],
242[200], <u>260</u>, 264[2], <u>281</u>
Randrup, A. , 162[45,46,49,50],
175[110], 176[110], <u>182</u>, <u>185</u>
Raper, C. , 137[96], 138[96], <u>151</u>
Rapp, J. P. , 65[87,88], <u>91</u>
Rasmussen, K. E. , 219[80],
220[80], <u>255</u>
Ravin, J. , 222[117], <u>256</u>
Ray, I. , 222[121], <u>257</u>
Raynaud, J.-P. , 249[214], <u>261</u>
Redwood, D. R. , 96[4], 104[42],
106[42], 118[101], <u>118</u>, <u>120</u>,
<u>123</u>
Reeves, T. J. , 98, <u>119</u>
Reichek, N. , 118[101], <u>123</u>
Reinke, D. , 233[186], <u>260</u>
Rembert, J. C. , 102[37], <u>120</u>
Remvig, J. , 219[80], 220[80], <u>255</u>
Reno, H. , 221[108], 226[162],
228[108], 231[162], 238[198],
<u>256</u>, <u>259</u>, <u>260</u>
Renyi, A. L. , 236[195], 237[195],
<u>260</u>
Renzini, V. , 87[118], <u>93</u>
Requin, S. , 193, <u>200</u>
Revoltella, R. , 41[40], 49[69],
<u>56</u>, <u>57</u>
Reynaud, G. , 229[171], 230, <u>259</u>
Rheinboldt, W. C. , 128[18], <u>147</u>
Rickels, K. , 206[14,15], 212[42],
<u>251</u>, <u>253</u>
Rimon, R. , 178[119], <u>186</u>
Rinzler, S. H. , 117[94], <u>123</u>
Riseman, J. E. F. , 107, <u>121</u>
Risley, E. A. , 4[2], 12[7], 19[2],
<u>26</u>
Risse, K. H. , 166[77], <u>184</u>
Ritzmann, L. W. , 109[67], <u>121</u>
Rivers, R. J. , 142[135], <u>153</u>
Roach, A. G. , 66[131], <u>94</u>
Roba, J. , <u>92</u>
Robak, O. H. , 219[80], 220[80], <u>255</u>

Robbins, B. G. , 61[5], <u>87</u>
Roberts, J. , 137[90,95], <u>151</u>
Roberts, M. , 33[18], <u>55</u>
Roberts, M. H. T. , 211[32], <u>252</u>
Robichaud, L. J. , 44[54], <u>56</u>
Robinson, G. , 127, <u>147</u>
Robison, G. A. , 220[93], 226[93],
<u>255</u>
Robson, R. D. , 139[109,110],
<u>152</u>
Rockey, J. H. , 34[24], <u>55</u>
Rodova, A. , 206[16], <u>251</u>
Roine, P. , 117[93], <u>123</u>
Roos, B. E. , 178[118,119], <u>186</u>
Rosen, M. R. , 142[132], <u>153</u>
Rosenbloom, A. L. , 223[128],
<u>257</u>
Rosenblueth, A. , 128, 131, <u>147</u>,
<u>148</u>
Rosenthale, M. E. , 18, <u>27</u>
Rosing, D. R. , 96[4], 104[42],
106[42], <u>118</u>, <u>120</u>
Ross, R. S. , 99[25], 100[25],
105[43], 106[43,50], <u>119</u>, <u>120</u>
Ross, S. B. , 236[195], 237[195],
<u>260</u>
Roth, F. E. , 47[64], 48[64], <u>57</u>
Roth, J. A. , 242[201], <u>260</u>
Roth, T. , 157[21], <u>181</u>
Rothberger, C. J. , 127, <u>147</u>
Rowles, G. , 86[111], <u>93</u>, 140[113],
<u>152</u>
Rubenson, A. , 86[107], <u>92</u>,
169[86], <u>184</u>
Rubin, A. A. , 223[134], <u>257</u>
Rubio-Chevannier, H. F. , 232[183],
<u>260</u>
Ruckart, R. , 161[43], <u>182</u>
Rudzik, A. D. , 190[7], 191[10],
192[7,10,15], 193[10], <u>199</u>,
<u>200</u>
Rumack, B. M. , 210[29], <u>252</u>
Ruskin, R. , 222[120], <u>257</u>
Russek, H. I. , 104, 105, <u>120</u>
Ryan, C. F. , 63[37], <u>89</u>
Rysanek, K. , 222[126], <u>257</u>

Thompson, K., 64[81], <u>91</u>
Thoms, R. K., 164[64], <u>183</u>
Thon, I. L., 32[11], <u>54</u>
Thurmond, A., 223[136], <u>257</u>
Tishler, M., 143[148], <u>153</u>
Tiwary, C. M., 223[128], <u>257</u>
Tobian, L., 62[17,19,20], <u>88</u>
Todd, A. H., 218[67], <u>254</u>
Tognoni, G., 212[37], 225[37], <u>253</u>
Toler, J. C., 142[138], <u>153</u>
Tomita, Y., 34[27], <u>55</u>
Tomiyasu, U., 117[95], <u>123</u>
Torchiana, M. L., 134[67,68,69], <u>150</u>, 231[180], <u>259</u>
Toru, M., 157[23], <u>181</u>
Toshinari, T., 65[83], <u>91</u>
Totaro, J. A., 234[189], 237[189], <u>260</u>
Tozzi, S., 47[64], 48[64], <u>57</u>
Trajkow, T., 64[66,67,68], <u>90</u>, <u>91</u>
Trautner, E. M., 219[75], <u>254</u>
Tretter, J. R., 215[51], <u>253</u>
Triggle, D. J., 62[22], 64[58], <u>88</u>, <u>90</u>
Troup, W., 112[78], <u>122</u>
Troyer, W. G., 97[10], <u>119</u>
Tuck, D., 224[138], <u>257</u>
Turek, I. S., 221[111], <u>256</u>
Turner, R. W., 218[67], <u>254</u>
Turpeinen, O., 117[93], <u>123</u>
Tye, N., 231[181], <u>259</u>

U

Udabe, R. U., 207[17], <u>251</u>
Udenfriend, S., 242[202], <u>261</u>
Ueda, H., 62[25], 63[38], <u>88</u>, <u>89</u>
Ueki, S., 214, 217[60], 228[60], <u>254</u>
Ungerstedt, U., 169, 170[87,90], <u>184</u>
Utiger, R. D., 221[98,99], <u>255</u>, <u>256</u>
Uvnas, B., 32[11], <u>54</u>

V

Vale, S., 223[133], <u>257</u>
Valzelli, L., 193[22], <u>200</u>
Van Arman, C. G., 4[2], 12, 19[2], 21[17,18,19], <u>26</u>, <u>27</u>
van Chappelle, F. J. V., 129[22], <u>148</u>
van der Burg, W. J., 216[53], 243[53], <u>253</u>
Van der Vis Melsen, M. J. E., 221[102], <u>256</u>
Van Dorsser, W., 236[192], <u>260</u>
VanDurme, J. P., 139, <u>152</u>
Van Pelt, R., 86[111], <u>93</u>
van Praag, H. M., 212[39], <u>253</u>
van Riezen, H., 216[53], 217[63], 243[53], 246[63], 248[63], <u>253</u>, <u>254</u>
Van Rossum, J. M., 175, 176[110], <u>185</u>
VanTyn, R. A., 130, <u>148</u>
Varga, E., 157[22], <u>181</u>
Varga, V., 157[16], <u>181</u>
Vargaftig, B. B., 217[64], <u>254</u>
Varma, D. R., 135, 137[97], <u>150</u>, <u>151</u>
Varner, L. L., 86[106], <u>92</u>
Vaughan, J. H., 41, <u>56</u>
Vaughan Williams, E. M., 132, 133, 137[64], 138[45,103,104], <u>148</u>, <u>149</u>, <u>151</u>
Vavra, I., 142[125], <u>152</u>
Vaynovsky, B., 83[105], <u>92</u>
Vaz, E. M., 42[44], <u>56</u>
Vaz, N. M., 42[44], <u>56</u>
Velduyzen, B., 63[39d], <u>89</u>
Vergara, L., 207[18,19], <u>251</u>, <u>252</u>
Verneire, P., 139[112], <u>152</u>
Vernier, V. G., 226[161], 227, <u>258</u>
Vetadzokoska, D., 64[66,67,68], <u>90</u>, <u>91</u>
Villeneuve, A., 158[26], <u>181</u>
Villeneuve, R., 158[26], <u>181</u>
Vilsanen, A. A., 40[36], <u>56</u>